Imaging of the Prostate

Imaging of the Prostate

Ethan J Halpern MD

Professor of Radiology and Urology
Co-Director, Prostate Diagnostic Imaging Center
Thomas Jefferson University
Philadelphia
USA

Dennis Ll Cochlin Mb BCh FRCR

Consultant Radiologist
and Director of General Ultrasound
University Hospital of Wales
Cardiff
UK

Barry B Goldberg MD

Professor of Radiology
Director, Division of Diagnostic Ultrasound
Director, Jefferson Ultrasound Research and Education Institute
Thomas Jefferson University
Philadelphia
USA

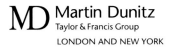
Martin Dunitz
Taylor & Francis Group
LONDON AND NEW YORK

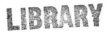
© 2002 Martin Dunitz Ltd, a member of the Taylor & Francis group

First published in the United Kingdom in 2002 by
Martin Dunitz Ltd,
The Livery House,
7-9 Pratt Street,
London NW1 0AE

Tel: +44 (0) 20 7482 2202
Fax: +44 (0) 20 7267 0159
E-mail: info@dunitz.co.uk
Website: http://www.dunitz.co.uk

A CIP record for this book is available from the British Library.

ISBN 1 84184 198 6

Although every effort has been made to ensure that all owners of copyright material have been acknowledged in this publication, we would be glad to acknowledge in subsequent reprints or editions any omissions brought to our attention.

Distributed in the USA by
Fulfilment Center
Taylor & Francis
7625 Empire Drive
Florence, KY 41042, USA
Toll Free Tel.: +1 800 634 7064
E-mail: cserve@routledge_ny.com

Distributed in Canada by
Taylor & Francis
74 Rolark Drive
Scarborough, Ontario M1R 4G2, Canada
Toll Free Tel.: +1 877 226 2237
E-mail: tal_fran@istar.ca

Distributed in the rest of the world by
Thomson Publishing Services
Cheriton House
North Way
Andover, Hampshire SP10 5BE, UK
Tel.: +44 (0)1264 332424
E-mail: salesordertandf@thomsonpublishingservices.co.uk

Composition by EXPO Holdings, Malaysia
Printed and bound in China by Imago

Dedicated to the memory of my beloved uncle
Dr. Yeheskel S. Halpern (1926-2001)
Professor of Microbiology Hebrew University – Hadassa Medical School
He devoted his life to biomedical research
and inspired my career in medicine

Contents

Contributors   ix

Preface   xi

Acknowledgements   xiii

I Anatomy

1 Anatomy of the prostate gland   3
Ethan J Halpern

II Prostate Cancer

2 Epidemiology and histopathology of prostate cancer   19
Ethan J Halpern

3 Gray-scale evaluation of prostate cancer   27
Ethan J Halpern

4 Color and power Doppler evaluation of prostate cancer   39
Ethan J Halpern

5 Ultrasound-guided biopsy of the prostate   51
Ethan J Halpern

6 Advanced sonographic techniques for detection of prostate cancer   65
Ethan J Halpern

7 CT evaluation of the prostate   77
Ethan J Halpern

8 Magnetic resonance evaluation of the prostate   87
Michael Bourne

9 Nuclear medicine evaluation and therapy of the prostate   101
Rakesh H Ganatra

III Benign disease of the prostate

10 Cysts and congenital anomalies of the prostate and ejaculatory ducts   115
Dennis Ll Cochlin

11 Benign prostatic hypertrophy   129
Dennis Ll Cochlin

12 Prostatitis   149
Dennis Ll Cochlin

13 Prostatic calculi and calcifications   163
Dennis Ll Cochlin

14 The seminal vesicles, ejaculatory ducts and vasa deferentia   171
Dennis Ll Cochlin

15 Imaging of male infertility   191
Dennis Ll Cochlin

16 Haematospermia   195
Dennis Ll Cochlin

IV Therapy

17 Image-guided therapy of prostatic disease   201
Ehab el-Gabry and Leonard G Gomella

18 Imaging for prostate cancer radiation therapy   211
Richard K Valicenti

Index   217

Contributors

Michael Bourne Mb BCh FRCR
Consultant Radiologist and
Director of MRI Services
University Hospital of Wales
Cardiff
UK

Dennis Ll Cochlin Mb BCh FRCR
Consultant Radiologist and
Director of General Ultrasound
University Hospital of Wales
Cardiff
UK

Rakesh H Ganatra Mb BCh FRCR
SPR in Nuclear Medicine
University Hospital of Wales
Cardiff
UK

Ehab el-Gabry MD
Research Fellow in Urologic Oncology
Department of Urology
Thomas Jefferson University
Philadelphia
USA

Leonard G Gomella MD
Bernard W.Goodwin Jr. Associate Professor of Prostate Caner
Director of Urologic Oncology, Kimmel Cancer Center
Thomas Jefferson University
Philadelphia
USA

Ethan J Halpern MD
Professor of Radiology and Urology
Co-Director, Prostate Diagnostic Imaging Center
Thomas Jefferson University
Philadelphia
USA

Richard K Valicenti MD MA
Associate Professor and Director of Clinical Research
Department of Radiation Oncology
Thomas Jefferson University
Philadelphia
USA

Preface

Although the prostate is a rather small gland, diseases of the prostate have a profound impact on public health in the male half of the population. Benign hyperplasia of the prostate is a nearly universal process in the aging population. Congenital and acquired pathological processes of the prostate may be an important element in the diagnosis of infertility. Cancer of the prostate is the most frequently diagnosed cancer in men. Imaging studies of the prostate are often requested for the diagnosis of these disease processes, to guide biopsy of the prostate, and for treatment of benign and malignant processes.

The ideal diagnostic study for prostate cancer would detect clinically significant cancers, and identify patients without cancer as normal. Various image processing techniques have been applied to clarify or quantify features that are present within the prostate. Unfortunately, current imaging technology cannot provide a tissue diagnosis to obviate a biopsy procedure. This diagnostic problem may be related, in part, to the unusual growth pattern of cancer within the prostate. Malignancy within the prostate is multifocal in 85% of cases, and often grows in an oblong shape along the capsule. The near ubiquitous presence of benign prostate hyperplasia in the mature prostate gland further distorts the appearance of the gland and complicates the process of imaging for cancer.

Nevertheless, technological advances in imaging of the prostate over the past decade have resulted in marked improvement in visualization of the prostate. Great strides have been made in non-invasive imaging of infertility. Cysts, stones and congenital anomalies that block the flow of semen may be diagnosed non-invasively. Recent studies suggest that newer ultrasound and magnetic resonance techniques may be useful in the diagnosis and staging of prostate cancer. Ultrasound and MR imaging of the stage and aggressiveness of prostate cancer may alter both diagnosis and treatment of this disease. Newer contrast-enhanced imaging techniques may be able to identify clinically significant cancer based upon the altered hemodynamics of neovascularity. A physician involved in the management of patients with prostate disease should be familiar with these techniques.

The motivation for writing this text is the rapid advance we have witnessed in imaging technology over the past decade. This textbook is the product of collaboration among radiologists and urologists in North America and Europe. An introductory chapter describes aspects of prostate anatomy that are relevant to imaging of disease. The greater part of the contents is organized into three sections to cover imaging of prostate cancer, benign disease and therapy. The most up to date techniques are described for both imaging and therapy. Numerous gray scale and color figures have been employed to illustrate specific imaging features in the prostate. This text should be of interest for those involved in the clinical care of prostate disease as well as those involved in research into new methods of diagnosis and treatment.

Acknowledgements

We recognize with appreciation the contributions of our contributing authors. We are indebted to Alan Burgess, our commissioning editor, for enabling this project, and to Charlotte Mossop, our project editor, for her expert editorial assistance. Most of all, we gratefully acknowledge the unwavering support and encouragement provided by our spouses – Sarah C Halpern, Margaret Cochlin and Phyllis R Goldberg – without whose assistance this endeavor would not have been possible.

Ethan J Halpern
Dennis Ll Cochlin
Barry B Goldberg

Section I

Anatomy

1

Anatomy of the prostate gland

Ethan J Halpern

In this chapter, we explore the three-dimensional anatomy of the prostate gland, with particular emphasis on the sonographic appearance. An understanding of normal prostate anatomy and common variations on both the macroscopic and microscopic levels is essential for diagnostic evaluation, biopsy, and treatment purposes. Vascular anatomy is covered in detail in Chapter 4.

Gross anatomy

The young adult prostate – from puberty until the onset of benign prostatic hyperplasia – is about the size of a walnut,

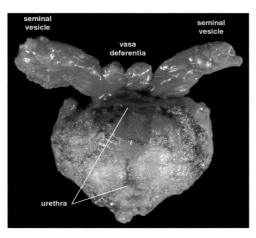

Figure 1.1
Surgical specimen of the prostate gland viewed from an anterior approach. The bladder has been removed from the base of the prostate. A seminal vesicle and vas deferens join on each side of midline to form the ejaculatory duct at the base of the prostate. The ejaculatory ducts traverse within the prostate and enter the urethra at the level of the veru montanum. (Obtained with the kind assistance of Dr Monica E deBaca.)

with a smooth, slightly firm texture (Figure 1.1). The process of benign prostatic enlargement with age affects almost all men, with considerable variability in age of onset and degree of gland enlargement. The normal adult prostate has average dimensions of 33 mm in height, 24 mm in thickness, and 41 mm in width.[1] Normal sonographic measurements are reported[2] as 20–40 mm in length, 21–34 mm in thickness, and 39–53 mm in width, with a volume of 12.9–37.1 cm^3. The base of the prostate refers to the more cranial aspect of the gland, closer to the bladder. The apex of the prostate is the most caudal portion of the gland, adjacent to the muscles of the pelvic floor. The length of the prostate is measured along the long axis of the urethra from base to apex (Figure 1.2). The short-axis diameter of the prostate is greatest in the transverse dimension at the base to mid-gland level (Figure 1.3). The transaxial diameter tapers from this level down toward the apex. Based upon a comparison of the author's experience with that of a European colleague, it is likely that prostatic volumes differ in various geographic locales, and are generally larger in the USA than in Europe (personal communication from Ferdinand Frauscher).

The prostate gland sits on the pelvic floor, and is bounded inferiorly and inferolaterally by the muscles of the pelvic floor (Figure 1.4). The symphysis pubis is anterior to the lower portion of the prostate (Figure 1.5). The fascial planes surrounding the prostate are a caudal continuation of the hypogastric sheath, and contain many neurovascular structures. Anterior to the prostate is the fascia of Zukerkandl, which contains the venous plexus of Santorini (Figure 1.6). The lateral pelvic fascia is found on either side of the prostate, and contains branches of the prostatic artery. The rectum lies posterior to the prostate, and is separated from the prostate by Denonvilliers fascia. Along the anterior wall of the rectum and the posterior and posterolateral aspect of the prostate are two ill-defined collections of vessels and neural structures known as the neurovascular bundles (Figure 1.7). In order to

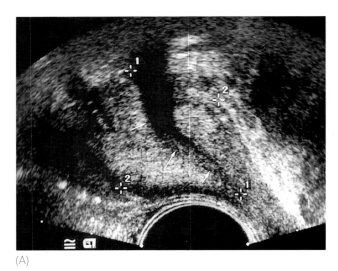

(A)

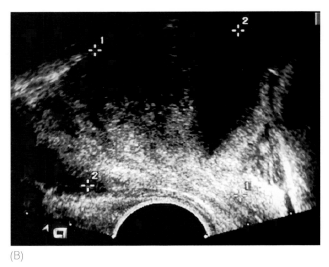

(B)

Figure 1.2
Midline, sagittal images of the prostate: (A) sagittal image of a normal prostate; (B) sagittal image of an enlarged prostate. The urethra is visualized along the long axis of the prostate in (A) (arrows) but is obscured by enlargement of the inner gland in (B).

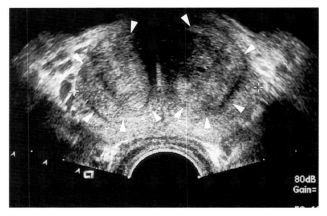

Figure 1.3
Transverse image of the enlarged prostate gland seen in Figure 1.2(B). Benign prostatic hyperplasia is manifest by enlargement of the inner gland in two distinct lobes, one on each side of midline (arrowheads). The maximum transverse diameter is obtained at the mid-gland level.

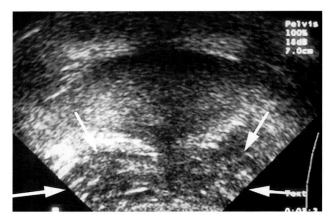

Figure 1.4
Coronal image of the prostate obtained from the transperineal approach. The muscles of the pelvic floor are seen as hypoechoic linear structures below the prostate (arrows).

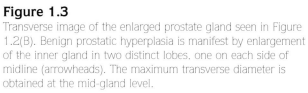

Figure 1.5
Coronal image obtained from the transperineal approach. The plane of imaging is slightly anterior to the prostate. The urethra is visualized entering the corpus spongiosum as it exists from the prostate (straight arrows). On either side of the urethra, a pubic bone is visualized just above the ischiocavernosus muscle as it becomes one of the corpora cavernosa (arrowheads).

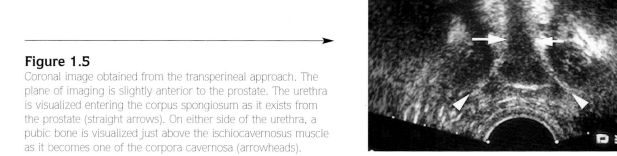

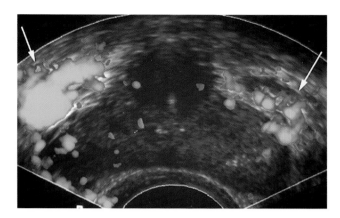

Figure 1.6
Transverse image of the prostate with power Doppler imaging. Large veins from the venous plexus of Santorini are visualized anterior to the prostate on both sides of the midline (arrows).

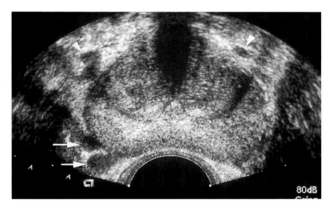

Figure 1.7
Transverse image of a prostate with mild benign prostatic hyperplasia. Two discrete vascular structures are visualized along the right posterolateral aspect of the gland (straight arrows). Although vessels in this position are often labeled as the neurovascular bundle, the neurovascular bundle is not usually a well-defined structure, and is not generally visualized by sonography. Veins from the plexus of Santorini are visualized anterior to the prostate (arrowheads).

preserve erectile function after prostatectomy, surgeons attempt to preserve these neurovascular bundles during surgery. Small perforating vessels and neural structures enter the prostate from the neurovascular structures in the adjacent fascial planes, and represent a potential pathway for spread of prostate cancer through the prostatic capsule.[3]

The urethra, seminal vesicles, and ejaculatory ducts

The prostatic urethra extends through the long axis of the prostate, and serves as a conduit for urine between the

bladder and distal urethra. The urethra is lined by transitional epithelium, which is surrounded by an inner longitudinal and an outer circular layer of smooth muscle. A posterior midline crest extends throughout the length of the prostatic urethra, with prostatic glands emptying into the prostatic sinuses on either side of this crista urethralis. The urethra is often best visualized when a Foley catheter is present (Figure 1.8). Along the posterior wall of the urethra, at the midportion of the prostatic urethra, is a raised ridge of tissue called the verumontanum. This tissue is visible endoscopically, but is not imaged by conventional sonography (Figure 1.9). The prostatic utricle is a small, midline, blind-ending pouch located

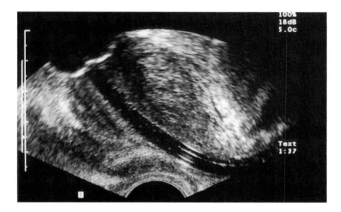

Figure 1.8
Sagittal image of the prostate with a Foley catheter in the urethra. The Foley balloon is within the bladder, resting upon the base of the prostate.

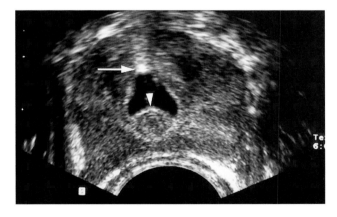

Figure 1.9
Transverse image of the prostate obtained during cystoscopy. The urethra has been distended with fluid. A wire is present at the anterior aspect of the distended urethra (straight arrow). The verumontanum is visualized along the posterior wall of the urethra (arrowhead). The verumontanum is not visible in the undistended urethra. (From Halpern EJ, Hirsch IH. Sonographically guided transurethral laser incision of a Müllerian duct cyst for treatment of ejaculatory duct obstruction. AJR 2000; 175: 777–8. Reprinted with permission.)

within the verumontanum. The prostatic urethra demonstrates an anterior concavity because it is angulated about 35° at the level of the verumontanum (Figure 1.10). The internal sphincter extends from the neck of the bladder into the base of the prostate, and surrounds the prostatic urethra above the verumontanum. Sonographically, the smooth muscle of the internal sphincter may present as a hypoechoic ring around the upper prostatic urethra (Figure 1.11).

The seminal vesicles and vasa deferentia are paired structures that lie along a depression at the base of the prostate posteriorly (Figure 1.12). The seminal vesicles are smooth

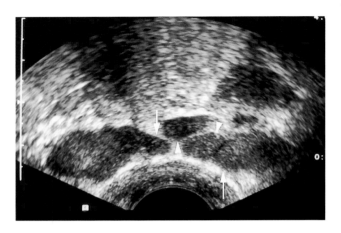

Figure 1.12
Transverse image above the prostate. The seminal vesicles are demonstrated as paired structures that taper toward the midline (straight arrows). The ampullary portion of the vas deferens is visualized coursing medial to the seminal vesicle on each side (arrowheads).

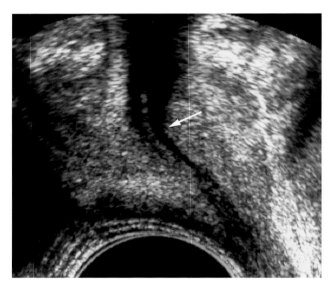

Figure 1.10
Sagittal image of the prostate. The urethra demonstrates a normal anterior concavity (arrow).

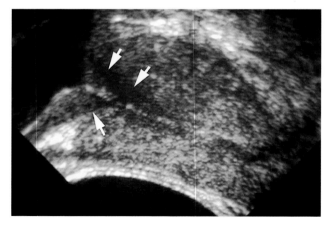

Figure 1.11
Sagittal image of the prostate. The urethra is visualized as a thin echogenic line, extending through the long axis of the gland. The hypoechoic internal sphincter extends from the bladder around the proximal prostatic urethra (arrows).

saccular organs, with a length of 27–50 mm and thickness of 12–15 mm.[4,5] Although there is a wide range in the normal size of the seminal vesicles, they should appear symmetric in size, and should taper toward the midline. As each seminal vesicle enters the base of the prostate, this tapered appearance often produces a 'beak sign'.[6] The vas deferens courses just above the seminal vesicle on each side, and dives caudally toward the prostate just medial to the ipsilateral seminal vesicle (Figure 1.13).

The seminal vesicle and vas deferens on each side join to form an ejaculatory duct. The ejaculatory ducts penetrate the posterior aspect of the base of the prostate on either side of the midline to join the intraprostatic portion of the urethra at the verumontanum, also known as the colliculus seminalis (Figure 1.14). The ejaculatory duct is sometimes visualized as a hypoechoic structure. This hypoechoic appearance is related to a thin surrounding layer of fibromuscular tissue that invaginates around the duct from the prostatic capsule. Occasionally, the ejaculatory duct will appear as an echogenic structure, or contain small echogenic foci corresponding to calcifications or stones (Figure 1.15). In a young patient without glandular enlargement, the course of the ejaculatory duct is parallel to the urethra beyond the verumontanum. The seminal vesicles and vas deferens supply the majority of volume in the ejaculate. The prostate itself contributes a small volume (about 0.5 cm^3) to the normal ejaculate (about 3.5 cm^3).

As the prostate enlarges with age, the normal anatomy of the urethra changes. Enlargement of the inner gland with benign prostatic hyperplasia occurs above the level of the verumontanum, and results in inferior displacement of the latter with mass effect upon the urethra (Figure 1.16). This process distorts the straight line connecting the ejaculatory ducts through the distal urethra. Enlargement of the prostate

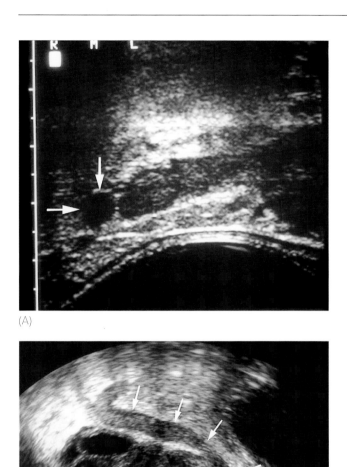

(A)

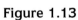

(B)

Figure 1.13

Relationship of the vas deferens to the seminal vesicle: oblique images along the long axis of the seminal vesicle. (A) A portion of the vas deferens coursing superior and lateral to the seminal vesicle (arrow). (B) The vas deferens as it courses toward the prostate, just medial to the seminal vesicle (arrow).

Figure 1.14

Course of the ejaculatory duct. (A) Transverse section of the prostate: the ejaculatory ducts are visualized as paired structures on either side of midline (arrows). (B) The course of a normal ejaculatory duct toward the verumontanum in a sagittal view of the prostate (arrows). (C, D) Transverse (C) and sagittal (D) views of ejaculatory ducts filled with echogenic concretions in a patient with diminished semen flow: the courses of these ejaculatory ducts are easily visualized (arrows).

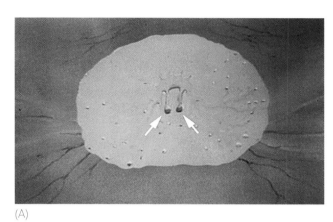

(A)

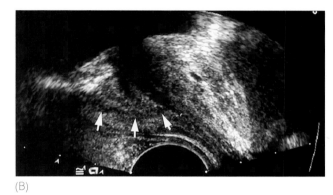

(B)

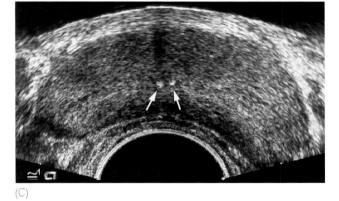

(C)

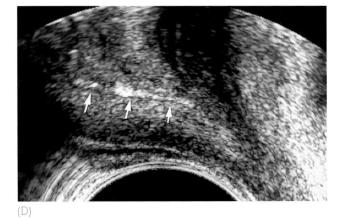

(D)

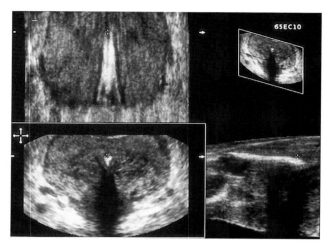

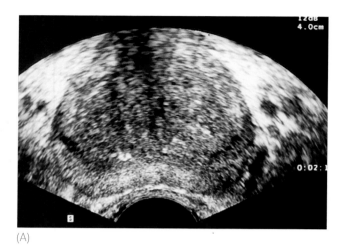

(A)

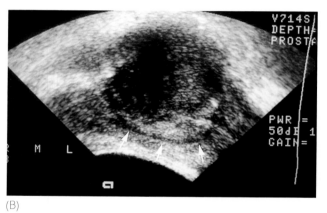

(B)

Figure 1.15

Three-dimensional sonography of the ejaculatory ducts in a patient with reduced semen flow. Coronal reconstruction (top left) demonstrates the paired ejaculatory ducts as echogenic structures due to inspissated debris and stones. Sagittal reconstruction (bottom right) demonstrates the full length of one of the ejaculatory ducts.

Figure 1.16

Enlargement of the prostate with benign prostatic hyperplasia. (A) Transverse image of the prostate: the urethra is compressed between two enlarged lobes of the transition zone, and is not visible. (B) Sagittal image of the prostate: the course of the ejaculatory duct is deviated posteriorly (arrows) by the presence of benign prostatic hyperplasia.

is often accompanied by ductal ectasia within the seminal vesicles (Figure 1.17), probably related to obstruction of the ejaculatory ducts. Prior to the advent of tissue ablation techniques, transurethral resection of the prostate was a common treatment of urinary obstruction related to benign prostatic hyperplasia. This procedure leaves a characteristic defect in the base of the prostate (Figure 1.18).

Anatomical variations are relatively common in the seminal vesicles and ejaculatory ducts.[5] Thickened muscle bundles surround the ejaculatory ducts in 6% of subjects, resulting in a more prominent hypoechoic appearance at sonography. Dilatation of the ductal structures within the seminal vesicles and ejaculatory system is noted in 5% of subjects. Although the ejaculatory duct usually forms as the seminal vesicle and vas deferens enter the prostate, the seminal vesicle and vas deferens will penetrate the prostate as separate structures in approximately 18% of subjects, and join to form the ejaculatory duct within the prostatic parenchyma. In another 12% of subjects, there is no prostatic glandular tissue posterior to a portion of the ejaculatory ducts. This variant may present as a hypoechoic stripe along the base of the prostate.

Congenital cysts of the prostate

A more complete discussion of prostatic cysts is found in Chapter 10. A short discussion of the cystic lesions is presented in this section to stress the embryological associations.

The seminal vesicles, vas deferens, and ejaculatory duct arise from the mesonephric (Wolffian) duct. Congenital anomalies of the seminal vesicle, including cysts and agenesis, may be associated with other Wolffian anomalies.[7] Cysts of the seminal vesicle are rare, and should be distinguished from the more common ductal ectasia of the seminal vesicles (Figure 1.19). Cysts of the seminal vesicles are associated with ipsilateral renal agenesis in two-thirds of cases.[8] Examination of the upper urinary tracts is suggested whenever a congenital anomaly of a seminal vesicle is found. Cysts of the ejaculatory duct are often associated with ejaculatory duct obstruction (Figure 1.20), although it is unclear whether these cysts are the cause or result of the obstruction.[9] Ejaculatory duct cysts arise on either side of the midline, but may appear to be in the midline. Because ejaculatory duct cysts communicate with the ejaculatory duct, aspiration of these cysts should demonstrate the presence of spermatazoa.

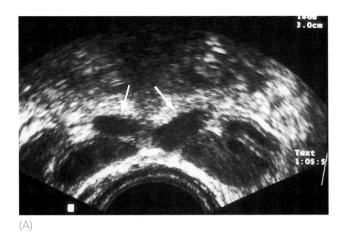

(A)

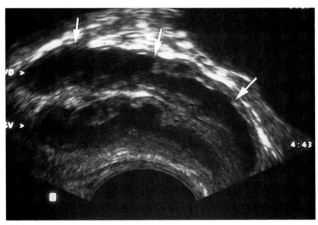

(B)

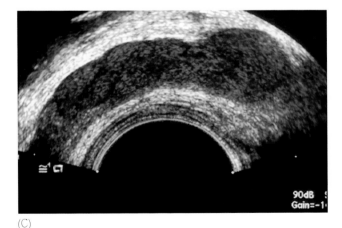

(C)

Figure 1.17

Ductal ectasia of the seminal vesicles. (A) Transverse view with ductal ectasia of the vasa deferentia (arrows) and seminal vesicles: dilated ducts appear as anechoic tubular structures. (B) Oblique view along the long axis of the vas deferens (arrow), with dilatation of both the vas deferens and seminal vesicle. (C) A different patient with ductal ectasia of the seminal vesicle. This seminal vesicle is filled with echogenic material. Echogenic debris within the dilated ducts was observed to move on real-time imaging.

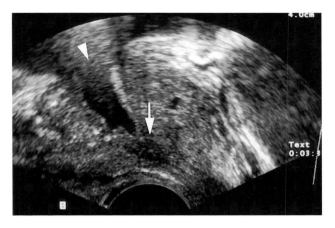

Figure 1.18

Sagittal image of the prostate with a TURP (transurethral resection of the prostate) defect. The defect extends from the level of the bladder (arrowhead) and ends just above the verumontanum (arrow).

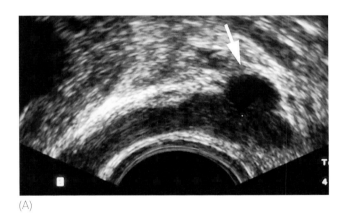

(A)

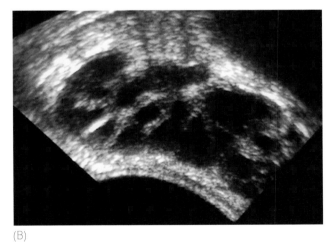

(B)

Figure 1.19

Cysts versus ductal ectasia of the seminal vesicle. (A) A single cyst along the seminal vesicle (arrow): this finding is often associated with other congenital anomalies in the urinary tract. (B) Ductal ectasia with multiple dilated tubular structures.

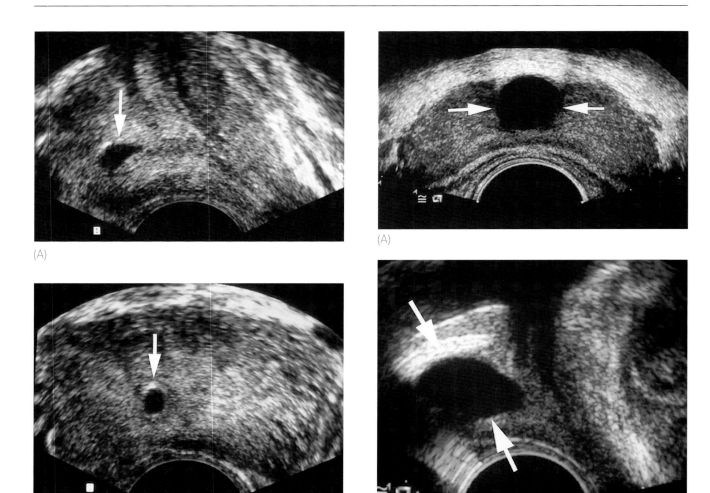

(A)

(B)

(C)

Figure 1.20
Ejaculatory duct cysts: (A) sagittal and (B) transverse images of a small ejaculatory duct cyst (arrow). The cyst demonstrates a characteristic beak pointing toward the verumontanum. (C) Sagittal image in a different patient, demonstrating a calcified stone within an ejaculatory duct cyst (arrows).

(A)

(B)

Figure 1.21
Müllerian duct cyst: (A) transverse and (B) sagittal images of a midline cyst at the base of the prostate. The round cyst extends slightly above the base of the prostate (arrows).

Other common midline cysts within the prostate arise from paramesonephric (Müllerian) ducts. The prostatic utricle, situated within the verumontanum, arises from the Müllerian tubercle. A utricular cyst may be defined as dilatation of the prostatic utricle to larger than 4 mm with loss of epithelial papillations.[5] Utricular cysts communicate with the urethra, and may result in post-void dribbling.[10] Utricular cysts are associated with other anomalies of the genitourinary system, including hypospadias, incomplete testicular descent, and renal agenesis.[11] Müllerian duct cysts are most commonly noted near the base of the prostate in the midline (Figure 1.21), but may extend well above the prostate (Figure 1.22). Müllerian duct cysts do not communicate with the urethra or ejaculatory ducts, and should not contain sperm. However, Müllerian duct cysts can cause ejaculatory duct obstruction.[12] When Müllerian cysts are located within

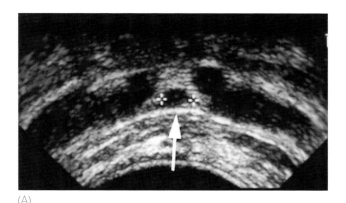

(A)

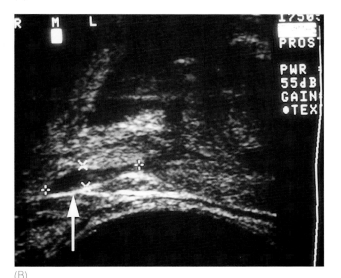

(B)

Figure 1.22
Müllerian duct cyst: (A) transverse and (B) sagittal images of a Müllerian duct cyst that is long and thin, and is completely above the prostate (arrows).

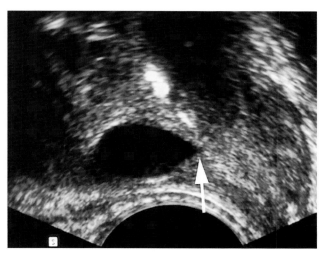

Figure 1.23
Sagittal image of the prostate demonstrates an asymptomatic midline cyst. The cyst is located in the base of the prostate, and demonstrates a beak pointing toward the verumontanum (arrow). On the basis of its location, this could represent either a Müllerian duct cyst or an ejaculatory duct cyst.

the prostate, they may be impossible to distinguish from ejaculatory duct cysts on the basis of imaging characteristics (Figure 1.23).[13] Müllerian duct cysts are not associated with significant congenital anomalies. Case reports have described endometrial carcinoma, clear cell carcinoma, and squamous cell carcinoma within utricular and Müllerian duct cysts.[14,15]

A historical perspective on prostate anatomy

The earliest description of lobar anatomy in the prostate was published in 1912 by Lowsley,[16] on the basis of an analysis of embryonic and fetal glands. This lobular anatomy, however, was never demonstrated in an adult prostate.[17] In 1948, a posterior lobe was proposed by Huggins and Webster[18] as the selective site of origin for prostate cancer. In 1953, on the basis of work with histologic sections from adults, children, and fetuses, Vernet[19] proposed a division of the prostate into three glandular zones: the caudal gland, the cranial gland, and the intermediate area. These zones were defined on the basis of the level of glandular duct openings into the urethra. The cranial gland was further subdivided into lobes. The intrasphincteric glands of Albarrán are contained within the internal sphincter along the upper portion of the urethra. The extrasphincteric glands were divided into two lateral undersphincteric lobes and a median lobe.

Subsequent work by McNeal[20-22] challenged these earlier systems of lobar classification and led to the contemporary zonal model of glandular anatomy in the prostate. This model is discussed in detail below. Several features of Vernet's model correspond to different aspects of the McNeal model.[17] The intrasphincteric glands of Albarrán correspond to the periurethral glands that are present above the level of the verumontanum. The two lateral undersphincteric lobes in Vernet's model correspond to the transition zone lobes in McNeal's model. The median lobe was inconsistently observed by Vernet, and does not exist in McNeal's zonal anatomy. Nonetheless, the term 'median lobe hypertrophy' persists in the common vernacular for benign prostatic hyperplasia that protrudes superiorly into the bladder (Figure 1.24). The intermediate gland in Vernet's description may correspond to McNeal's central zone. The caudal gland in Vernet's description may correspond to McNeal's peripheral zone.

Over the past 30 years, McNeal's model of zonal anatomy in the prostate has come to be accepted as the standard. This model is supported both by characteristic cytologic

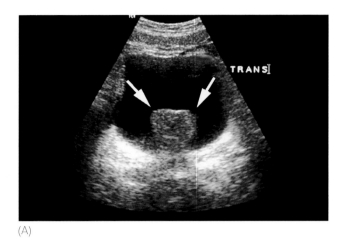

(A)

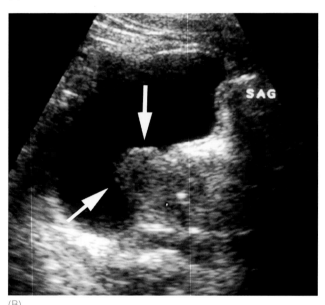

(B)

Figure 1.24

Transverse and sagittal images of the prostate obtained through a transabdominal approach. The prostate is enlarged and extends into the bladder (arrows). This appearance is often described as median lobe hypertrophy.

appearances of the different glandular zones and by histochemical techniques that allow assessments of glandular and stromal functions.[17]

McNeal's zonal anatomy

Approximately one-third of the prostate is composed of nonglandular tissue in the anterior fibromuscular stroma.[23,24] Few pathologic processes involve this fibromuscular stroma, which extends in a plane anterior to the prostatic urethra. The remaining two-thirds of the prostatic volume, located lateral and posterior to the urethra, consists of glandular tissue.

The internal sphincter of the bladder extends around the proximal prostatic urethra from the bladder neck to the verumontanum. McNeal refers to this muscle as the preprostatic sphincter because of its location proximal to the openings of the major glandular components of the prostate. The preprostatic urethra measures approximately 15 mm. The remainder of the prostatic urethra, including the verumontanum as part of the distal urethra, also measures approximately 15 mm. A thin distal smooth sphincter extends from the verumontanum to the prostatic apex, and merges with the external striated sphincter below the prostate. Contained within the preprostatic sphincter are lateral line ducts along the upper urethra with limited glandular development. The limited glandular development may be related to growth restriction by the well-developed preprostatic sphincter.[23] These *periurethral glands* account for 1% of the glandular tissue in the prostate.

The central and peripheral zones compose the bulk of the glandular tissue along the posterior aspect of the prostate. The *central zone* consists of glandular tissue that surrounds the ejaculatory ducts as they course toward the verumontanum. Ducts of the central zone account for 25% of the glandular tissue of the prostate, and empty into the urethra at the verumontanum on either side of the ejaculatory ducts. Central zone tissue exists entirely above the level of the verumontanum. The central zone forms a cone of tissue that sits atop the peripheral zone (Figure 1.25). Ducts of the *peripheral zone* drain into the distal urethra on either side of the verumontanum and the crista urethralis. The peripheral zone composes approximately 70% of the glandular tissue within the prostate.

The transition zone consists of two lobes of glandular tissue on either side of the urethra that drain into the urethra at the verumontanum just above the ejaculatory duct openings. Glands of the transition zone are situated above the level of the verumontanum. Histologically, transition zone glands are identical to peripheral zone glands. In the absence of benign prostatic hyperplasia, transition zone glands compose no more than 5% of the prostatic glandular volume.

A short-axis section of the prostate below the level of the verumontanum will demonstrate anterior fibromuscular stroma anteriorly and peripheral zone glandular tissue posteriorly. A short-axis section of the prostate above the level of the verumontanum should demonstrate periurethral tissue, transition zone tissue, central zone tissue and peripheral zone tissue.

The distinction between central and peripheral zones is based upon microscopic glandular appearance as well as the different locations where their ducts enter along the urethra.[23] Histologic sections of tissue from the central zone have large acini with irregular contours, and prominent stromal ridges projecting into the gland lumens. The peripheral zone glands have narrow ducts that terminate in small, simple acini. Because of the location of the central zone

3. Villers A, McNeal JE, Redwine EA et al. The role of perineural space invasion in the local spread of prostatic adenocarcinoma. J Urol 1989; 142: 763–8.

4. Aboul-Azm TE. Anatomy of the human seminal vesicles and ejaculatory ducts. Arch Androl 1979; 3: 287–92.

5. Villers A, Terris MK, NcNeal JE, Stamey TA. Ultrasound anatomy of the prostate: the normal gland and anatomical variations. J Urol 1990; 143: 732–8.

6. Lee F, Torp-Pederson ST, Siders DB et al. Transrectal ultrasound in the diagnosis and staging of prostatic carcinoma. Radiology 1989; 170: 609–15.

7. Carvalho HA, Paiva JLB, Santos VHV et al. Ultrasonic recognition of a cystic seminal vesicle with ipsilateral renal agenesis. J Urol 1986; 135: 1267–8.

8. Heaney JA, Pfister RC, Meares EM. Giant cyst of the seminal vesicle with renal agenesis. AJR 1987; 149: 139–40.

9. Littrup PJ, Lee F, McLeary RD et al. Transrectal ultrasound of the seminal vesicles and ejaculatory ducts: clinical correlation. Radiology 1988; 168: 626–8.

10. Shabsigh R, Lerner S, Fishman IJ, Kadmon D. The role of ultrasonography in the diagnosis and management of prostatic and seminal vesicle cysts. J Urol 1989; 141: 1206–9.

11. Nghiem HT, Kellman GM, Sandberg SA, Craig BM. Cystic lesions of the prostate. Radiographics 1990; 10: 635–50.

12. Halpern EJ, Hirsch IH. Sonographically guided transurethral laser incision of a müllerian duct cyst for treatment of ejaculatory duct obstruction. AJR 2000; 175: 777–8.

13. Lucey DT, McAninch JW, Bunts RC. Genital cysts of the male pelvis: case report of müllerian and ejaculatory duct cysts in the same patient. J Urol 1973; 109: 440–3.

14. Szemes GC, Rubin DJ. Squamous cell carcinoma in a müllerian duct cyst. J Urol 1968; 100: 40–3.

15. Novak RW, Raines RB, Sollee AN. Clear cell carcinoma in a müllerian duct cyst. Am J Clin Pathol 1981; 76: 339–41.

16. Lowsley OS. The development of the human prostate gland with reference to the development of other structures at the neck of the urinary bladder. Am J Anat 1912; 13: 299–349.

17. Villers A, Steg A, Boccon-Gibod L. Anatomy of the prostate: review of different models. Eur Urol 1991; 20: 261–8.

18. Huggins C, Webster WO. Duality of human prostate in response to estrogen. J Urol 1948; 59: 258–66.

19. Vernet GS. Pathologia Urogenital: Biologia y Pathologia de la Prostata, Madrid: Vol 1, Book 2. Editorial Paz-Montalvo, 1953.

20. McNeal JE. Regional morphology and pathology of the prostate. Am J Clin Pathol 1968; 49: 347–57.

21. McNeal JE. Origin and evolution of benign prostatic enlargement. Invest Urol 1978; 15: 340–5.

22. McNeal JE. Anatomy of the prostate: an historical survey of divergent views. Prostate 1980; 1: 3–13.

23. McNeal JE. The zonal anatomy of the prostate. Prostate 1981; 2: 35–49.

24. McNeal JE. Normal and pathologic anatomy of prostate. Urology 1981; 17(Suppl): 11–16.

25. Coakley FV, Hricak H. Radiologic anatomy of the prostate gland: a clinical approach. Radiol Clin North Am 2000; 38: 15–30.

26. McNeal JE. Origin and development of carcinoma in the prostate. Cancer 1969; 23: 24–33.

27. McNeal JE, Price HM, Redwine EA et al. Stage A versus stage B carcinoma of the prostate: morphologic comparison and biologic significance. J Urol 1988; 139: 61–5.

28. McNeal JE, Redwine EA, Freiha FS, Stamey TA. Zonal distribution of prostatic adenocarcinoma. Correlation with histologic pattern and direction of spread. Am J Surg Pathol 1988; 12: 897–906.

29. Stamey TA. Making the most out of six systematic sextant biopsies. Urology 1995; 45: 2–12.

Section II

Prostate cancer

2

Epidemiology and histopathology of prostate cancer

Ethan J Halpern

A basic understanding of both the epidemiology and histopathology of prostate cancer is essential for the sonographer who evaluates the prostate. The epidemiology of this disease defines those patients who are at increased risk, and should be screened for cancer of the prostate. An understanding of the histopathologic growth patterns of prostate cancer is useful in planning the biopsy strategy.

Epidemiology

Cancer of the prostate is the single most commonly diagnosed malignancy in men. It is estimated that in the year 2001, 198 100 men will have been diagnosed with cancer of the prostate in the USA with 31 500 expected deaths.[1] The incidence of prostate cancer increases exponentially with age. The American Cancer Society recommends a digital rectal examination and a PSA (prostate-specific antigen) blood test once a year to screen for prostate cancer in men 50 years of age and older. For men with increased risk for cancer of the prostate, including African-Americans or those with a strong family history of prostate cancer, screening should commence at age 45. Different subspecialty groups have their own recommendations for PSA screening that may differ from those suggested by the American Cancer Society.

Among risk factors, age is the most important.[2] Eighty percent of cancer in the prostate is diagnosed after the age of 65. It is estimated that 40% of men in their 70s and 80% of men in their 80s harbor prostate cancer. Although the incidence of asymptomatic cancer in the prostate increases with age, so does the incidence of death from prostate cancer.

The risk associated with family history depends upon the number of close relatives affected with prostate cancer. The risk of cancer may increase by a factor of 2–5 with an affected first-degree relative,[3] and increases by a factor of 5–8 with

two affected first-degree relatives. The relative risk is higher if the affected relative contracted the disease at an early age. Early-onset prostate cancer may be related to an autosomal dominant allele. This autosomal dominant allele is associated with only 9% of all prostate cancer, but with 45% of prostate cancer in men under the age of 55.[4] Nonetheless, over 80% of cases of prostate cancer are diagnosed in people with no known affected first-degree relatives.

The incidence of clinically significant prostate cancer varies with race. In the USA, African-American men have a higher incidence of prostate cancer.[5] Prostate cancer in African-American men tends to be diagnosed at a later stage, and has a lower survival rate even when the survival rate is adjusted for stage at diagnosis. Furthermore, although the mortality rate from prostate cancer has decreased in the entire population, this improvement is less noticeable in the African-American population. Interestingly, the rate of microscopic, clinically insignificant cancer of the prostate is equal in different ethnic groups. Nonetheless, Black men and Scandinavian men do have a higher incidence of clinically apparent disease.

Other environmental risk factors may be associated with prostate cancer. Analysis of eating habits in different countries suggests that high dietary fat is associated with increased risk of prostate cancer.[6,7] Reduced sun exposure and elevated levels of testosterone are associated with increased rates of prostate cancer. Prostate cancer is uncommon in countries near the equator with high levels of sun exposure. Prostate cancer is also less common in Oriental populations that tend to have a lower content of dietary fat and lower levels of testosterone. It is possible that dietary fat may increase the risk of prostate cancer through the production of testosterone. Testosterone is necessary for the growth of normal prostate, and is also essential for the early growth phase of most prostate cancer.[8] For this reason, anti-androgen therapy is often effective in slowing or stopping the progression of prostate cancer.

Screening for cancer of the prostate

With respect to screening for cancer of the prostate, the serum level of PSA is the single non-invasive test with the highest sensitivity for prostate cancer.[9] PSA is found in normal prostate as well as in malignant prostate tissue. However, the concentration of PSA is much higher in malignant prostate tissue. The probability of cancer increases with the serum PSA level, and may reach 50% for PSA values above 10 ng/ml. Nonetheless, 25% of men with prostate cancer have a serum PSA value of less than 4 ng/ml. Furthermore, PSA generally increases as the prostate enlarges with age.[10,11] Various strategies have been used to increase the sensitivity and/or specificity of the PSA test, including lowering of the cutoff value or the use of age-adjusted PSA.[12] PSA velocity is computed based upon the change in serum PSA over time. A PSA velocity above 0.75 ng/ml/year may be more accurate in predicting cancer than a single PSA measurement.[13] PSA density is computed as a ratio of the total serum PSA to the sonographically estimated gland volume. In selected populations, the PSA density may more accurately distinguish benign prostatic hyperplasia from prostate cancer.[14,15] More recently, fractionated PSA with a reported value of percentage of free PSA has been useful to improve specificity of cancer detection in subjects with total PSA values between 4 and 10 ng/ml.[16]

Digital rectal examination is relatively insensitive for the detection of prostate cancer. Fewer than half of all cancers in the prostate can be detected with digital rectal examination.[17] Approximately half of cancers detected by digital rectal examination are at an advanced stage, when treatment is unlikely to be effective. Furthermore, digital rectal examination is a subjective examination prone to inter-observer disagreement and dependent upon the experience of the examiner.[18] Nonetheless, it remains an integral part of the standard physical examination. The findings of an abnormal digital rectal examination should be used to guide the sonographic examination of the prostate and the biopsy procedure.

Sonographic screening for cancer of the prostate remains a controversial topic. Conventional sonography with or without color or power Doppler may be useful to select sites for directed biopsy and increase the positive biopsy rate. Nonetheless, conventional sonography is insensitive to many isoechoic cancers, and often lacks sufficient discriminatory power to distinguish malignancy from benign inflammatory change.[19] For these reasons, sonography should not be used at present as a screening examination for prostate cancer. Rather, sonographically directed biopsy should serve as a diagnostic test for the presence of prostate cancer among patients in specific high-risk categories as defined by PSA, digital rectal examination, or other evidence for the presence of prostatic malignancy.

Histopathology

The vast majority of cancers that arise within the prostate are adenocarcinomas, and over 85% are multifocal.[20] Two-thirds of these malignancies arise in the peripheral zone. Since the central zone and peripheral zone are indistinguishable by sonography, we define the outer gland as that portion of the prostate outside the sonographically visible surgical capsule, including both the central and peripheral zones. Just over three-quarters of all prostatic malignancies arise in the outer gland.[21] Fewer than one-quarter of all prostatic malignancies arise within the sonographically identified inner gland, which is composed primarily of transition zone material. Furthermore, these inner gland cancers generally spread into the outer gland before they metastasize. A recent series of whole-mount radical prostatectomy specimens reviewed at Thomas Jefferson University demonstrated multiple foci of malignancy in approximately 85% of glands with an average of three malignant foci in each prostate.[22] Just over two-thirds of all lesions were localized to the outer gland (Figure 2.1).

Both the surgical capsule and the prostatic capsule act as relative barriers to the spread of prostatic malignancy. The surgical capsule lies between the inner gland and outer gland, and represents the tissue plane of resection for open prostatectomy. It may be visualized sonographically by a linear deposition of corpora amalacea or calcifications. The prostatic capsule is not a true epithelial capsule, but rather a thin layer of fibrous tissue that extends from the anterior fibromuscular stroma to surround the prostate. As a consequence of these barriers, prostate cancer tends to spread along the prostate capsule in the transverse and cranio-caudal directions. The long axis of tumor growth does not usually extend through the surgical capsule between the inner gland and outer gland. On the basis of this understanding of the growth pattern of prostatic cancer, Stamey has recommended a modified approach

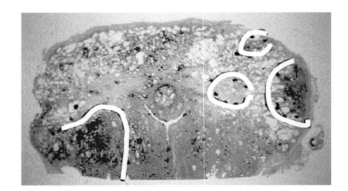

Figure 2.1

Whole-mount section from a radical prostatectomy specimen. The circled areas contain malignant foci. Multiple malignant foci are identified in 85% of prostate glands removed for cancer. Of the four malignant areas identified in this section, two are in the outer gland along the capsule, and two are in the inner gland. (Courtesy of Peter A McCue, MD.)

to sextant biopsy of the prostate. The modified sextant specimens are obtained along the prostatic capsule at the base, mid-gland, and apex of the prostate in a pattern that will more efficiently sample tumor growing along the capsule.[23]

Capsular invasion refers to infiltration of tumor into the thin layer of tissue that surrounds the prostate. *Capsular penetration* refers to extension of tumor outside the prostate gland into the surrounding fascial planes. The diagnoses of capsular invasion and capsular penetration are made from the pathological specimen removed at surgery, but can be suggested by sonography or magnetic resonance imaging (MRI) when there is irregularity of the glandular margins, or loss of the visible fat planes around the prostate (Figure 2.2). The layer of fibrous tissue that surrounds the prostate is perforated by the ejaculatory ducts as they enter the base of the prostate (Figure 2.3), and is incomplete at the prostatic apex. These anatomic facts explain the greater propensity for prostate cancer to spread outside the organ into the seminal vesicles or out of the apex of the gland. Extracapsular spread of tumor increases the risk of post-prostatectomy recurrence.

Perineural invasion of prostate cancer is sometimes noted on needle-biopsy cores. The neural tissue enters the prostate

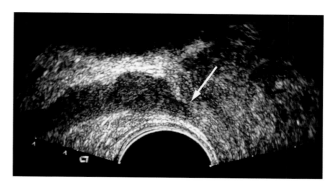

Figure 2.3
Sagittal sonogram demonstrates the seminal vesicle as it enters the base of the prostate (arrows). A thin layer of fibromuscular tissue surrounding the prostate, commonly called the capsule of the prostate, invaginates around the ejaculatory duct. This invagination may provide a pathway for extracapsular spread of prostate cancer. A second area of potential weakness in the capsule of the prostate is the apex of the gland, where the capsule may be incomplete.

through the capsule from the neurovascular bundles that course along the posterolateral aspect of the prostate (Figure 2.4). The presence of perineural invasion may be helpful to the pathologist in determining that biopsy tissue is truly malignant. Furthermore, since these nerves must perforate the capsule of the prostate, perineural invasion represents a potential pathway for extracapsular spread of prostate cancer (Figure 2.5). A pathologic diagnosis of perineural invasion from a biopsy core does not confirm extracapsular spread, but does increase the risk for it.

Cancer volume and stage are important prognostic indicators. Larger tumors have a higher rate of high-grade cancer,

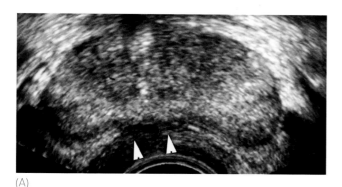

(A)

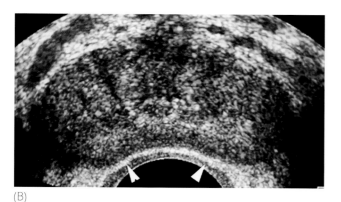

(B)

Figure 2.2
Transverse sonography of the prostate to demonstrate fat planes around the gland. (A) Focal loss of the posterior fat planes to the right of midline, related to capsular penetration by a Gleason 7 cancer (arrowheads). Thinning of the fat planes is commonly related to prostatic enlargement by benign prostatic hyperplasia. (B) A normal posterior fat plane (arrowheads).

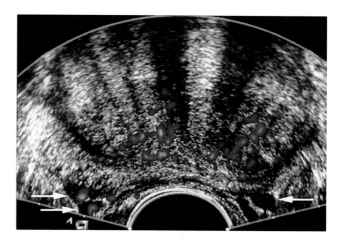

Figure 2.4
Transverse sonogram of the prostate with power Doppler imaging demonstrates vessels bilaterally along the posterolateral aspect of the gland (arrows). The presence of blood flow is demonstrated by Doppler signal within the right-sided neurovascular bundle, and within the enlarged transition zone.

Figure 2.5

Transverse sonogram of the prostate in a patient with a Gleason 6 cancer at the right base. The area of cancer appears as a hypoechoic bulge of the prostate contour (arrows). Power Doppler demonstrates flow within the neurovascular bundles (arrowheads) as well as flow extending into the area of cancer. Vessels and nerves traveling along the posterior and posterolateral aspect of the prostate send small branches into the prostate through the capsule. These neurovascular bundle branches represent a potential pathway for spread of malignancy outside of the prostate.

capsular penetration, and distant metastases. A tumor volume under 0.5 cm^3 Is often termed insignificant, especially in older subjects. When comparing cancers of the inner and outer gland, inner gland tumors are less likely to metastasize until they reach a larger size, and often will not metastasize until after they have spread into the outer gland. The TNM (tumor, node, metastasis) staging system has generally replaced the Whitmore–Jewett staging system for prostate cancer (Figure 2.6).[24] In the TNM

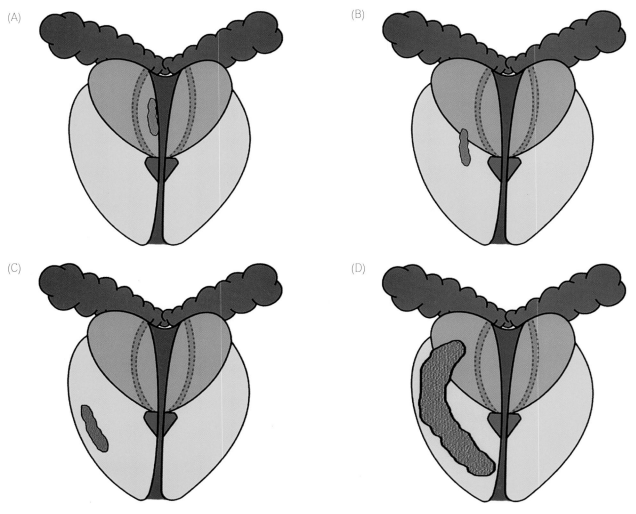

(A)

(B)

(C)

(D)

Figure 2.6

For caption, see opposite.

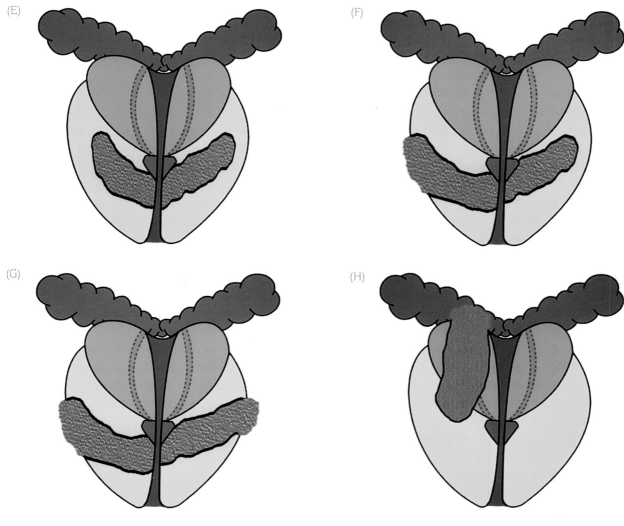

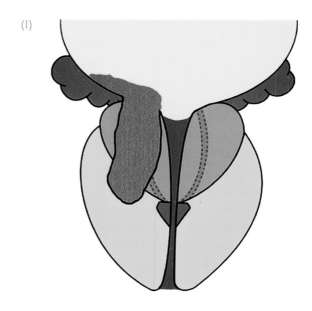

Figure 2.6

TNM staging system for prostate cancer. Stage T1 lesions are not palpable. Stage T2 lesions are palpable, but confined to the prostate. Stage T3 lesions extend beyond the gland. (A, B) Stage T1 lesions are found incidentally on transurethral resection (T1a and T1b: (A)) or on needle biopsy for an elevated PSA (T1c: (B)). (C) Stage T2a involves less than 50% of one side of the gland. (D) Stage T2b involves over 50% of one side of the gland. (E) Stage T2c involves both sides of the gland. (F) Stage T3a extends through the capsule on one side. (G) Stage T3b extends through the capsule on both sides. (H) Stage T3c involves the seminal vesicles. (I) Stage T4 extends into adjacent organs other than the seminal vesicles. TNM stage T2 lesions correspond to stage B lesions in the Whitmore–Jewett system. TNM stage T3 lesions correspond to stage C1 lesions in the Whitmore–Jewett system. TNM stage T4 lesions correspond to stage C2 lesions in the Whitmore–Jewett system. Cancer that extends into nodal chains (TNM stage: N1, N2, N3) or distant organs (TNM stage: M1) is classified as stage D in the Whitmore–Jewett system. (Adapted from Rifkin MD, Dahnert W, Kurtz AB. Stage of the art: endorectal sonography of the prostate gland. AJR 1990; 154: 691–700. Reprinted with permission. Additional artwork by Jon D'Agostino.)

system, T1 cancer is not palpable and is incidentally discovered on transurethral resection. T1c cancer is discovered on biopsy that is obtained for an elevated PSA. T2 cancer is palpable but confined to the prostate. T3 tumor extends beyond the prostate. T3c represents extension into the seminal vesicles. T4 tumor invades adjacent organs or muscles. Nodes are classified by their number and size.

Cancer grade is generally reported with the Gleason scoring system.[25] Each biopsy core that contains malignant tissue can be described by the percent or length of the biopsy core that is involved with tumor, and by a Gleason score. The Gleason score is based upon the microscopic glandular pattern. For each tissue core, the dominant (primary) and secondary glandular architectural patterns are graded based upon the orderliness of gland formation. The Gleason grade varies from 1 for a well-differentiated pattern with well-defined gland formation to a grade of 5 for complete loss of the glandular pattern (Figure 2.7). The Gleason score or Gleason sum is simply the sum of grades assigned to the primary and secondary patterns. When there is only a small amount of cancer tissue in the core, it may not be possible to define a Gleason score, and only the Gleason pattern is reported. A Gleason pattern of 4 or 5 suggests high-grade malignancy. The logic behind use of the Gleason score (sum) is related to the observation that prognosis is tied to both the primary and secondary patterns. Nonetheless, since the primary pattern has greater prognostic significance than the secondary pattern, a Gleason score of 7 (4 + 3) will behave more aggressively than a Gleason score of 7 (3 + 4). Treatment options may be viewed differently for these two Gleason 7 cancers, depending upon the primary Gleason pattern.

The diagnosis and histologic grading of prostate cancer depends upon the glandular pattern that is observed microscopically. When individual prostatic cells appear cytologically atypical but remain in a normal glandular pattern, the diagnosis of prostatic intraepithelial neoplasia (PIN) is assigned. PIN is often classified as low-grade or high-grade, depending upon the cytological appearance. High-grade PIN is often present along with cancer of the prostate. Although it is likely that high-grade PIN may progress to prostate cancer, this progression has never been proven with a longitudinal study of individual PIN foci. For this reason, PIN is not called carcinoma in situ. It is generally accepted that a patient with high-grade PIN on biopsy of the prostate has a risk of 30–50% for finding prostate cancer on subsequent biopsy.[26,27]

The diagnosis of prostate cancer from a biopsy core may be uncertain when only minimal malignant tissue is observed. The differential diagnosis of minimal adenocarcinoma includes high-grade PIN as well as 'atypical small acinar proliferation'. The latter is a pathologic description used for the presence within a biopsy core of small glandular formations suspicious, but not diagnostic, for carcinoma. The benign entities most commonly confused with minimal adenocarcinoma are atypical adenomatous hyperplasia (adenosis) and atrophy.[28] Special immunohistochemical stains against basal-cell-specific high-

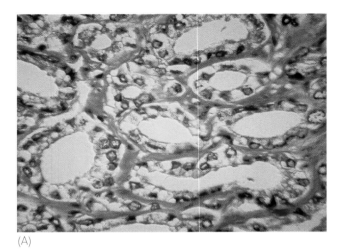

(A)

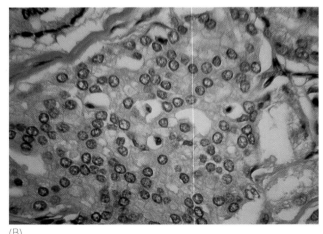

(B)

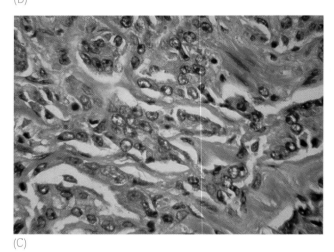

(C)

Figure 2.7

Gleason grading system for prostate cancer. The Gleason sum for each biopsy core is computed as a sum of two patterns: a primary and a secondary glandular pattern. (A) A cancer with a well-differentiated glandular pattern, rated as Gleason 4 (sum of 2 + 2). (B) An intermediate pattern, rated as Gleason 6 (sum of 3 + 3). (C) A poorly differentiated glandular pattern with a Gleason score of 8 (sum of 4 + 4). (Courtesy of Pamela R Edmonds, MD.)

molecular-weight cytokeratins may be useful in this differential diagnosis.[29] Various criteria have been described to distinguish atypical small acinar proliferation.[30] A diagnosis of atypical small acinar proliferation is associated with increased risk of adenocarcinoma on repeat biopsy (as high as 50%).[31,32]

In addition to the size, stage, and grade of prostate cancer, microvascular density provides an independent prognostic marker for the aggressiveness of the disease and propensity to metastasize. Microvascular density is not observed on the standard H&E staining performed on all prostatectomy specimens. Special stains for endothelial cells are required for the quantification of microvascular density (Figure 2.8). Studies of microvessel density within the prostate demonstrate a clear association of increased microvessel density with the presence of cancer,[33] with metastases,[34] with the stage of disease,[35–37] and with disease-specific survival.[38,39] The recent literature also suggests that quantitative assessment of microvascular density may actually provide important data to guide therapeutic decisions.[40] From the sonographic viewpoint, the increased microvessel density associated with clinically significant prostate cancer represents a potential method for improved diagnosis of prostate cancer.

Another potentially useful histologic criteria in the diagnosis of prostate cancer is the DNA ploidy. The presence of non-diploid DNA patterns in prostatic adenocarcinoma is associated with early disease relapse and shortened patient survival.[41–44] DNA ploidy analysis of needle-biopsy specimens of prostate cancer may be a more sensitive and specific indicator of final tumor grade at radical prostatectomy than the original needle biopsy grade.[45]

Summary

Adenocarcinoma of the prostate is the single most common cancer diagnosed in the male population, with a marked preponderance in older age groups. Although many small, low-grade cancers may not be clinically significant, larger tumors with higher histologic grades and increased microvascular density are clinically significant and should be treated. A basic understanding of the histologic growth patterns of prostate cancer is invaluable to guide the biopsy strategy for improved early detection of prostate cancer.

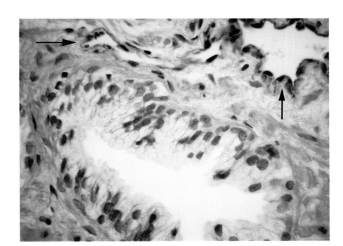

(A)

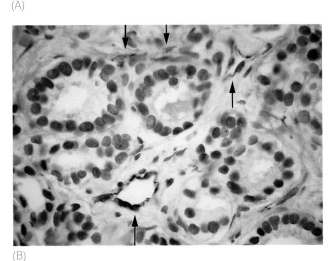

(B)

Figure 2.8

Endothelial cell staining with CD31. Endothelial cells stain brown. (A) Normal prostate tissue with a solitary gland and adjacent vessels (arrows). (B) A Gleason 6 prostate cancer with crowded glands and many smaller vessels (arrows). Images are at 400× magnification. (Courtesy of Pamela R Edmonds, MD.)

References

1. Greenlee RT, Hill-Harmon MB, Murray T, Thun M. Cancer statistics, 2001. CA Cancer J Clin 2001; 51: 15–36.
2. Pienta KJ, Esper PS. Risk factors for prostate cancer. Ann Intern Med 1993; 118: 793–803.
3. Steinberg GD, Carter BS, Beaty TH et al. Family history and the risk of prostate cancer. Prostate 1990; 17: 337–47.
4. Carter BS, Beaty TH, Steinberg GD et al. Mendelian inheritance of familial prostate cancer. Proc Natl Acad Sci USA 1992; 89: 3367–71.
5. Baquet CR, Horm JW, Gibbs T, Greenwald P. Socioeconomic factors and cancer incidence among Blacks and Whites. J Natl Cancer Inst 1991; 83: 551–7.
6. Carroll KK, Khor HT. Dietary fat in relation to tumorigenesis. Prog Biochem Pharmacol 1975; 10: 308–53.
7. Giovannucci E, Rimm EB, Colditz GA et al. A prospective study of dietary fat and risk of prostate cancer. J Natl Cancer Inst 1993; 85: 1571–9.
8. Montie JE, Pienta KJ. A review of the role of androgenic hormones in the pathogenesis of benign prostatic hypertrophy and prostate cancer. Urology 1994; 43: 892–9.
9. Gann PH, Hennekens CH, Stampfer MJ. A prospective evaluation of plasma prostate-specific antigen for detection of prostatic cancer. JAMA 1995; 273: 289–94.

10. Oesterling JE, Cooner WH, Jacobsen SJ et al. Influence of patient age on the serum PSA concentration. An important clinical observation. Urol Clin North Am 1993; 20: 671–80.

11. Collins GN, Lee RJ, McKelvie GB et al. Relationship between prostate specific antigen, prostate volume, and age in the benign prostate. Br J Urol 1993; 71: 445–50.

12. Oesterling JE, Jacobsen SJ, Cooner WH. The use of age-specific reference ranges for serum prostate specific antigen in men 60 years old or older. J Urol 1993; 150: 1837–9.

13. Carter HB, Pearson JD, Metter EJ et al. Longitudinal evaluation of prostate-specific antigen levels in men with and without prostate disease. JAMA 1992; 267: 2215–20.

14. Bretton PR, Evans WP, Borden JD, Castellanos RD. The use of prostate specific antigen density to improve the sensitivity of prostate specific antigen in detecting prostate carcinoma. Cancer 1994; 74: 2991–5.

15. Benson MC, Whang IS, Olsson CA et al. The use of prostate specific antigen density to enhance the predictive value of intermediate levels of serum prostate specific antigen. J Urol 1992; 147: 817–21.

16. Catalona WJ, Smith DS, Wolfert RL et al. Evaluation of percentage of free serum prostate-specific antigen to improve specificity of prostate cancer screening. JAMA 1995; 274: 1214–20.

17. Epstein JI, Walsh PC, Carmichael M, Brendler CB. Pathologic and clinical findings to predict tumor extent of nonpalpable (stage T1c) prostate cancer. JAMA 1994; 271: 368–74.

18. Smith DS, Catalona WJ. Interexaminer variability of digital rectal examination in detecting prostate cancer. Urology 1995; 45: 70–4.

19. Halpern EJ, Strup SE. Using gray scale, color and power Doppler sonography to detect prostatic cancer. AJR 2000; 174: 623–7.

20. Byar DP, Mostofi FK. Carcinoma of the prostate: prognostic evaluation of certain pathologic features in 208 radical prostatectomies. Cancer 1972; 30: 5–13.

21. McNeal JE, Redwine EA, Freiha FS, Stamey TA. Zonal distribution of prostatic adenocarcinoma. Correlation with histologic pattern and direction of spread. Am J Surg Pathol 1988; 12: 897–906.

22. Halpern EJ, McCue PA, Aksnes AK et al. Contrast-enhanced sonography of the prostate with Sonozoid – correlation with whole mount prostatectomy specimens. Radiology (in press).

23. Stamey TA. Making the most out of six systematic sextant biopsies. Urology 1995; 45: 2–12.

24. Montie JE. 1992 staging system for prostate cancer. Semin Urol 1993; 11: 10–13.

25. Gleason DF. Histologic grading and clinical staging of prostatic carcinoma. In: Urologic Pathology: The Prostate (Tannenbaum M, ed). Philadelphia: Lea & Febiger, 1977: 171–97.

26. Brawer MK, Bigler SA, Sohlberg OE et al. Significance of prostatic intraepithelial neoplasia on prostate needle biopsy. Urology 1991; 38: 103–7.

27. Weinstein MH, Epstein JI. Significance of high grade prostatic intraepithelial neoplasia (PIN) on needle biopsy. Hum Pathol 1993; 24: 624–9.

28. Thorson P, Humphrey PA. Minimal adenocarcinoma in prostate needle biopsy tissue. Am J Clin Pathol 2000; 114: 896–909.

29. Helpap B, Kollermann J, Oehler U. Limiting the diagnosis of atypical small glandular proliferations in needle biopsies of the prostate by the use of immunohistochemistry. J Pathol 2001; 193: 350–3.

30. Iczkowski KA, Bostwick DG. Criteria for biopsy diagnosis of minimal volume prostatic adenocarcinoma: analytic comparison with nondiagnostic but suspicious atypical small acinar proliferation. Arch Pathol Lab Med 2000; 124: 98–107.

31. Iczkowski KA, Bassler TJ, Schwob VS et al. Diagnosis of 'suspicious for malignancy' in prostate biopsies: predictive value for cancer. Urology 1998; 51: 749–57.

32. Ouyang RC, Kenwright DN, Nacey JN, Delahunt B. The presence of atypical small acinar proliferation in prostate needle biopsy is predictive of carcinoma on subsequent biopsy. BJU Int 2001; 87: 70–4.

33. Bigler SA, Deering RE, Brawer MK. Comparison of microscopic vascularity in benign and malignant prostate tissue. Hum Pathol 1993; 24: 220–6.

34. Weidner N, Carroll PR, Flax J et al. Tumor angiogenesis correlates with metastasis in invasive prostate carcinoma. Am J Pathol 1993; 143: 401–9.

35. Fregene TA, Khanuja PS, Noto AC et al. Tumor-associated angiogenesis in prostate cancer. Anticancer Res 1993; 13: 2377–82.

36. Brawer MK, Deering RE, Brown M et al. Predictors of pathologic stage in prostate carcinoma, the role of neovascularity. Cancer 1994; 73: 678–87.

37. Bostwick DG, Wheeler TM, Blute M et al. Optimized microvessel density analysis improves prediction of cancer stage from prostate needle biopsies. Urology 1996; 48: 47–57.

38. Lissbrant IF, Stattin P, Damber JE, Bergh A. Vascular density is a predictor of cancer-specific survival in prostatic carcinoma. Prostate 1997; 33: 38–45.

39. Borre M, Offersen BV, Nerstrom B, Overgaard J. Microvessel density predicts survival in prostate cancer patients subjected to watchful waiting. Br J Cancer 1998; 78: 940–4.

40. Brawer MK. Quantitative microvessel density. A staging and prognostic marker for human prostatic carcinoma. Cancer 1996; 78: 345–9.

41. Adolfsson J, Ronstrom L, Hedlund P-O et al. The prognostic value of modal deoxyribonucleic acid in low grade, low stage untreated prostate cancer. J Urol 1990; 144: 1404–7.

42. Dejter SW, Cunningham RE, Noguchi PD et al. Prognostic significance of DNA ploidy in carcinoma of prostate. Urology 1989; 33: 361–6.

43. Humphrey PA, Walther PJ, Currin SM, Vollmer RT. Histologic grade, DNA ploidy, and intraglandular tumor extent as indicators of tumor progression in clinical stage B prostatic carcinoma. Am J Surg Pathol 1991; 15: 1165–70.

44. Lieber MM, Murtaugh PA, Farrow GM et al. DNA ploidy and surgically treated prostate cancer. Important independent association with prognosis for patients with prostate carcinoma treated by radical prostatectomy. Cancer 1995; 75: 1935–43.

45. Ross JS, Sheehan CE, Ambros RA et al. Needle biopsy DNA ploidy status predicts grade shifting in prostate cancer. Am J Surg Pathol 1999; 23: 296–301.

3

Gray-scale evaluation of prostate cancer

Ethan J Halpern

Sonographic evaluation of the prostate may be performed via a transabdominal, transrectal, or transperineal approach. The transabdominal approach through a full urinary bladder is useful to measure the overall size of the gland, but lacks fine anatomic detail for the detection of focal lesions (Figure 3.1). Transperineal imaging is a useful technique for biopsy of patients in whom the transrectal approach is not possible (Figure 3.2). The transperineal technique is discussed further in Chapter 5. The transrectal approach, however, is the mainstay of prostate imaging (Figure 3.3). Transrectal imaging provides a unique window immediately adjacent to the prostate that allows high-frequency imaging at close range. It provides superior image quality for the diagnosis of pathologic processes. Furthermore, since most cancers of the prostate arise within the peripheral zone, the posterior transrectal approach is ideal for sonographic guidance of prostate biopsy procedures.

Gray-scale examination technique

Transrectal examination may be performed with the patient in the lithotomy or lateral decubitus position. A digital rectal examination should be performed prior to insertion of the ultrasound transducer. Lubricant is placed on the transducer tip. Special anesthetic techniques may be required in patients with stenosis or tenderness of the rectal sphincter, and in

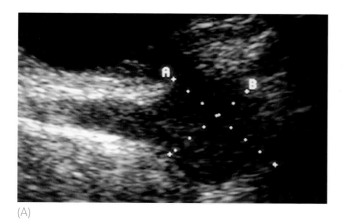

(A)

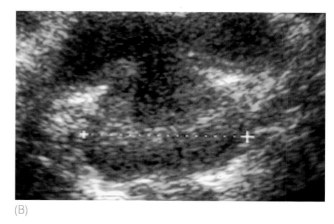

(B)

Figure 3.1
Sagittal and transverse images of the prostate obtained from the transabdominal approach through a partially distended urinary bladder. (A) Sagittal and AP (anteroposterior) measurements of the gland. The apex of the gland is obscured by posterior acoustical shadowing from the symphysis pubis. A seminal vesicle is demonstrated extending superiorly from the base of the gland. (B) A transverse measurement of the gland. The outer gland is more echogenic than the inner gland. Because the outer gland is far from the transducer, the transabdominal approach is limited in its ability to evaluate focal lesions in the outer gland.

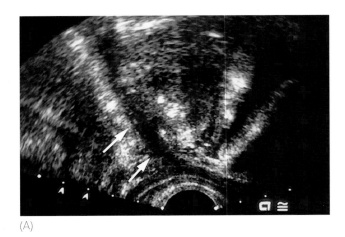

(A)

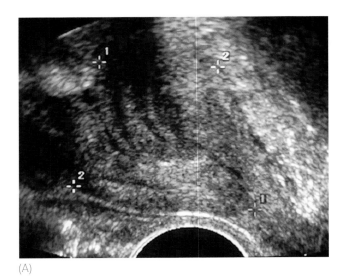

(A)

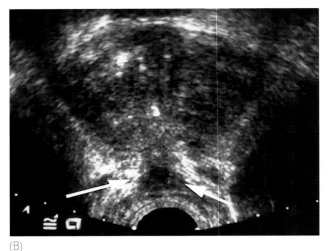

(B)

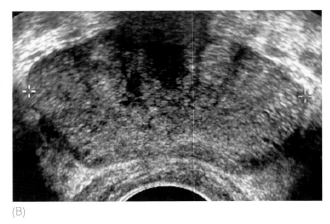

(B)

Figure 3.2

Sagittal and coronal images of the prostate obtained with a transperineal approach. (A) Sagittal midline image. As the urethra extends anteriorly along the perineum, it courses within the corpus spongiosum (arrows). (B) Coronal image of the prostate near the apex. At this level, the urethra is observed to extend out of the prostate (arrows). Calcifications are observed within the parenchyma of the prostate. Visualization of the prostatic parenchyma is slightly better than with the transabdominal approach. However, evaluation of the outer gland is limited, particularly at the base of the prostate, which is furthest from the perineum.

Figure 3.3

Sagittal and transverse images of the prostate obtained from the transrectal approach. (A) Sagittal midline section with sagittal and AP measurements of the gland. (B) A transverse measurement of the gland. The outer gland is immediately adjacent to the transducer, and details of the gray-scale anatomy are well visualized with a high-frequency transducer.

patients who will have multiple biopsy specimens obtained. These are discussed in more detail in Chapter 5. Asking the patient to 'bear down' during the process of probe insertion may facilitate insertion of the probe into the rectum. Once the probe is inserted into the rectum, the patient should not experience any further pain from the imaging procedure.

Transrectal sonography may be performed with a biplane probe that allows imaging in both the transverse and sagittal planes. Alternatively, an end-fire endocavitary probe may be used to image in an oblique transverse plane (actually an oblique plane between the coronal and transverse planes).

The end-fire probe is rotated by 90° to image in the orthogonal sagittal plane. Older side-fire systems may require two probes: one for the transverse plane and a second for the sagittal plane. The close proximity of the ultrasound probe in the rectum to the prostate allows high-resolution imaging. In order to take advantage of this geometry, a high-frequency probe with a wide scan sector should be employed. Transrectal probes are commercially available with transmit frequency ranges of 6–10 MHz. Higher-frequency probes should provide better resolution along the axis of propagation of sound waves. When measuring the prostate, a lower frequency may be useful to define the more anterior aspect of the gland. Lower frequencies in the range of 5–6 MHz are also useful for transperineal scanning. A wideband transducer with an adjustable frequency range from 6 to 10 MHz will allow optimal imaging for both measurement of the gland and gray-scale evaluation. Harmonic imaging is now available on several transrectal probes, but has not been proven to improve the detection of cancers. Harmonic imaging of the prostate is generally reserved for contrast-enhanced imaging (see Chapter 6). A wide scanning angle is important in order to visualize the entire transverse or craniocaudal dimension of the prostate at one time. An optimal scanning sector should allow close to 180° of visualization.

Three-dimensional (3D) volumetric acquisition of sonographic images of the prostate provides imaging capability in multiple planes following a single scan sweep that is performed over a few seconds.[1] 3D sonography may provide more accurate estimates of prostatic volume,[2] but 3D imaging systems may be more cumbersome for biopsy applications as compared with standard 2D systems. We have applied 3D volumetric acquisition to assist in localization of radioactive seed implants within the prostate (Figure 3.4).[3] 3D gray-scale sonography does not result in significant clinical improvement in the detection and staging of prostate cancer.[4]

Gray-scale sonography of the prostate begins with measurement of the prostate in the transverse and sagittal planes. A midline sagittal image demonstrating the urethra is used to obtain measurements in the craniocaudal and anteroposterior (AP) dimensions. A transverse image at the mid-gland level is used to measure the maximum transverse diameter (see Figure 3.3b). Three techniques have been described for the estimation of prostatic volume with conventional 2D ultrasound systems. Volume may be calculated from measurements in a single plane (ellipsoid method), or in two orthogonal planes (volumetric extension of the ellipsoid method by rotating the ellipse), or by planimetric measurements of contiguous cross-sections (planimetry method). The ellipsoid methods assume that the prostate has an ellipsoid shape, although this is not universally accurate. When using

measurements in two orthogonal planes, the volume of the prostate is computed based upon a formula for a prolate ellipse (length × width × height × 0.52). It is well known that measurements of prostate volume often vary by 10–20%.[5] However, in experienced hands, the prolate ellipsoid equation is accurate for estimation of prostatic volume, with a coefficient of correlation of approximately 0.80.[6] Planimetry is a time-consuming technique in which the outline of the prostate is identified on multiple transverse images, and is not suited to everyday use.

Gray-scale appearance of prostate cancer

Early reports of sonographic detection of prostate cancer suggested that most cancers were echogenic.[7–10] Subsequent studies demonstrated that most cancers were either isoechoic or hypoechoic on gray-scale sonography,[11–13] and that there is a great overlap in the sonographic appearance of benign and malignant lesions.[14] In the author's experience, cancer of the prostate rarely presents as an echogenic focus (Figure 3.5). Cancers of the prostate that were found in the early 1980s tended to be larger (and at a higher stage) than those that are generally detected today. It is likely that the larger lesions described as echogenic cancers in earlier studies were diffuse cancers that overlapped with other pathologic processes such as benign prostatic hyperplasia and chronic prostatitis. Hyperplastic processes and prostatitis are quite common in the prostate, and may result in areas of calcification and increased echogenicity. Alternatively, a minority of cancers may appear echogenic due to reactive changes in the adjacent prostatic parenchyma.

Several studies have suggested that there is no difference between prostate cancer that is visible or invisible on gray-scale sonography with respect to tumor grade and stage,[15] and that the sonographic gray-scale appearance is of no clinical consequence.[16] However, a review of 400 patients staged with the TNM classification for cancer of the prostate found that sonographically detected, non-palpable cancers were more likely to extend outside the prostate than T1c cancers detected only by an elevated PSA.[17] Sonographically detected stage T2 cancers are similar to palpable T2 cancers in terms of grade, extension, and prognosis.[17] An analysis of cancers detected by digital rectal examination, PSA, and sonography demonstrated that each of these diagnostic tests detected a similar proportion of clinically significant disease.[18] The percentage of clinically insignificant cancers detected by sonography was much lower than the incidence of clinically insignificant prostate cancer found incidentally at cystoprostatectomy.[18] A recent study suggests that sonographically visible tumor on gray-scale imaging is more likely to be hypervascular on Doppler imaging, and to have a significantly higher Gleason score.[19]

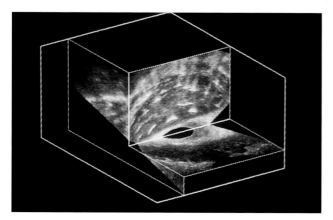

Figure 3.4
Three-dimensional volume acquisition of the prostate after radioactive seed implantation. A sagittal slice through the volume demonstrates the position of multiple bright pellets within the prostate.

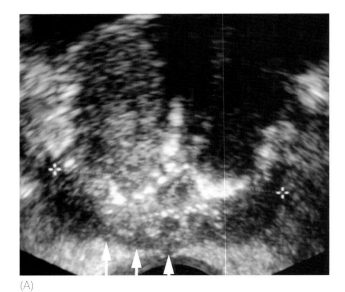

(A)

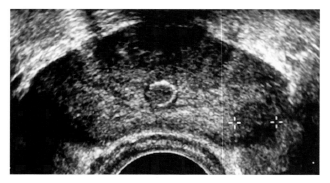

(B)

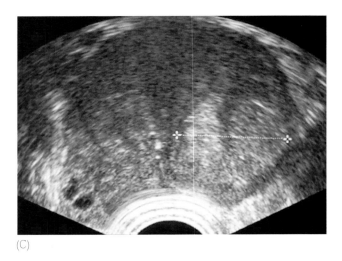

(C)

Figure 3.5

Transverse images of the prostate with echogenic lesions. (A) An enlarged prostate with inner gland enlargement characteristic of benign prostatic hyperplasia. The outer gland appears more echogenic in the midline and to the right of the midline (arrows). Biopsy specimens obtained from these echogenic areas were positive for cancer. (B) A focal hyperechoic area bridging the inner and outer gland at the left base (calipers). This focus was found to correspond to a Gleason 6 cancer. The echogenic appearance of cancer is rare, and may be related to chronic inflammation or a fibrotic response within the prostate to the presence of a cancer. (C) A large focal hyperechoic mass in the left side of the prostate. Multiple biopsies of this mass demonstrated chronic prostatitis.

It is now generally accepted that most cancers of the prostate are isoechoic or hypoechoic to surrounding parenchyma in the outer portion of the gland (Figure 3.6). The more hypoechoic and easily visualized tumors are often larger and of higher histologic grade (Figure 3.7). Diffusely infiltrating cancers may be more difficult to identify, since they may present with a diffuse echotexture abnormality, no loss of

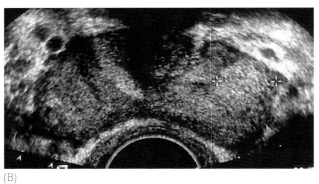

Figure 3.6

Transverse image of the prostate, with classical hypoechoic appearance of a Gleason 6 cancer in the left mid-gland (calipers).

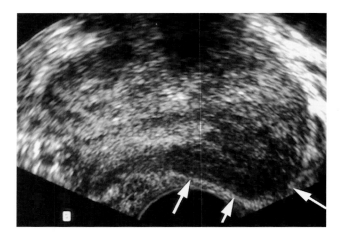

Figure 3.7

Transverse image of the prostate, with a large hypoechoic mass in the left mid-gland (arrows). The mass results in a posterior bulge of the left side of the prostate. Biopsy demonstrated a Gleason 7 cancer corresponding to the sonographic abnormality.

symmetry, and no focal, definable mass (Figure 3.8). Cystic lesions are most often related to a benign process such as cystic hyperplasia (Figure 3.9). Cancers are rarely identified prospectively during examination of the inner portion of the gland, because they are masked by the typically heterogeneous echotexture pattern characteristic of benign prostatic hyperplasia. However, when cancer is suspected and cannot be identified

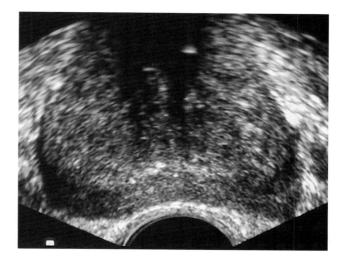

Figure 3.8
Transverse image of the prostate demonstrates enlargement of the inner gland and a diffusely hypoechoic appearance to the outer gland. The appearance was found to represent infiltrating carcinoma that involved all parts of the peripheral zone. Prostatitis can present with a similar appearance.

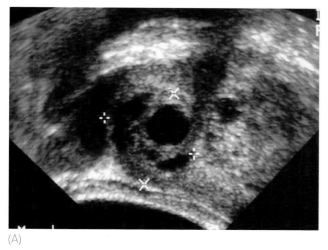

(A)

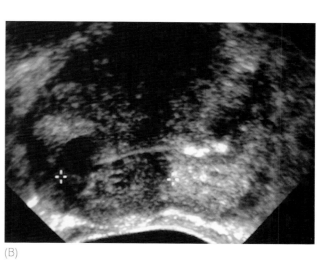

(B)

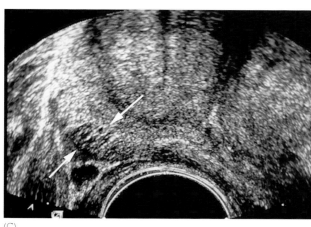

(C)

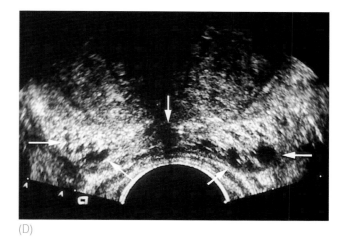

(D)

Figure 3.9
Cystic lesions in the prostate. (A) Sagittal image of a focal mass in the right base containing two obvious cystic areas (calipers). (B) Transverse image of the same lesion, with a mild bulge of the prostate contour that was palpable on digital rectal examination. Multiple biopsies of this lesion demonstrated cystic hyperplasia. (C, D) Images from two separate patients demonstrate small areas of cystic dilatation in the outer gland (arrows). Needle biopsy demonstrated normal prostate. Small areas of cystic dilatation are commonly seen, and are rarely associated with cancer.

on biopsy of the outer gland, focal hypoechoic lesions of the inner gland must be carefully evaluated (Figure 3.10).

The transverse imaging plane is preferred for evaluation of pathologic processes because it allows comparison of symmetry from side to side. In addition to symmetry in echotexture, changes in contour may provide a clue to the presence of a cancer (Figure 3.11). A contour bulge is often palpated on digital rectal examination, and is most easily evaluated in the transverse plane. When evaluating a contour abnormality, it is important to apply as little pressure as possible with the probe. Normal prostate tissue has a firm texture, but is easily deformed by probe pressure. A curvilinear echogenic line of calcification or corpora amylacea identifies the surgical capsule that divides the outer gland from the inner gland. A contour bulge related to asymmetric enlargement of the inner gland within the confines of the surgical capsule is most often related to benign prostatic hyperplasia. Asymmetric thickening or bulging of outer gland parenchyma should be regarded as suspicious for neoplasm.

After searching for hypoechoic lesions and focal bulges in the contour of the gland, the sonographer should survey the margin of the prostate and the fat planes around the prostate. The prostatic contour is generally smooth and well defined because of a very thin layer of smooth muscle and fibrous tissue that extends posteriorly around the gland from the anterior fibromuscular zone. Although this layer is not a true capsule, we refer to it as the prostatic capsule for the purposes of our discussion. This capsule is only a few cell layers thick, and while it is not sonographically visible, it is responsi-

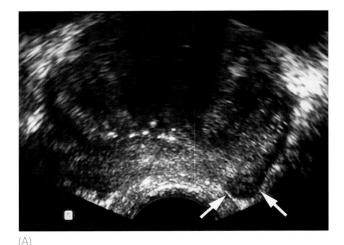

(A)

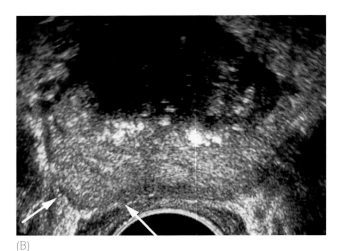

(B)

Figure 3.11

Abnormalities of contour. (A) Transverse image of the prostate, with a focal posterior bulge of the left mid-gland (arrows) corresponding to a small focus of cancer. (B) Transverse image in a different patient, with a large area of thickening in the right base. The contour bulge of the outer gland in this area corresponded to a Gleason 7 cancer (arrows).

ble for the smooth margin of the prostate. When this capsule is infiltrated by tumor, capsular invasion may result in loss of the smooth, well-defined margin of the gland on sonography. The periprostatic fat planes are generally visible as a uniformly bright layer outside the prostate, although an enlarged prostate may thin the periprostatic fat (Figure 3.12). A focal area of loss of the periprostatic fat plane is suspicious for capsular penetration by cancer (Figure 3.13). While a simple bulge in the prostatic contour is often associated with a benign process, a contour bulge in association with loss of the periprostatic fat plane is highly suspicious for invasive malignancy.

Whenever possible, gray-scale evaluation should be performed in two orthogonal planes to verify findings seen in

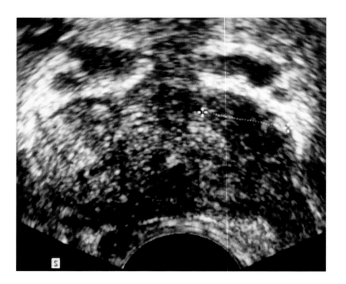

Figure 3.10

Transverse image at the base of the prostate demonstrates a focal hypoechoic lesion in the inner gland (calipers). Such areas are often associated with benign hyperplasia in the transition zone. In this patient, the focal lesion corresponded to a Gleason 7 cancer. (Reproduced with permission.[20])

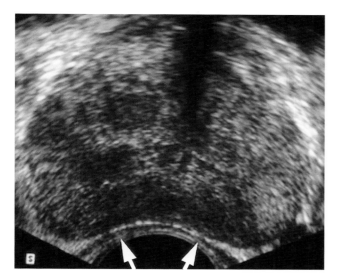

Figure 3.12

Transverse image of the prostate in a patient with diffusely infiltrating Gleason 7 cancer throughout the outer gland. There is enlargement of the inner gland, with thinning of the bright periprostatic fat planes (arrows). Although the periprostatic fat planes are thinned, there is no focal area with definite loss of these planes. No extracapsular spread was found at surgery.

the transverse orientation (Figure 3.14). As a general principle of sonography, any true mass should be visible in two orthogonal imaging planes. For transrectal imaging of the prostate, the preferred second plane is in the sagittal orientation. Unfortunately, cancer of the prostate is often difficult to visualize in the sagittal plane, and may be impossible to visualize in two planes. The transverse plane is generally more useful for defining subtle lesions, because comparison of the two sides of the gland permits the identification of

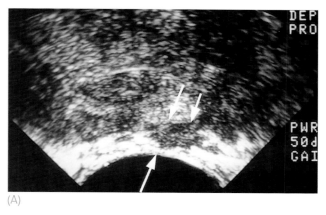

(A)

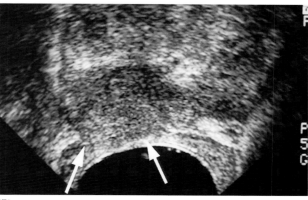

(B)

Figure 3.13

Transverse images of the prostate with capsular penetration by prostate cancer. (A) A focal irregularity in the posterior wall of the prostate, with invasion of hypoechoic material through the periprostatic fat planes (arrows). The cancer was found to invade the rectal wall. (B) A large hypoechoic bulge along the right side of the prostate, with loss of the periprostatic fat (arrows). This cancer was found to have invaded through the prostatic capsule.

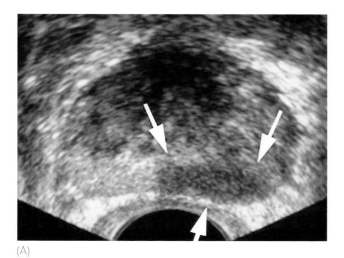

(A)

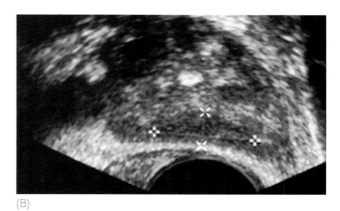

(B)

Figure 3.14

Transverse (A) and sagittal (B) images of the prostate with a Gleason 7 cancer. A classical hypoechoic appearance of the cancer is noted and measured in two orthogonal planes (arrows and calipers).

subtle areas of asymmetry. Whenever possible, measurements of focal lesions should be obtained in both the transverse and sagittal planes in order to define the size in three dimensions.

Seminal vesicles

A sagittal, transverse or oblique plane of imaging may be required to identify the long axis of the seminal vesicles. The ejaculatory duct, which extends from the seminal vesicle into the prostate, perforates the thin prostatic capsule and creates a potential pathway for spread of cancer outside the prostate. When tumor spreads along the ejaculatory duct, it may result in thickening of the seminal vesicle as it approaches the prostate. It is therefore important to demonstrate a symmetric tapered appearance of the two seminal vesicles as they approach the base of the prostate (Figure 3.15). Although the size of the normal seminal vesicle may vary considerably, any asymmetry in the two seminal vesicles should be noted. Ductal ectasia of the seminal vesicles is commonly seen in older men, and may be related to compression of the ejaculatory duct by benign prostatic hyperplasia (Figure 3.16). When ductal ectasia is present, and especially when it is present unilaterally, a conscious effort should be made to identify the site of obstruction. Since a malignancy can result in obstruction of the ejaculatory duct, it may be useful to biopsy the area where an ejaculatory duct appears obstructed.

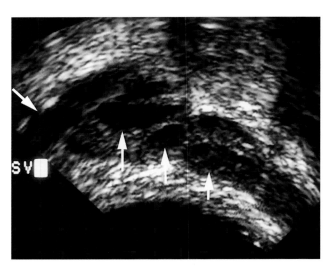

Figure 3.16
Long-axis view of a seminal vesicle demonstrates ductal ectasia. Dilated tubular areas are seen throughout the seminal vesicle (arrows). Ductal ectasia is often seen in elderly men. It has been suggested that this finding may be related to decreased frequency of ejaculation, but it may also result from obstruction by benign prostatic hyperplasia, ejaculatory duct stones, or an obstructing cancer. The finding of ductal ectasia should always lead to a search for the cause of obstruction. Unilateral ductal ectasia is more concerning than bilateral ductal ectasia. Bilateral ductal ectasia is most often related to benign prostatic hyperplasia.

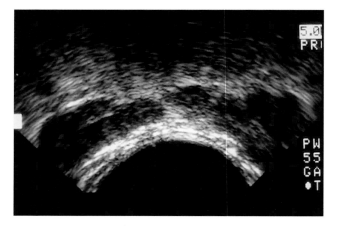

Figure 3.15
Normal tapered appearance of the seminal vesicles. A transverse image of the seminal vesicles demonstrates that each seminal vesicle tapers to a point as it approaches the midline. Extension of prostatic cancer through the ejaculatory duct directly into the seminal vesicle may result in a loss of this normal tapered appearance.

Gray-scale evaluation after prostatectomy

Transrectal sonography may be requested after prostatectomy in order to determine whether there is a local recurrence. Sonography is requested most often for evaluation and biopsy of a palpable postoperative abnormality, but may also be requested on the basis of an elevated prostate-specific antigen (PSA) suspicious for local recurrence. The normal post-prostatectomy appearance demonstrates a urethrovesical anastomosis with a smooth, tapered appearance from the bladder neck to the urethral sphincter (Figure 3.17).[21] Ideally, there should be no residual tissue in the prostatic bed after radical prostatectomy. Post-prostatectomy scans may demonstrate portions of the seminal vesicles that have not been removed. The more superior and lateral portions of the seminal vesicles are often not removed at surgery. Biopsy of residual seminal vesicle tissue may be useful, since residual tumor may be present within the seminal vesicles.

Recurrent tumor in the prostate bed can present as a focal solid nodule (Figure 3.18) or as a complex solid and cystic lesion (Figure 3.19).[22] When the recurrence is small, biopsy may be needed to distinguish a focal recurrence from post-

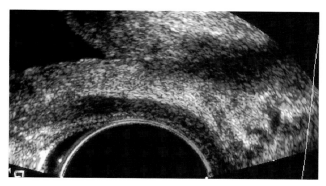

Figure 3.17
Sagittal view of the urethra after prostatectomy. The bladder neck tapers smoothly into the urethra. A small amount of fibrous tissue is seen around the urethra, with no discrete mass.

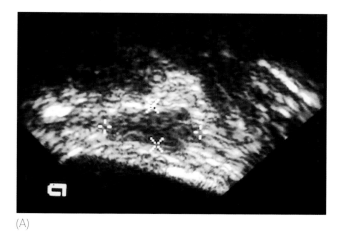

(A)

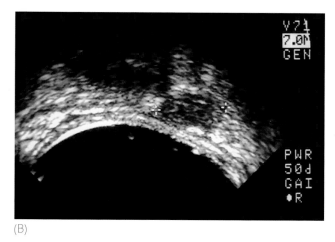

(B)

Figure 3.18
Post-prostatectomy scan demonstrates a focal solid nodule in the prostatic bed. Sagittal (A) and transverse (B) measurements of the nodule were obtained. Needle biopsy demonstrated recurrent cancer.

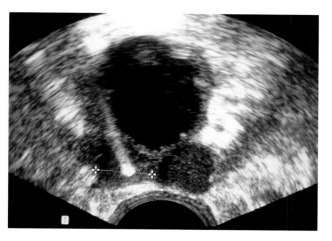

Figure 3.19
Post-prostatectomy scan demonstrates a complex mass in the prostatic bed. Biopsies of the cystic areas yielded fibrous tissue. However, biopsy of the hypoechoic area adjacent to the rectum (calipers) demonstrated recurrent cancer. A small amount of post-biopsy air is present within the recurrent cancer.

operative scarring. Locally recurrent masses are found most frequently in the perianastomotic area, but can also be found in adjacent structures.[23] Local recurrence may appear as a focal hypoechoic nodule, as asymmetric thickening or fullness of the anastomosis, or as loss of the retroanastomotic fat plane.[24–26] A variable amount of the bladder neck is removed during prostatectomy. In order to match the bladder to the distal urethra for reanastomosis, the surgeon may need to suture the inferior portion of the bladder to reduce the outflow orifice. Postoperative changes in the bladder may simulate the appearance of a mass just above the urethral anastomosis (Figure 3.20).

Gray-scale sonography for radiation therapy

In order to plan for adequate levels of radiation to all parts of the prostate, accurate measurements must be obtained for the prostate contour and volume. Traditionally, helical computed tomography (CT) has been the method of choice for planning of both external-beam radiation therapy and radioactive-seed implantation (brachytherapy). Radioactive-seed implants were performed under fluoroscopic guidance. However, sonography may be used to image the entire prostate, to compute gland volumes (Figure 3.21) and to demonstrate the position of seed implants (see Figure 3.6). Recently, sonography has been used as a replacement for fluoroscopy during seed implantation for brachytherapy (Figure 3.22). A major issue when planning brachytherapy is pubic arch interference with seed placement. An overlap of

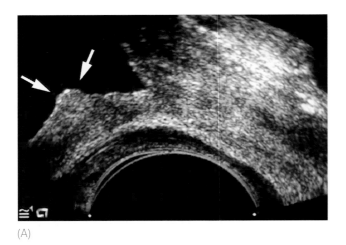

(A)

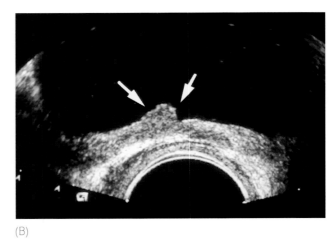

(B)

Figure 3.20

Post-prostatectomy changes in the bladder neck. (A) Sagittal image of the bladder neck after prostatectomy. A focal nodule of soft tissue is visible (arrows), and is confirmed on the transverse image (B). This patient had a rising PSA, but repeated biopsy of this area demonstrated only normal transitional mucosa. A variable amount of the bladder neck is removed during prostatectomy. In order to approximate the bladder for anastamosis with the urethra, the bladder neck must be reconstructed. Suturing of the bladder neck may result in a pseudomass above the urethral anastamosis.

more than one-third of the prostate by the pubic arch on transverse CT sections suggests that there will be pubic arch interference during seed implantation.[27] It has recently been demonstrated that transrectal sonography performed in the lithotomy position can be more accurate than CT for this assessment, and may avoid the need for additional hormonal therapy to shrink the prostate prior to brachytherapy.[26]

Concluding remarks

Finally, it is important to realize that many cancers are not visible on gray-scale sonography. A large number of cancers are isoechoic (Figure 3.23), and many hypoechoic foci correspond to benign processes (Figure 3.24). The appearance of prostatitis is often indistinguishable from that of cancer (Figure 3.25). Furthermore, in a recent prospective study, gray-scale sonography was minimally better than random chance in defining the presence of cancer during sextant biopsy.[29]

Figure 3.21

Three-dimensional sonography of the prostate. The contour of the prostate is clearly visualized in multiple planes. This type of 3D data acquisition may provide more accurate estimates of prostate volume. The extra effort required for this type of imaging may not be justified for routine evaluation, but may be useful in specific circumstances.

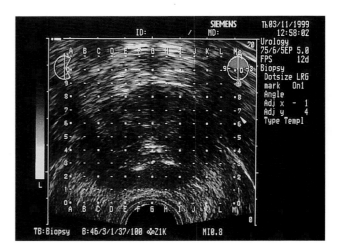

Figure 3.22

Transverse sonogram of the prostate with superimposed brachytherapy grid. The grid is used to target seeds into specific locations within the prostate under real-time sonographic guidance. (Courtesy of Dr Adam P Dicker.)

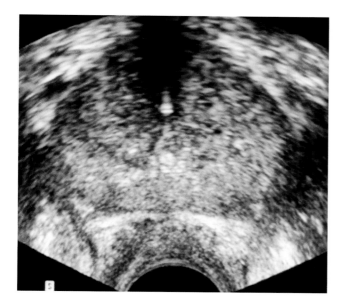

Figure 3.23

Transverse image of the prostate with a Gleason 7 cancer in the lateral aspect of the right mid-gland. Sonography demonstrates a normal echogenic appearance to the outer gland, particularly on the right side. Approximately half of cancers detected within the prostate are isoechoic and invisible by conventional sonography.

Given the relatively low sensitivity of gray-scale sonography, this technique is not recommended as a screening test for prostate cancer. Nonetheless, when a gray-scale abnormality is clearly present, directed biopsy of the site is warranted, since biopsy of these areas is more likely to yield malignant tissue, when compared with biopsy results from adjacent sites. Furthermore, tumor grade tends to be higher in biopsy

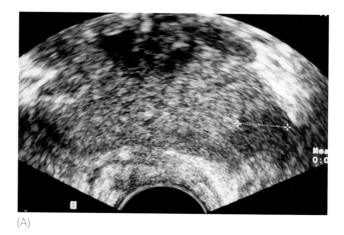

(A)

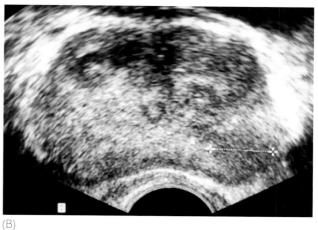

(B)

Figure 3.25

Two patients with hypoechoic lesions on the left side of the base of the prostate (calipers): (A) a Gleason 6 cancer; (B) an area of focal prostatitis. The two lesions cannot be distinguished on the basis of conventional sonography.

cores from visible lesions. The preferred use of gray-scale imaging is to direct both systematic and targeted biopsies of the prostate in patients who are referred because of an elevated PSA or abnormal digital rectal examination.

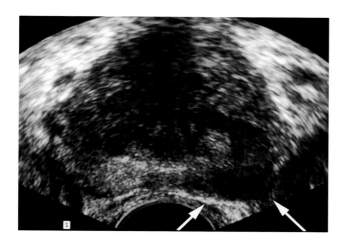

Figure 3.24

Hypoechoic lesion in the left mid-gland in a patient with an elevated PSA. The appearance is classic for cancer. However, multiple biopsy cores of this lesion (arrows) demonstrated only prostatitis.

References

1. Hamper UM, Trapanotto V, DeJong MR et al. Three-dimensional US of the prostate: early experience. Radiology 1999; 212: 719–23.

2. Elliot TL, Downey DB, Tong S et al. Accuracy of prostate volume measurements in vitro using three-dimensional ultrasound. Acad Radiol 1996; 3: 401–6.

3. Dicker AP, Rawool NM, Halpern EJ. Three-dimensional multiplanar transrectal ultrasound imaging for visualization of radioactive seeds for prostate brachytherapy. Radiology 1998; 209(P): 209.

4. Sedelaar JP, van Roermund JG, Van Leenders GL et al. Three-dimensional grayscale ultrasound: evaluation of prostate cancer compared with benign prostatic hyperplasia. Urology 2001; 57: 914–20.

5. Sehgal CM, Broderick GA, Whittington R et al. Three-dimensional measurement by US and volumetric assessment of the prostate. Radiology 1994; 192:274–8.

6. Gonzalez LL, Galan LM, Borda PA et al. A reliability analysis of transrectal echographic estimation of prostatic volume. Actas Urol Esp 1999; 23: 10–13.

7. Resnick MI, Willard JW, Boyce WH. Ultrasonic evaluation of prostatic nodule. J Urol 1978; 120: 86–9.

8. Rifkin MD, Kurtz AB, Choi HY, Goldberg BB. Endoscopic ultrasonic evaluation of the prostate using a transrectal probe: prospective evaluation and acoustic characterization. Radiology 1983; 149: 265–71.

9. Fritzsche PJ, Axford PD, Ching VC et al. Correlation of transrectal sonographic findings in patients with suspected and unsuspected prostatic disease. J Urol 1983; 130: 272–4.

10. Abu-Yousef MM, Narayana AS. Prostatic carcinoma: detection and staging using suprapubic US. Radiology 1985; 156: 175–80.

11. Lee F, Gray JM, McLeary RD et al. Transrectal ultrasound in the diagnosis of prostate cancer: location, echogenicity, histopathology and staging. Prostate 1985; 7: 117–29.

12. Dahnert WF, Hamper UM, Eggleston JC et al. Prostatic evaluation by transrectal sonography with histopathologic correlation: the echopenic appearance of early carcinoma. Radiology 1986; 158: 97–102.

13. Lee F, Gray JM, McLeary RD et al. Prostatic evaluation by transrectal sonography: criteria for diagnosis of early carcinoma. Radiology 1986; 158: 91–5.

14. Rifkin MD, Friedland GW, Shortliffe L. Prostatic evaluation by transrectal endosonography: detection of carcinoma. Radiology 1986; 158: 85–90.

15. Ferguson JK, Bostwick DG, Suman V et al. Prostate-specific antigen detected prostate cancer: pathological characteristics of ultrasound visible versus ultrasound invisible tumors. Eur Urol 1995; 27: 8–12.

16. Sanders H, El-Galley R. Ultrasound findings are not useful for defining stage T1c prostate cancer. World J Urol 1997; 15: 336–8.

17. Ohori M, Wheeler TM, Scardino PT. The New American Joint Committee on Cancer and International Union Against Cancer TNM classification of prostate cancer. Clinico-pathologic correlations. Cancer 1994; 74: 104–14.

18. Ohori M, Wheeler TM, Dunn JK et al. The pathological features and prognosis of prostate cancer detectable with current diagnostic tests. J Urol 1994; 152: 1714–20.

19. Cornud F, Hamida K, Flam T et al. Endorectal color Doppler sonography and endorectal MR imaging features of nonpalpable prostate cancer: correlation with radical prostatectomy findings. AJR 2000; 175: 1161–8.

20. Halpern EJ, Mc Cue IA, Aksnes AK et al. Contrast-enhanced US of the prostate with sonazoid: Comparison with whole-mount prostatomy specimens in 12 patients. Radiology 2002; 222: 361–6.

21. Wasserman NF, Kapoor DA, Hildebrandt WC et al. Transrectal US in evaluation of patients after radical prostatatectomy. Part I. Normal postoperative anatomy. Radiology 1992; 185: 361–6.

22. Wasserman NF, Kapoor DA, Hildebrandt WC et al. Transrectal US in evaluation of patients after radical prostatectomy. Part II. Transrectal US and biopsy findings in the presence of residual and early recurrent prostatic cancer. Radiology 1992; 185: 367–72.

23. Leventis AK, Shariat SF, Slawin KM. Local recurrence after radical prostatectomy: correlation of US features with prostatic fossa biopsy findings. Radiology 2001; 219: 432–9.

24. Salomon CG, Flisak ME, Olson MC et al. Radical prostatectomy: transrectal sonographic evaluation to assess for local recurrence. Radiology 1993; 189: 713–19.

25. Kapoor DA, Wasserman NF, Zhang G, Reddy PK. Value of transrectal ultrasound in identifying local disease after radical prostatectomy. Urology 1993; 41: 594–7.

26. Saleem MD, Sanders H, Abu El Naser M, El-Galley R. Factors predicting cancer detection in biopsy of the prostatic fossa after radical prostatectomy. Urology 1998; 51: 283–6.

27. Wallner K, Chiu-Tsao ST, Roy J et al. An improved method for computerized tomography: planned transperineal [125]iodine prostate implants. J Urol 1991; 146: 90–5.

28. Strang JG, Rubens DJ, Brasacchio RA et al. Real-time US versus CT determination of pubic arch interference for brachytherapy. Radiology 2001; 216: 387–93.

29. Halpern EJ, Strup SE. Using gray scale, color and power Doppler sonography to detect prostatic cancer. AJR 2000; 174: 623–7.

4

Color and power Doppler evaluation of prostate cancer

Ethan J Halpern

Doppler sonography is used to identify blood flow within the prostate. As an adjunct to gray-scale sonography, Doppler techniques assist in the identification of suspicious lesions within the prostate. Numerous studies have suggested that color and power Doppler imaging may improve the detection of prostate cancer.[1–6] Nonetheless, the application of Doppler imaging to the diagnosis of prostate cancer remains controversial. Doppler imaging requires additional expertise and examination time, as well as more expensive equipment than conventional gray-scale sonography. A survey of urologists who perform biopsy of the prostate suggests that most of these physicians utilize sonography to guide placement of systematic biopsies, but do not attempt targeted biopsy of suspicious areas.[7] However, as Doppler systems improve, there is increasing evidence that color and power Doppler imaging may assist in the detection of clinically significant prostate cancer. Furthermore, the presence of increased Doppler flow in patients with prostate cancer is associated with increased Gleason grade, seminal vesicle invasion, and overall higher rate of post-therapy relapse.[8] It is therefore reasonable to use gray-scale imaging to guide a systematic biopsy for the detection of cancer, and to supplement systematic biopsy with Doppler-guided targeted biopsy of suspicious areas.

Arterial anatomy

The arterial supply of the prostate derives predominantly from the prostaticovesicle artery, a branch of the internal iliac artery.[9] Each prostaticovesicle artery divides into two branches: the inferior vesical artery and the prostatic artery. Both the inferior vesical artery and the prostatic artery supply peri-urethral arteries that enter the base of the prostate and course parallel to the urethra. These peri-urethral arteries create a hypervascular zone around the urethra (Figure 4.1). Each prostatic artery also supplies multiple ipsilateral capsular arteries that course along the lateral and posterolateral aspects of the prostate (Figure 4.2). The prostatic artery supplies the neurovascular bundle on the posterolateral aspect of the prostate on each side.

Capsular arteries supply multiple branches that perforate into the prostate in a radial orientation in the transverse plane (Figure 4.3). These perforating branches create a symmetric spoke wheel pattern in the normal young subject (Figure 4.4). Power Doppler may be more sensitive than color Doppler in depicting the course and continuity of these vessels within the prostate.[10] Minor additional arterial branches to the apex of the prostate are derived from the middle hemorrhoidal and internal pudendal arteries, which themselves are branches of the internal iliac arteries.[9] Spectral Doppler tracings may be obtained from periprostatic and intraprostatic vessels. Arterial flow patterns around the prostate demonstrate sharp systolic peaks with minimal diastolic flow. As the capsular arteries radiate toward the center of the prostate, Doppler flow patterns demonstrate a greater level of diastolic flow (Figure 4.5). Unfortunately, evaluation of spectral Doppler flow patterns has not proven useful for the detection and characterization of prostate cancer.

Cancer detection

Doppler detection of prostate cancer is based upon a pattern of increased flow associated with cancer. Three patterns have been described: diffuse flow (Figure 4.6), focal flow (Figure 4.7) and surrounding flow (Figure 4.8). Flow patterns associated with prostate cancer are characterized by

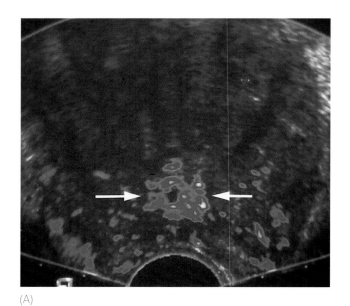

(A)

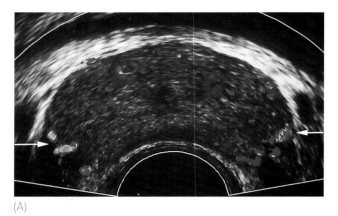

(A)

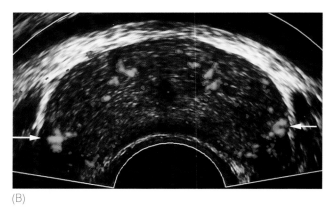

(B)

Figure 4.2
Transverse image of the prostate. Doppler demonstrates normal capsular arteries along the posterolateral aspect of the gland (arrows). (A) Color (frequency) Doppler. (B) Power (amplitude) Doppler.

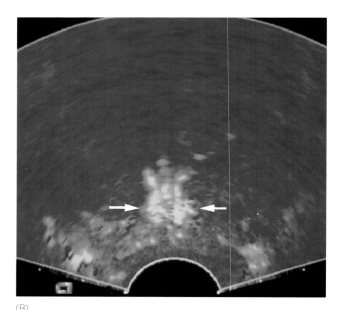

(B)

Figure 4.1
Transverse power Doppler image of the prostate demonstrates enlargement of the inner gland secondary to benign prostatic hyperplasia, with prominent flow around the urethra (arrows). (A, B) Different adjustments of the power Doppler gain setting: in (A), the power gain is adjusted to demonstrate flow within vessels, but to suppress color over other areas; in (B), the gain is increased so that there is a low level of color over the entire image. The higher gain adjustment demonstrated in (B) is often recommended in order to standardize power Doppler gain settings and to maximize sensitivity for slow flow in small vessels. However, the higher gain settings also obscure the underlying gray-scale image, making it more difficult to correlate the location of increased Doppler flow with gray-scale findings.

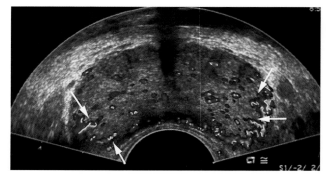

Figure 4.3
Transverse power Doppler image of the prostate. Capsular arteries are visualized with perforating arteries that extend toward the center of the gland (arrows).

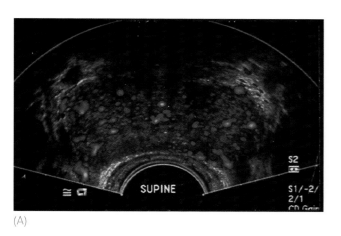
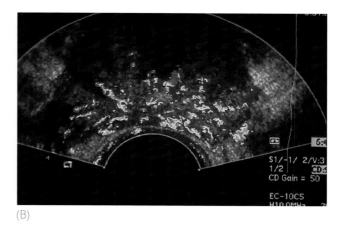

(A)   (B)

Figure 4.4

Transverse power Doppler image of the prostate. Perforating arteries create a radial pattern of flow toward the center of the gland.
(A) A normal subject. (B) There is greater flow in a subject with prostatitis.

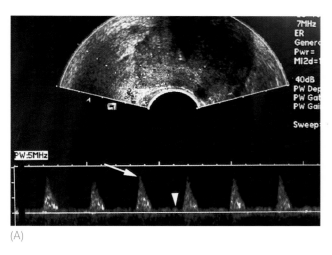
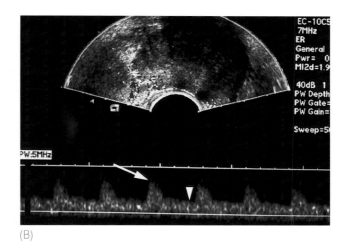

(A)   (B)

Figure 4.5

Spectral Doppler tracings of the arterial supply to the prostate. (A) Spectral tracing of a capsular artery along the outside of the prostate with strong systolic flow (arrow), but little diastolic flow (arrowhead). (B) Spectral tracing from a perforating artery within prostatic parenchyma. The perforating artery has antegrade flow in both systole (arrow) and diastole (arrowhead).

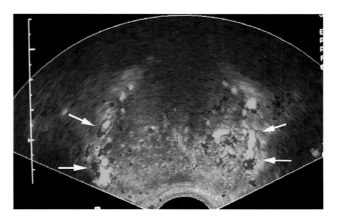

Figure 4.6

Transverse power Doppler image of the prostate. Normal capsular arteries are visualized bilaterally (arrows). Diffusely increased flow within the left side of the gland corresponds to a Gleason 7 cancer that extends from the left base to the left mid-gland.

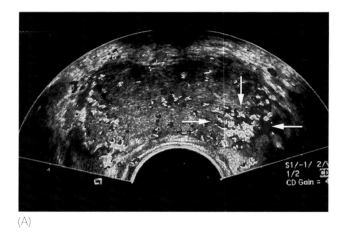

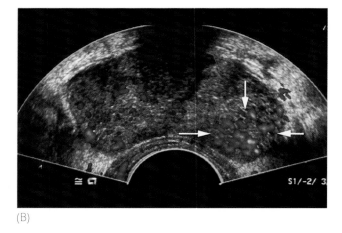

(A)   (B)

Figure 4.7

Transverse images of the prostate, with increased flow in the left base. In (A), there is a focal area of increased color Doppler signal within the left base (arrows) corresponding to the site of cancer. In (B), there is a focal area of increased power Doppler signal within the left base (arrows). This patient had a Gleason 7 cancer bilaterally at the base of the prostate.

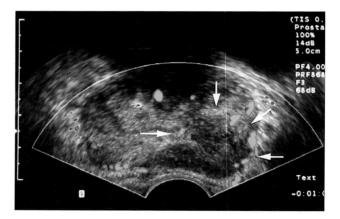

Figure 4.8

Transverse image of the prostate demonstrates a classic hypoechoic lesion in the left mid-gland corresponding to a cancer. Power Doppler demonstrates increased flow in a pattern surrounding the hypoechoic cancer (arrows).

asymmetric flow to the region of tumor, with increased number and size of vessels. Theoretically, vessels supplying a neoplasm should demonstrate irregular orientation, as opposed to the regular radial orientation of normal capsular arteries. Multiple studies have suggested that color Doppler improves both the sensitivity and positive predictive value of prostate biopsy.[1–6] Nonetheless, color Doppler detection of cancer is not sufficiently sensitive to exclude patients from biopsy.[11,12] Recent studies suggest that power Doppler offers an extended dynamic range,[13] and may be even more sensitive than color Doppler for the detection of prostate cancer.[14–16] The author's personal experience suggests that

focal areas with increased color or power Doppler flow are 4–5 times more likely to contain cancer than adjacent areas without flow, but that conventional color and power Doppler imaging are not yet sufficiently sensitive to exclude a patient from biopsy.[17]

Several factors complicate the detection of cancer based upon Doppler imaging. The presence of benign prostatic hyperplasia within the adult prostate usually distorts the expected radial pattern of perforating vessels, even in the absence of malignancy (Figure 4.9). Benign prostatic hyperplasia of the transition zone often presents as nodular hyperplasia on both sides of the midline with increased flow on

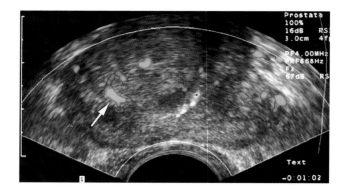

Figure 4.9

Transverse image of a prostate with benign prostatic hyperplasia. The enlarged inner gland demonstrates several areas of increased flow with power Doppler imaging. A large vessel is visualized coursing around the inner gland on the right side (arrow). The normal radial pattern of flow toward the center of the gland is not present.

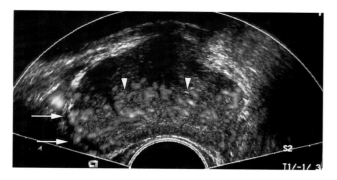

Figure 4.10

Transverse power Doppler image of the prostate in a patient with mild benign prostatic hyperplasia. Increased flow is identified in the right outer gland (arrows), with a normal radial distribution of the vessels. Diffusely increased flow is demonstrated in the hyperplastic inner gland (arrowheads).

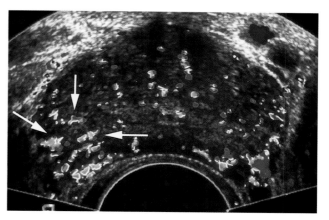

Figure 4.11

Transverse color Doppler image of the prostate. Increased flow is identified in the right mid-gland (arrows). Biopsy of this area revealed benign hyperplasia. The Doppler pattern demonstrates a normal radial orientation of perferating vessels, but the increased flow is indistinguishable fro that of cancer.

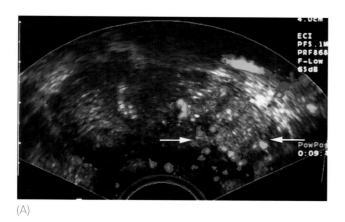

(A)

(B)

Figure 4.12

Transverse power Doppler images of the prostate in two patients with prostatitis. (A) Diffusely increased flow at the left base of the gland (arrows). (B) Increased flow surrounding a hypoechoic area of prostatitis in the right mid-gland (arrows).

both sides of midline (Figure 4.10). Focal areas of benign hyperplasia with increased Doppler flow may be found in the outer gland as well (Figure 4.11). Prostatitis may present with a pattern of increased blood flow that is indistinguishable from neoplasm (Figure 4.12).[18] Increased flow is also seen with focal infection or an abscess of the prostate (Figure 4.13). Ejaculation results in diffusely increased flow throughout the prostate that persists for up to 24 hours.[19]

Technical factors

Technical factors are an important consideration for Doppler evaluation of the prostate. Patient positioning is a critical factor influencing the Doppler flow pattern of the prostate. When patients are studied in the left lateral decubitus position, there is a significant tendency to observe increased flow along the left side of the gland. A recent study of normal volunteers who were imaged in both right and left decubitus positions demonstrated increased flow lateralizing to the base of the gland on the dependent side (Figures 4.14 and 4.15).[20] A more symmetric flow pattern was observed with subjects in a supine position. Thus, Doppler evaluation should be performed with the patient in a supine position.

The frequency of insonation used to create a Doppler image will impact the visualized distribution of flow. Lower frequency of insonation will provide better penetration for visualization of flow deep within the prostate. Higher

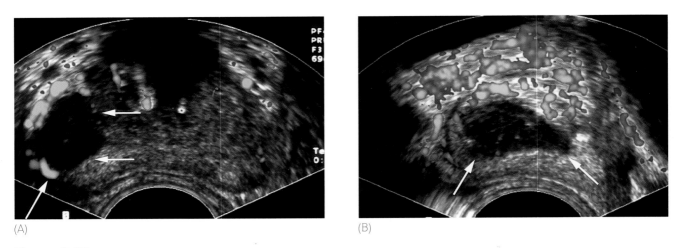

(A)   (B)

Figure 4.13

Transverse (A) and sagittal (B) power Doppler images of the prostate. A hypoechoic abscess is present along the right side of the gland (arrows) with increased flow around the abscess.

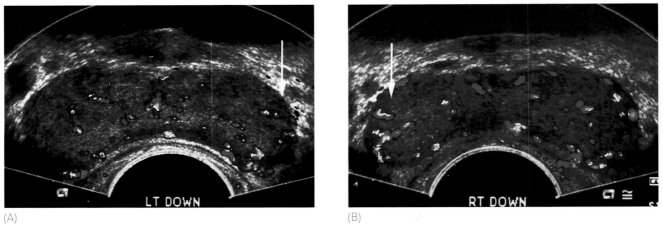

(A)   (B)

Figure 4.14

Color Doppler transverse images of the prostate of a normal volunteer. (A) was obtained in the left-side-down decubitus position, and demonstrates slightly more flow on the left side of the gland (arrow). (B) was obtained in the right-side-down decubitus position, and demonstrates slightly more flow on the right side of the gland (arrow). (Reproduced with permission.[20])

frequency provides increased sensitivity to flow in the peripheral zone of the prostate, and may demonstrate smaller vessels (Figure 4.16). This frequency trade-off should be considered when imaging the prostate. Probe pressure will also affect the Doppler signal. While probe pressure is necessary to maintain adequate acoustic coupling between the transducer and the prostate, this pressure can result in reduced blood flow to the posterior aspect of the prostate (Figure 4.17). Doppler sensitivity for flow is greatest at the depth of the focal zone (Figure 4.18). The focal zone position should be properly adjusted to visualize

flow in the peripheral zone, but also to demonstrate flow along the anterolateral portion of the gland – a site of frequently missed cancer. This may require repeat scanning with different focal zone settings. Flow sensitivity settings should be adjusted to keep the wall filter as low as possible without filling the image with clutter. Visualization of intraprostatic flow can be altered by changes in flow sensitivity settings (Figure 4.19). Finally, care should be exercised in preparing the probe for a prostate study. The presence of air within the condom can create artifactual areas of asymmetry in flow (Figure 4.20).

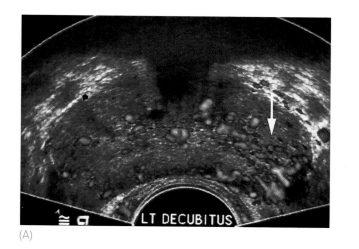

(A)

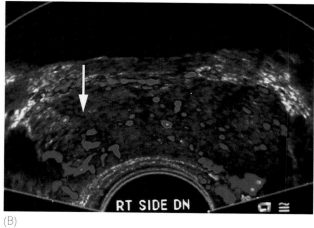

(B)

Figure 4.15
Power Doppler transverse images of the prostate of a second normal volunteer. (A) was obtained in the left-side-down decubitus position, and demonstrates more flow on the left side of the gland (arrow). (B) was obtained in the right-side-down decubitus position, and demonstrates more flow on the right side of the gland (arrow). (Reproduced with permission.[20])

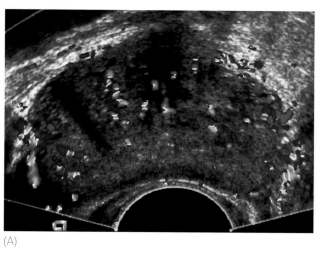

(A)

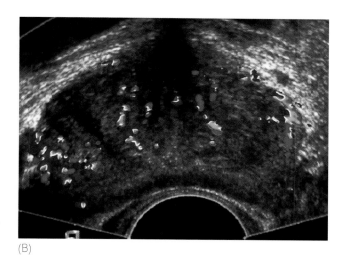

(B)

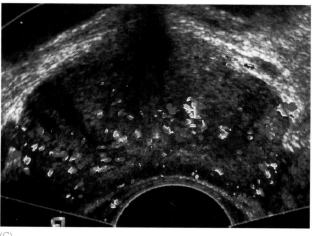

(C)

Figure 4.16
Transverse color Doppler images of the prostate. The identical scan was performed with a Doppler frequency of 5 MHz (A), 6 MHz (B), and 9 MHz (C). As the frequency is increased, more flow is appreciated in the near field of the transducer in the peripheral zone of the prostate. Higher Doppler frequencies also provide better spatial resolution for the display of small vessels.

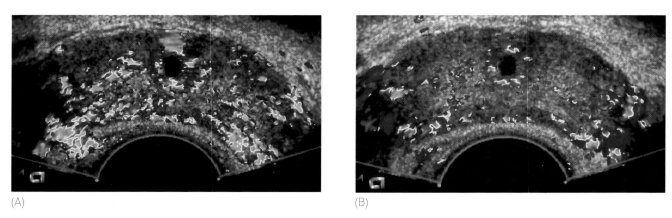

(A) (B)

Figure 4.17
Transverse color Doppler images of a normal volunteer. (A) was obtained with minimal pressure applied to the prostate: substantial color flow is demonstrated with a radial pattern of vessels coursing toward the urethra. (B) was obtained several seconds later with greater probe pressure applied to the prostate: the gland is mildly deformed by the probe pressure, and the degree of color flow is reduced.

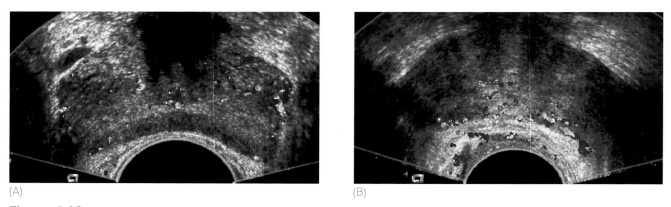

(A) (B)

Figure 4.18
Transverse color Doppler images of a normal volunteer. (A) was obtained with a transmit focal zone in the more anterior aspect of the prostate: very little flow is seen in the near field. (B) was obtained after the focal zone was moved into the near field: more flow is apparent in the near field of the transducer.

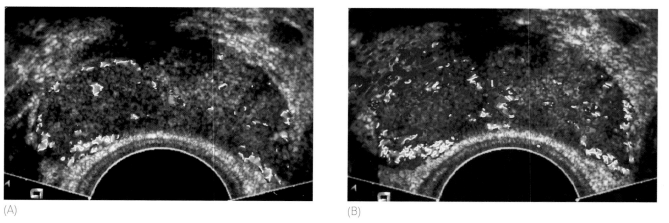

(A) (B)

Figure 4.19
Transverse color Doppler images of a normal volunteer. (A) was obtained with the default color sensitivity settings: it demonstrates capsular flow with a small amount of intraparenchymal flow. (B) was obtained with low flow settings: the lower wall filter and higher pulse repetition frequency demonstrate more color signal.

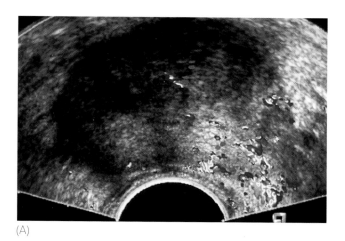

(A)

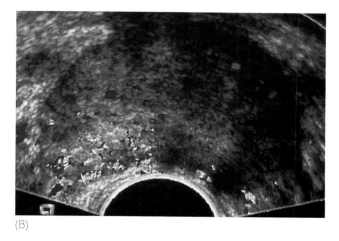

(B)

Figure 4.20

Transverse color Doppler image of a prostate. In (A), flow can be seen on the left side of the gland only. In (B), which was obtained after the transducer was rotated 180°, flow can be seen on the right side of the gland. A small amount of air or debris between the probe and the condom may result in shadowing in the gray-scale image and loss of color flow on the Doppler image.

Venous anatomy

The prostatic venous plexus represents a continuation of the deep dorsal vein of the penis. Right- and left-sided deep venous branches of the deep dorsal vein of the penis form the lateral venous plexus around the prostate. The venous plexus anterior to the prostate is known as the deep plexus of Santorini. The plexus of veins around the prostate drain into the pudendal, obturator, and vesical venous plexus, and ultimately into the internal iliac vein. There is also communication with the prevertebral plexus of Batson. It has been hypothesized that the high frequency of metastatic disease from prostate cancer to the spine may be related to venous drainage from periprostatic veins into Batson's plexus. Venous flow patterns around the prostate may demonstrate continuous or mildly phasic flow (Figure 4.21).

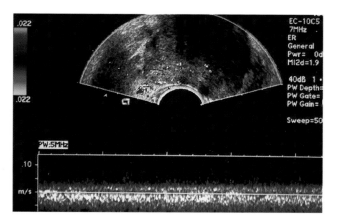

Figure 4.21

Spectral Doppler tracing of a vein along the side of the prostate demonstrates a continuous flow pattern.

Microvascular considerations

The theoretical basis for detection of prostate cancer with Doppler imaging is related to anatomic changes in the microvascular bed. There is strong pathologic evidence to suggest that the vascular supply to malignant prostate tissue differs from the vascular anatomy of normal prostate tissue. Studies of microvessel density within the prostate demonstrate a clear association of increased microvessel density with the presence of cancer,[21] with metastases,[22] with the stage of disease,[23–25] and with disease-specific survival.[26,27] There is also evidence suggesting that quantitative assessment of microvascular density may actually provide important data to guide therapeutic decisions.[28] When microvessels are stained and counted in whole-mount prostatectomy specimens, the number of vessels per square millimeter in areas with malignancy is approximately twice as great as that in benign tissue.[29] These vessels demonstrate greater tortuosity and a more homogeneous distribution as compared with microvessels in benign tissue.[30] On the basis of increased microvessel tortuosity and decreased vascular tone in neovessels, one might expect to find increased Doppler flow within areas of malignancy. However, conventional Doppler imaging is limited in its resolution to vessels that are of the order of 1mm in size. The microvessels in tumor neovasculature are of the order of 10–50 μm in size. Thus, conventional Doppler will only image the feeding vessels to the microvascular bed.

Few studies have been performed to demonstrate the relationship between Doppler flow and microvascular density. A recent study of tumor blood flow in a mouse model demonstrated a highly significant correlation between power Doppler imaging and microvascular density.[31] One study in humans has compared microvascular density with the presence of malignancy in biopsy cores from the prostate.[32] Although malignant cores did demonstrate greater microvessel density, there was no difference in microvessel density between malignant cores from areas with increased Doppler flow and malignant cores from areas with no detectable Doppler flow. Furthermore, the overall vascular volume within the microvascular bed was similar in malignant and benign tissue. Further clinical investigation will be required to elucidate the relationship between microvessel density and color/power Doppler imaging.

Color versus power

In order to understand the potential for imaging of blood flow within prostate cancer, we must first review some basic principles of Doppler imaging.[33,34] Both color (frequency shift) and power (amplitude) Doppler Images are derived from an autocorrelation function. The intensity of the power Doppler display is related to the R_0 term of the autocorrelation function. The R_0 term represents the total energy in the Doppler signal. The color displayed in a color Doppler representation of flow is related to the R_1 term of the autocorrelation function. The R_1 term corresponds to the velocity of flow. Thus, the signal in a power Doppler display depends upon the number of moving red blood cells, and is relatively independent of the direction and velocity of flow. The color Doppler signal depends upon the flow velocity.

Power Doppler displays increased dynamic range relative to color Doppler, and may therefore be more sensitive to small amounts of flow. It is theoretically possible to compute the volume of flowing blood within tissue from the power

Doppler signal.[35] If the total volume of moving blood is similar in benign and malignant tissue, however, color Doppler may be better suited to demonstrate altered flow velocity resulting from arteriovenous shunting or rapid flow in tortuous, low-resistance vessels. Again, it is important to understand that neither color nor power Doppler has sufficient resolution to visualize microvascularity. Imaging of neovasculature may be possible with contrast-enhanced imaging (see Chapter 6). Conventional color and power Doppler techniques, however, do reflect flow patterns in larger vessels that may themselves be altered by changes in the microvascular circulation (Figure 4.22).

Given the choice between color and power Doppler imaging, which technique should be chosen? Several small series have suggested that power Doppler may be more sensitive for the detection of malignancy.[16] One recent analysis of patients prior to radical prostatectomy suggested that color pixel density is the single best Doppler measure to discriminate malignant prostate tissue, and that the intensity of the power Doppler signal may be inversely related to the presence of cancer.[36] The author's personal experience, however, suggests that both color and power Doppler display similar flow patterns in any individual patient, and both techniques may identify an isoechoic cancer that is invisible with gray-scale sonography (Figures 4.23 and 4.24). With respect to directed biopsy of the prostate, power Doppler is complicated to a greater extent than color Doppler by flash artifact during the biopsy. In the final analysis, a clear superiority for either of these two Doppler methodologies has not yet been established. Nonetheless, careful attention to technical factors and use of a high-quality ultrasound unit may be more important than the choice of color versus power Doppler technology.

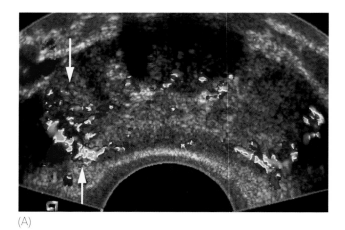

(A)

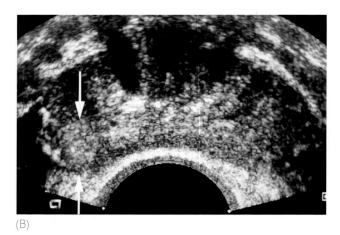

(B)

Figure 4.22
Transverse images of a prostate with a Gleason 6 cancer in the right mid-gland. (A) A color Doppler image demonstrates increased flow on the right side of the gland (arrows). Linear patterns of color flow suggest an increased number of large vessels. (B) A contrast-enhanced gray-scale image obtained during infusion of a microbubble agent demonstrates a round focus of increased parenchymal enhancement corresponding to the cancer in this area (arrows).

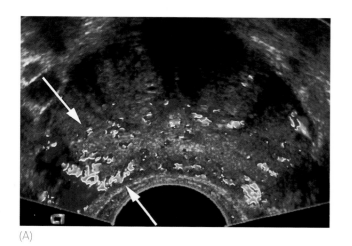

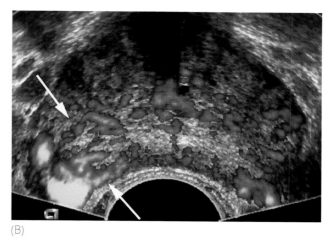

(A)

(B)

Figure 4.23

Transverse images of a prostate with a Gleason 7 lesion in the right mid-gland. Gray-scale images were normal. (A) Increased color Doppler flow at the site of a positive biopsy (arrows). (B) Increased power Doppler flow in the identical distribution (arrows).

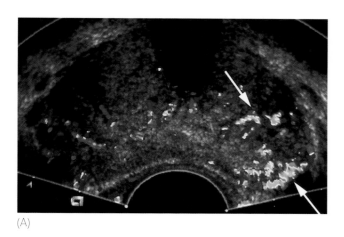

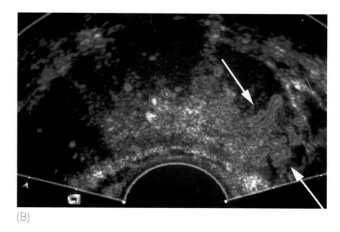

(A)

(B)

Figure 4.24

Transverse images of a prostate with a Gleason 6 lesion in the left base to mid-gland. Gray-scale images were normal. (A) Increased color Doppler flow in the left mid-gland (arrows). (B) Increased power Doppler flow in this area (arrows).

References

1. Rifkin MD, Sudakoff GS, Alexander AA. Prostate: Techniques, results, and potential applications of color Doppler US scanning. Radiology 1993; 186: 509–13.

2. Kelly IMG, Lees WR, Rickards D. Prostate cancer and the role of color Doppler US. Radiology 1993; 189: 153–6.

3. Newman JS, Bree RL, Rubin JM. Prostate cancer: diagnosis with color Doppler sonography with histologic correlation of each biopsy site. Radiology 1995; 195: 86–90.

4. Lavoipierre AM, Snow RM, Frydenberg M et al. Prostatic cancer: role of Doppler imaging in transrectal sonography. Am J Radiol 1998; 171: 205–10.

5. Shigeno K, Igawa H, Shirna H et al. The role of colour Doppler ultrasonography in detecting prostate cancer. BJU Int 2000; 86: 229–33.

6. Cornud F, Hamida K, Flam T et al. Endorectal color Doppler sonography and endorectal MR imaging features of nonpalpable prostate cancer: correlation with radical prostatectomy findings. AJR 2000; 175: 1161–8.

7. Plawker MW, Fleisher JM, Vapnek EM, Macchia RJ. Current trends in prostate cancer diagnosis and staging among United States urologists. J Urol 1997; 158: 1853–8.

8. Ismail M, Petersen RO, Alexander AA et al. Color Doppler imaging in predicting the biologic behavior of prostate cancer: correlation with disease-free survival. Urology 1997; 50: 906–12.

9.   Neumaier CE, Martinoli C, Derchi LE et al. Normal prostate gland: examination with color Doppler US. Radiology 1995; 196: 453–7.

10. Leventis AK, Shariat SF, Utsunomiya T, Slawin KM. Characteristics of normal prostate vascular anatomy as displayed by power Doppler. Prostate 2001; 46: 281–8.

11. Cornud F, Belin X, Piron D et al. Color Doppler-guided prostate biopsies in 591 patients with an elevated serum PSA level: impact on Gleason score for nonpalpable lesions. Urology 1997; 49: 709–15.

12. Bree RL. The role of color Doppler and staging biopsies in prostate cancer detection. Urology 1997; 49(Suppl 3A): 31–4.

13. Rubin JM, Bude RO, Carson PL et al. Power Doppler US: a potentially useful alternative to mean frequency-based color Doppler US. Radiology 1994; 190: 853–6.

14. Downey DB, Fenster A. Three-dimensional power Doppler detection of prostatic cancer. AJR 1995; 165: 741.

15. Sakarya ME, Arslan H, Unal O et al. The role of power Doppler ultrasonography in the diagnosis of prostate cancer: a preliminary study. Br J Urol 1998; 82: 386–8.

16. Okihara K, Kojima M, Nakanouchi T et al. Transrectal power Doppler imaging in the detection of prostate cancer. BJU Int 2000; 85: 1053–7.

17. Halpern EJ, Strup SE. Using gray-scale and color and power Doppler sonography to detect prostatic cancer. AJR 2000; 174: 623–7.

18. Patel U, Rickards D. The diagnostic value of colour Doppler flow in the peripheral zone of the prostate, with histological correlation. Br J Urol 1994; 74: 590–5.

19. Keener TS, Winter TC, Berger R et al. AJR 2000; 175: 1169–72.

20. Halpern EJ, Frauscher F, Forsberg F et al. High frequency Doppler US of the prostate effect of patient positioning. Radiology 2002; 222: 634–90.

21. Bigler SA, Deering RE, Brawer MK. Comparison of microscopic vascularity in benign and malignant prostate tissue. Hum Pathol 1993; 24: 220–6.

22. Weidner N, Carroll PR, Flax J et al. Tumor angiogenesis correlates with metastasis in invasive prostate carcinoma. Am J Pathol 1993; 143: 401–9.

23. Fregene TA, Khanuja PS, Noto AC et al. Tumor-associated angiogenesis in prostate cancer. Anticancer Res 1993; 13: 2377–82.

24. Brawer MK, Deering RE, Brown M et al. Predictors of pathologic stage in prostate carcinoma, the role of neovascularity. Cancer 1994; 73: 678–87.

25. Bostwick DG, Wheeler TM, Blute M et al. Optimized microvessel density analysis improves prediction of cancer stage from prostate needle biopsies. Urology 1996; 48: 47–57.

26. Lissbrant IF, Stattin P, Damber JE, Bergh A. Vascular density is a predictor of cancer-specific survival in prostatic carcinoma. Prostate 1997; 33: 38–45.

27. Borre M, Offersen BV, Nerstrom B, Overgaard J. Microvessel density predicts survival in prostate cancer patients subjected to watchful waiting. Br J Cancer 1998; 78: 940–4.

28. Brawer MK. Quantitative microvessel density. A staging and prognostic marker for human prostatic carcinoma. Cancer 1996; 78: 345–9.

29. Bigler SA, Deering RE, Brawer MK. Comparison of microscopic vascularity in benign and malignant prostate tissue. Hum Pathol 1993; 24: 220–6.

30. Kay PA, Robb RA, Bostwick DG. Prostate cancer microvessels: a novel method for three-dimensional reconstruction and analysis. Prostate 1998; 37: 270–7.

31. Donnelly EF, Geng L, Wojcicki WE et al. Quantified power Doppler US of tumor blood flow correlates with microscopic quantification of tumor blood vessels. Radiology 2001; 219: 166–70.

32. Louvar E, Littrup PJ, Goldstein A et al. Cancer 1998; 83: 135–40.

33. Bude RO, Rubin JM. Power Doppler sonography. Radiology 1996; 200: 21–3.

34. Flemming F. Principles of Doppler Imaging. RSNA Categorical Course in Diagnostic Radiology Physics: CT and US Cross-sectional Imaging, 2000: 65–75.

35. Rubin JM, Bude RO, Fowlkes JB et al. Normalizing fractional moving blood volume estimates with power Doppler US: defining a stable intravascular point with the cumulative power distribution function. Radiology 1997; 205: 757–65.

36. Moskalik AP, Rubin MA, Wojno KJ et al. Analysis of three-dimensional Doppler ultrasonographic quantitative measures for the discrimination of prostate cancer. J Ultrasound Med 2001; 20: 713–22.

5

Ultrasound-guided biopsy of the prostate

Ethan J Halpern

Needle biopsy of the prostate is generally performed to establish or exclude the diagnosis of cancer. In most clinical practices, the positive biopsy rate ranges from 1 in 3 to 1 in 4 patients referred for biopsy. On the basis of an estimated 198 100 new cases of prostate cancer in the USA for 2001,[1] the number of people in the USA subjected to biopsy of the prostate will be in the range of 600,000–800,000.

For a variety of reasons, ultrasound is the preferred technique to guide biopsy of the prostate. Palpable masses are generally visible with ultrasound and can be directly targeted for biopsy. Furthermore, the depth of such palpable abnormalities is more accurately assessed with ultrasound guidance as compared with digital rectal examination. Using sonographic guidance, biopsies can be distributed throughout the prostate in a standard geometric pattern. The risk of damage to midline structures and the bladder is minimized by direct visualization with ultrasound. Sonographically guided biopsies can be positioned along the periphery of the gland, where most cancers are located, without damage to adjacent neurovascular structures. Finally, ultrasound may detect areas of abnormality that are not palpable by digital examination. Such areas may be preferentially targeted for biopsy.

Indications for biopsy

Among patients referred for biopsy of the prostate, the most frequent request is as follow-up for an elevated prostate-specific antigen (PSA) blood test. Expanded screening with serum PSA has increased greatly the number of patients referred for biopsy. Among patients in whom prostate cancer is detected, the rate of organ-confined disease is increased by screening with serum PSA.[2] Given a serum PSA value above

4.0 ng/ml, the positive predictive value for prostate cancer is in the range of 17–28%.[3–6] The positive predictive value of PSA increases at higher levels. A PSA value above 10 ng/ml has a positive predictive value of 42–64%.[7]

Several variations of the PSA examination have been used to improve patient selection for biopsy of the prostate. The use of age-adjusted PSA has been advocated to allow for the expected rise in PSA with increasing size of the prostate in older patients.[8] In order to normalize the PSA for different-size glands, PSA density may be computed as a ratio of the serum PSA to the size of the prostate. Among patients with a serum PSA in the range of 4–10 ng/ml, PSA density may be useful for selecting patients for biopsy.[9,10] For a given serum level of PSA, the proportion of free PSA relative to PSA bound to other macromolecules tends to be lower in subjects with cancer of the prostate.[11] Finally, a PSA velocity above 0.75 ng/ml/year may be more accurate in predicting cancer than a single PSA measurement.[12]

Before the advent of PSA testing, an abnormal digital rectal examination was the primary indication for biopsy of the prostate. The normal rectal examination of the prostate should demonstrate a smooth gland contour with a moderately firm texture similar to that of a tennis ball. Focal bulges of the prostatic contour and/or hard palpable masses are acceptable indications for biopsy.

Patients with the diagnosis of prostatic intraepithelial neoplasia on core biopsy are at increased risk for the presence of cancer on repeat biopsy, and should have a second biopsy regardless of serum PSA.[13,14] A previous biopsy with atypical small acinar proliferation is also associated with an increased risk of cancer on repeat biopsy (up to 50%).[15,16] Repeat biopsy is generally recommended in these patients after an interval of approximately three to six months. In patients with a history of prostate cancer, biopsy may be requested to document the presence of active tumor after radiation therapy, or to evaluate a soft tissue mass in the prostatic bed after prostatectomy.

The most controversial indication for biopsy of the prostate is for follow-up of an abnormal sonographic finding. Ultrasound is often used to assess the prostate of a patient with urinary tract symptoms for the diagnosis of benign prostatic hyperplasia or prostatitis. Ultrasound is also used to guide various ablation procedures for treatment of benign prostatic disease. A focal hypoechoic echotexture abnormality or focal bulge in the gland contour may be found on such an examination, prompting concern for the possibility of malignancy. Although there are no standard guidelines to follow in this circumstance, the sonographer's judgement of the abnormality should be interpreted in conjunction with other clinical and laboratory findings. A clearly present mass deserves definitive follow-up, including a biopsy procedure if the mass persists after treatment for other conditions such as prostatitis. Subtle gray-scale or color Doppler abnormalities with no other cause for suspicion of cancer present a more difficult problem. The specificity of ultrasound in these situations may be quite low, and the risks/costs of biopsy may not be justified. The author's preference is to explain this dilemma to the patient and referring physician. In many cases, the decision whether to perform a biopsy is then based upon the personal preferences of the patient and physician. Often, such patients may be best served by follow-up with serial assessment of the serum PSA.

Preparation and follow-up for biopsy

An explanatory letter should be sent to each patient approximately 2 weeks prior to the biopsy encounter. This letter should include instructions related to anticoagulation and a preparatory enema. A recent history of anticoagulation may be a contraindication to biopsy. If a patient has been taking warfarin, it may be wise to check the prothrombin time prior to performing a biopsy. Biopsy should not be performed with an INR (International Normalized Ratio) greater than 1.5. Other anticoagulants – including aspirin, non-steroidal anti-inflammatory drugs, and some herbal medications (*Ginkgo biloba*) – should be stopped 1 week prior to biopsy. Such medications may be restarted 24–48 hours after the biopsy procedure, provided the patient is not experiencing urinary or rectal bleeding. The patient should be instructed to take a cleansing enema prior to the biopsy procedure. The use of an enema reduces the amount of fecal contents within the rectum. A clean rectum provides a superior acoustic window for imaging the prostate, and may reduce the risk of infection.

Without antibiotic prophylaxis, the rate of bacteriuria after transrectal needle biopsy of the prostate may be as high as 8%, with a clinical rate of urinary tract infections of 5% and a hospitalization rate of 2%.[17] Antibiotic prophylaxis should be given to all patients prior to transrectal biopsy in order to reduce the risk of subsequent infection.[18,19] Antibiotics are not needed for transperineal biopsy. There is considerable variability among physicians in the choice of antibiotics for prophylaxis.[20] Nonetheless, antibiotic prophylaxis has become the standard of care for transrectal prostate biopsy. Most centers prefer an oral fluoroquinolone, such as ciprofloxacin. Ideally, the antibiotic should be administered at least 30–60 minutes before biopsy in order to have adequate serum levels at the time of biopsy. The antibiotic is then continued for 3 days. This regimen seems adequate in most situations for prophylaxis against post-biopsy prostatitis, cystitis, or septicemia. The standard prophylaxis regimen used at the Jefferson Prostate Diagnostic Center is ofloxacin 300 mg prior to the procedure, and then continued twice daily for three days.

Bacteremia is common after manipulation of the prostate.[21] Although there are no randomized, controlled human trials to definitively establish that antibiotic prophylaxis provides protection against endocarditis, intravenous antibiotic prophylaxis is recommended during biopsy of the prostate for patients in the moderate- or high-risk AHA (American Heart Association) categories.[22] The high-risk category includes patients with bioprosthetic and homograft heart valves, a prior history of endocarditis, complex congenital heart disease, or surgically constructed systemic pulmonary shunts. The moderate-risk category includes those patients with other congenital cardiac malformations, acquired valve dysfunction (e.g. rheumatic heart disease), hypertrophic cardiomyopathy, or mitral valve prolapse with regurgitation or thickened leaflets. AHA recommendations for moderate-risk patients include ampicillin 2 g or vancomycin 1 g intravenously prior to the procedure. Intravenous gentamycin (1.5 mg/kg) is added to this regimen for high-risk patients.

A focused clinical history should be obtained from every patient prior to biopsy. The reason for biopsy must be assessed. If there is a palpable abnormality on digital rectal examination, that abnormality should be identified on repeat examination prior to biopsy. A history of previous biopsy may alter the current biopsy strategy. If previous biopsies yielded normal tissue and the serum PSA continues to rise, it may be appropriate to obtain biopsy material from the inner gland. If a previous biopsy demonstrated the presence of suspicious cells, it may be appropriate to obtain multiple cores from the site of the prior suspicious biopsy. Major medical problems that might interfere with the procedure must be investigated.

Written informed consent should be obtained from all patients prior to biopsy. The consent should include a complete explanation of the risks and benefits of the procedure. Life-threatening complications, including severe hemorrhage[23,24] and sepsis, occur in less than 1% of patients, but pain and mild complications are common.[25] Spread of tumor into the biopsy track has been reported after both transrectal[26] and transperineal[27] biopsy, although its clinical significance is uncertain. Mild complications such as hematuria and hematospermia are reported at rates of 23.6% and 45.3%, respectively.[28] Fever, usually of low grade, may be seen in up to 5% of biopsies. In one study, 19% of subjects complained of significant complications, the most common being painful or difficult voiding (13%) and hematuria (11%).[29]

In order to ascertain that all patients are able to void after the biopsy, a urine specimen should be obtained before each patient is discharged. A small amount of hematuria is common, and should not be of great concern as long as the urine appears to clear toward the end of the stream. The patient should be instructed to drink plenty of fluids. Delayed urinary retention is relatively uncommon, but may present several hours after the procedure. Delayed retention can be related to accumulation of clotted blood within the bladder (Figure 5.1). If urinary retention becomes painful, the physician should be ready to insert a Foley catheter. When a catheter is necessary, it is generally left in place for 2–3 days.

Each patient should be given written discharge instructions, with a telephone number to call in case of complications. Since most complications occur within the first few hours, the author's preference is to perform all biopsies in the morning. Patients are instructed to avoid strenuous activity for 24 hours, to take prophylactic antibiotics, and to drink plenty of fluid.

Acetaminophen (paracetamol) may be used for post-biopsy pain. Patients should not take aspirin or other non-steroidal anti-inflammatory drugs for at least 24 hours, or until all bleeding stops. They are asked to call back and report any fevers or chills, increase in hematuria, urinary retention, dysuria, or increasing pain that is not relieved by acetaminophen (paracetamol).

Analgesia

Prostate biopsy is an uncomfortable procedure, but need not be painful. Almost all patients can be managed with topical or local anesthesia. Patients with anal strictures may be more difficult to manage. General anesthesia should be reserved only for those patients who cannot tolerate the physical or emotional stress of biopsy while awake.

Transperineal biopsy should be preceded by local anesthesia with 1% or 2% lidocaine. A 25-gauge needle is used to anesthetize the skin and subcutaneous tissues of the perineum. Deeper anesthesia is obtained under ultrasound guidance by injecting lidocaine along the expected biopsy tract with a spinal needle. It is useful to infiltrate local anesthetic into the tissues down to the level of the prostate. A total of 10–20 ml of local anesthetic agent may be used.

Transrectal biopsy is often performed without anesthesia. In a recent survey of patients undergoing transrectal biopsy of the prostate, 6% of patients judged that the procedure

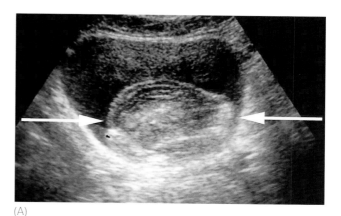

(A)

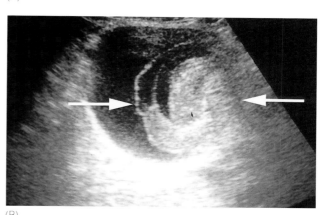

(B)

Figure 5.1

Transabdominal images of the urinary bladder after prostate biopsy. The patient complained of urinary retention that began several hours after the biopsy procedure. (A) Transverse image of the bladder obtained with the patient in supine position. A hematoma is present within the bladder (arrows). (B) This image demonstrates that the hematoma moves to a dependent position when the patient assumes a decubitus position. This large blood clot formed after biopsy, and necessitated placement of a Foley catheter to relieve the bladder outlet obstruction.

should have been performed under general anesthesia, while 19% would not agree to undergo it again without some form of anesthesia.[30] Topical anesthetic gel is a simple technique to provide analgesia for prostate biopsy.[31] Lidocaine gel may be used as the lubricant at the time of digital rectal examination, and again at the time of probe insertion. A short delay is required before the analgesic effect of lidocaine gel is apparent. However, since several minutes are required for a diagnostic examination of the prostate, the analgesic effect is usually present at the time biopsy specimens are obtained. Although the biopsy procedure may be less painful after administration of lidocaine gel, many patients continue to feel discomfort with each biopsy.[32]

Transrectal injection of lidocaine into the region of the neurovascular bundles has been reported to provide excellent anesthesia for the transrectal biopsy procedure.[33,34] When a large number of biopsy cores are to be obtained, infiltration of local anesthetic around the posterolateral aspect of the prostate may be used in addition to topical gel. A 22- to 25-gauge 15 cm spinal needle is used with injection of 2% lidocaine around the neurovascular bundle on each side of the prostate, into the plane between the rectum and the prostate. Injection is performed under direct sonographic visualization. Anesthetic is injected bilaterally at the level where the seminal vesicles join the prostate, and again, bilaterally, at a point midway between the base and apex of the prostate. In order to achieve adequate anesthesia and to minimize the risk of systemic side-effects, it is important to avoid injection into the periprostatic vessels. Anesthetic is readily visualized by sonography when it is properly injected into the plane between the prostate and the rectum. A total of 10 ml of local anesthetic is generally sufficient.

The utility of transrectal lidocaine remains somewhat controversial. One recent randomized study of this procedure concluded that transrectal lidocaine injection did not diminish the pain associated with biopsy,[35] while a second similar study demonstrated significant pain reduction with periprostatic anesthesia.[36] Our experience at the Jefferson Prostate Diagnostic Center, however, suggests that many patients do benefit from this technique. Patients who complain of extreme pain from a transrectal biopsy procedure performed without anesthetic often find that the same biopsy procedure is almost painless after proper administration of a local nerve block. Unfortunately, injection of lidocaine adjacent to the prostate may produce areas of focal hyperemia on color/power Doppler evaluation, and may interfere with Doppler evaluation of the prostate. In order to avoid lidocaine-induced hyperemia during Doppler-directed biopsy, injection of transrectal lidocaine should be limited to the level of the seminal vesicles. A single injection of 5 ml of lidocaine on each side of the midline between the rectum and the seminal vesicle will usually provide sufficient analgesia for biopsy of the entire prostate.

Biopsy approaches

There are three basic approaches to ultrasound-guided biopsy of the prostate: transrectal ultrasound and biopsy, transrectal ultrasound with transperineal biopsy, and transperineal ultrasound and biopsy. Transrectal ultrasound and biopsy is generally the preferred technique. A full gray-scale and Doppler examination requires no more than 5–10 minutes, with an additional 5–10 minutes for biopsy. The transperineal approach may be required when there is no rectum, or after various types of rectal surgery.[37] In contrast to transrectal biopsy, transperineal biopsy is performed as a sterile technique and requires additional time and technical

expertise. All three approaches may be performed in an outpatient setting.

A digital rectal examination should always be performed prior to inserting a probe into the rectum. The digital examination serves as a roadmap for scanning, and alerts the sonographer to potential problems such as masses, strictures, or hemorrhoids prior to probe insertion. Sphincter tone is assessed at the time of the digital rectal examination, and palpable abnormalities of the prostate are noted. A combination of sonographic findings and digital rectal examination findings should be used to guide the biopsy procedure for the prostate.[38]

Transperineal approach

Transperineal evaluation and biopsy of the prostate was widely used before the introduction of transrectal ultrasound. Infectious complications are rare, since transperineal examination is performed with sterile technique. With the patient in the lithotomy position, the area of the perineum is shaved and cleaned with an antiseptic solution. The scrotum is taped up or held up with a towel so that it does not fall into the sterile field. Local anesthesia is administered as described above.

An end-fire transducer is positioned on the perineum. The transducer frequency should be adjusted to allow sufficient penetration to visualize the prostate (generally 5–6 MHz). The position of the transducer on the perineum is critical. When the transducer is positioned too far anteriorly, the pubic symphysis blocks visualization of deeper structures. If the transducer is positioned too far posteriorly, it will fall into the rectum, and the sterile field will be contaminated. When the transducer is positioned anteriorly along the perineum, the corpora of the penis are visualized (Figure 5.2). The corpus spongiosum may be followed posteriorly into the prostate, with the urethra visualized as a hypoechoic structure (Figure 5.3). When the transducer is angled posteriorly from a position where the corpora were visualized, the prostate becomes visible. A full urinary bladder is helpful to demarcate the base of the prostate. Coronal and sagittal images of the prostate are obtained for measurements (Figure 5.4). Visualization of the prostate is more limited than with the transrectal approach, and it may be difficult to distinguish inner gland from outer gland (Figure 5.5). Seminal vesicles are poorly visualized from this approach.

Transperineal biopsy of the prostate may be performed in the coronal or sagittal orientation (Figure 5.6). The author's preference is for the coronal orientation, because this allows the midline structures to be visualized and thus avoided during biopsy. As with the transrectal approach, biopsy cores should be obtained from the peripheral aspect of the gland. It is important to clearly identify the boundary of the gland prior to biopsy. Focal lesions are rarely identified from the

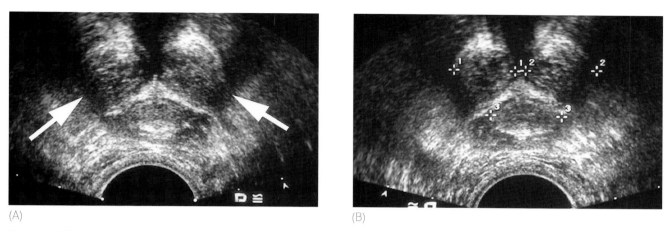

(A)   (B)

Figure 5.2
Coronal image obtained through the perineum, anterior to the prostate. (A) Demonstrates the ischiocavernosi muscles (arrows) as they form the two corpora cavernosa and join the corpus spongiosum. The corpus spongiosum is closest to the transducer, and is flattened by transducer pressure. (B) Demonstrates calipers around each of the three corpora.

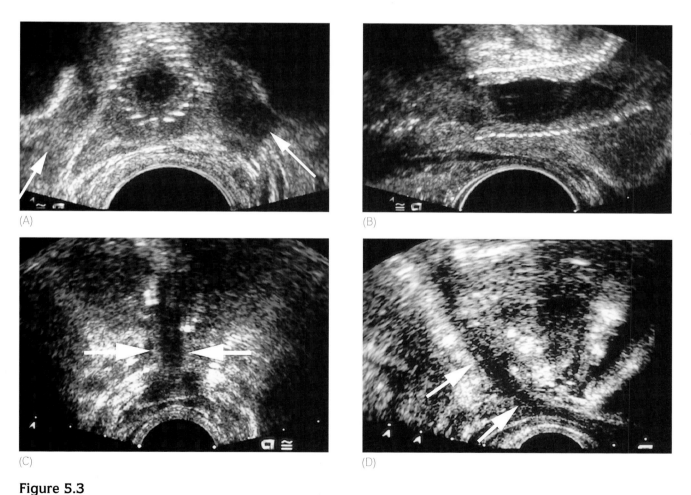

(A)   (B)

(C)   (D)

Figure 5.3
Transperineal images of the urethra as it enters the prostate. In (A) and (B), a urethral stent marks the location of a dilated urethra. (A) Coronal image demonstrating the short axis of the urethra. The stent is visible as an echogenic ring. The ischiocavernosi muscles are visible on either side of the stent (arrows). (B) Sagittal image along the long axis of the urethral stent extending from the apex of the prostate into the corpus spongiosum. (C, D) A normal urethra: (C) coronal image showing the urethra as it turns superiorly to enter the apex of the prostate (arrows); (D) sagittal image tracing the course of the urethra back into the prostate (arrows).

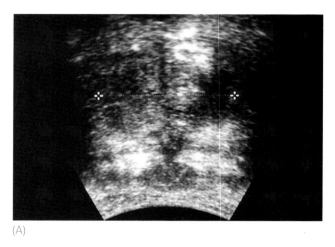

(A)

Figure 5.4
Transperineal measurement of the prostate. (A) Coronal image
with a transverse measurement. (B) Sagittal image with cranio-
caudal and antero-posterior measurements. A full urinary
bladder is useful to help identify the base of the prostate.

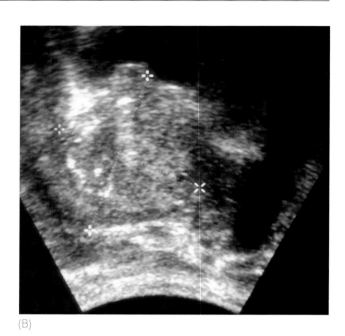

(B)

Figure 5.5
Transperineal image of the prostate in a patient with diffusely
infiltrating Gleason 7 cancer. A midline sagittal image
demonstrates the urethra (arrows). It is not possible to distinguish
inner gland from outer gland on this image. Furthermore, the
presence of cancer is not visualized on this image.

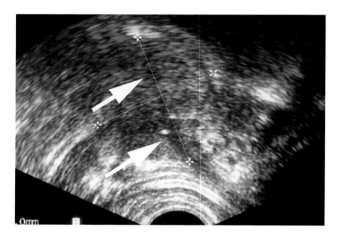

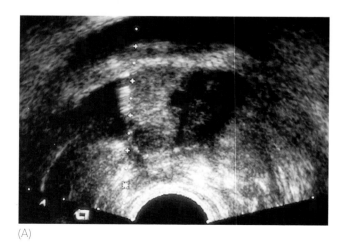

(A)

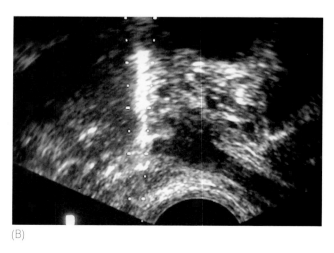

(B)

Figure 5.6
Transperineal biopsy of the prostate: (A) biopsy performed in the coronal plane; (B) biopsy performed in the sagittal plane.

transperineal approach (Figure 5.7). Six core biopsy specimens should be obtained: three on either side of the midline – posteriorly, anteriorly, and at a mid-level between these first two sets. If the prostate is large, biopsy specimens may be repeated at each site, with a first specimen obtained closer to the apex, and with a deeper specimen toward the base of the gland.

Although transperineal biopsy is generally performed in patients without a rectum, a transperineal biopsy approach may be performed with transrectal sonography. A transperineal guide is attached to the shaft of a side-fire transrectal

transducer to guide needle placement into the prostate (Figure 5.8). Transrectal visualization of the prostate is generally superior to transperineal visualization (Figure 5.9). The perineum is cleaned to provide a sterile field for biopsy. This combined transrectal/transperineal approach may be useful in

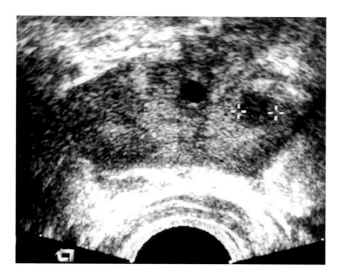

Figure 5.7
Transperineal image of the prostate in the coronal plane. This unusually clear image demonstrates a focal hypoechoic lesion on the left side of the gland (calipers). Biopsy of this lesion demonstrated a Gleason 7 cancer.

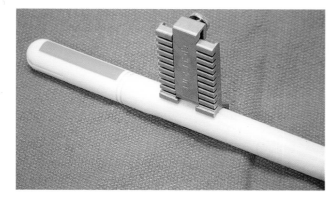

Figure 5.8
Transperineal biopsy guide for transrectal sonography. A guide is attached to the side of a transducer. The transducer is placed within the rectum to allow optimal imaging of the prostate. The guide remains on the patient's perineum to guide a transperineal biopsy of the prostate.

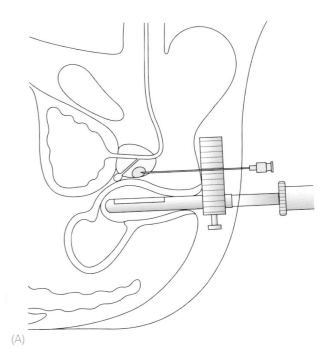

(A)

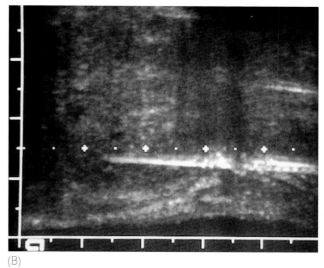

(B)

Figure 5.9
Transperineal biopsy with transrectal sonography. (A) Schematic demonstrating the position of the transrectal probe within the rectum. The guide is placed on the perineum in order to direct a transperineal biopsy of the prostate. (B) Demonstrates the needle as it is placed into the prostate from a transperineal approach. This technique allows optimal transrectal imaging of the prostate with transperineal biopsy.

patients who have had recent rectal surgery or creation of an ileo-anal pouch.[39] The trajectory of a biopsy needle introduced from the transperineal approach will extend parallel to the capsule of the prostate. On the basis of the known growth pattern of prostate cancer along the prostatic capsule, there is therefore a theoretical advantage to the transperineal biopsy approach over the transrectal approach.[40] Nonetheless, given the greater technical difficulty and patient pain with transperineal biopsy, the transrectal approach to imaging and biopsy has evolved as the standard of care.

Transrectal approach

Transrectal ultrasound with biopsy is the more conventional approach. Because the probe is positioned immediately adjacent to the posterior aspect of the prostate, the image quality obtained with the transrectal approach is superior to that obtained with the transperineal approach. The patient may be positioned in either the decubitus or lithotomy position. Although the decubitus position may be slightly more comfortable for the patient, the lithotomy position is preferred for detection of asymmetry in Doppler flow patterns.[41] Transrectal ultrasound is generally accomplished without sedation, although the procedure is facilitated by the use of local analgesics as described above.

Transrectal sonography may be performed with end-fire or side-fire probes (Figure 5.10). Both types of probes provide imaging in the sagittal plane. When a side-fire probe is used, a true axial plane may be obtained. End-fire probes provide imaging in an oblique plane that lies between the axial and coronal planes (Figure 5.11). Transrectal imaging should be performed in the sagittal plane as well as a coronal/axial plane. Imaging in the coronal/axial plane allows a side-to-side comparison for symmetry of the gland, and clearly demonstrates the neurovascular bundle and the lateral margin of the gland (Figure 5.12). Older side-fire systems require the use of two different probes for sagittal and axial imaging. More advanced side-fire systems may have two side-fire transducer elements built into a single probe, and may display both sagittal and transverse images simultaneously.

When a side-fire probe is used, biopsy of the prostate is usually guided in the sagittal imaging plane so that the biopsy needle can be observed as it courses into the prostate. The transverse imaging plane of a side-fire probe will only visualize the needle in cross-section, and will not visualize the depth of needle penetration. When an end-fire probe is used, biopsy may be performed in either the sagittal (Figure 5.13) or axial/coronal planes (Figure 5.14). Imaging within the sagittal plane clearly identifies the cranio-caudal position of the needle within the prostate. Imaging in the axial/coronal plane visualizes the position of the needle relative to the capsule of the prostate, and allows the operator to direct the biopsy along a peripheral course parallel to the capsule.

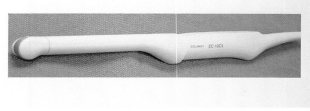

(A)

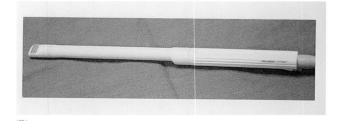

(B)

Figure 5.10
End-fire versus side-fire probes for transrectal imaging. (A) End-fire probe. Such a probe may be used for a variety of endocavitary purposes. In order to switch from transverse to sagittal planes, the probe is simply rotated by 90°. (B) Side-fire probe. The side-fire transducer provides a true transverse image. A side-fire transducer is preferred for brachytherapy, since multiple parallel images of the prostate can be obtained in a true transverse orientation by slowly withdrawing the transducer from the rectum.

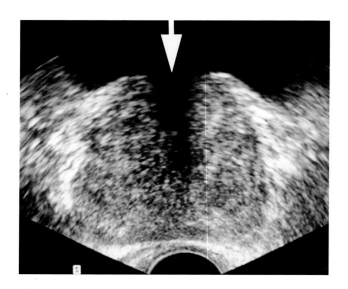

Figure 5.11
Transverse image of the prostate obtained with an end-fire probe. The end-fire probe provides an angled plane of imaging that lies between the true transverse and coronal planes. Posteriorly, the outer gland is demonstrated at the mid-gland level. The anterior portion of this same scan demonstrates the bladder neck (arrow), which is at the base of the prostate.

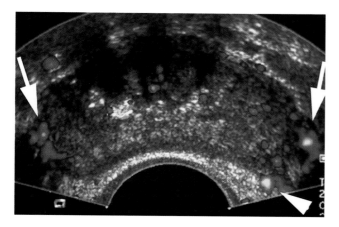

Figure 5.12
Transverse power Doppler sonography of the prostate allows comparison of symmetry on the two sides, and demonstrates vascular structures on both sides of the prostate. Capsular arteries are seen bilaterally (arrows). The left-sided neurovascular bundle is visualized (arrowhead).

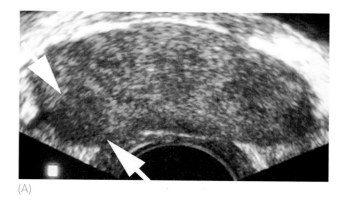

(A)

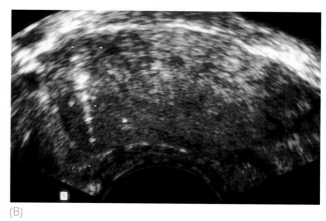

(B)

Figure 5.14
Biopsy of the prostate in the axial/coronal plane. (A) Transverse image of the prostate, with a focal hypoechoic lesion in the posterolateral aspect of the gland, on the right side (arrows). (B) Biopsy needle passing through the lesion which proved to be a Gleason 7 cancer.

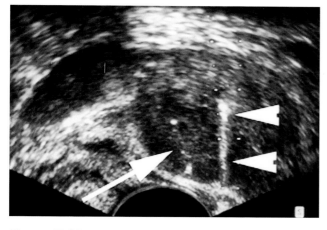

Figure 5.13
Sagittal biopsy of the prostate. The sagittal image along the left lateral aspect of the prostate demonstrates a relative hypoechoic area extending from base to mid-gland. A left base specimen had already been taken (visible needle tract – arrow). A biopsy needle is present within the hypoechoic lesion in the left mid-gland (arrowheads). Biopsy cores demonstrated Gleason 7 cancer in the left base and mid-gland.

After the transrectal probe has been covered with a clean condom, a biopsy guide is generally attached along the side of the probe (Figure 5.15). When biopsy is performed in the sagittal plane, the biopsy guide is positioned along the anterior aspect of the transducer so that the needle will pass through the anterior rectal wall to the prostate. In order to obtain specimens from both the right and left sides of the gland, the transducer is simply angled to the right side and to the left side. When biopsy is performed in the transverse plane, the biopsy guide is positioned along the lateral aspect of the transducer. Biopsies are obtained from the side of the prostate that is ipsilateral to the biopsy guide. In order to obtain biopsies from both the right and left sides of the gland, the transducer must be rotated 180°. Rotation of the transducer may be uncomfortable for some patients.

The biopsy needle

In order to obtain a core of tissue from the prostate, a spring-loaded automatic biopsy gun is used. Two types of automatic core biopsy systems are available: a completely disposable system and a reusable gun with disposable needles. Both systems function in a similar fashion. The needle consists of an inner, notched cannula and an outer hollow cannula (Figure 5.16). The inner cannula is fired first into the prostate, and a

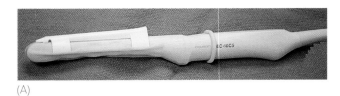

(A)

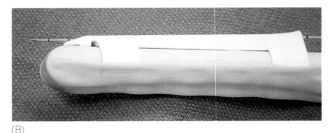

(B)

Figure 5.15

Preparation of the transrectal probe. (A) A condom covers the transrectal probe. A needle guide is attached along the transducer before the transducer is placed into the patient. (B) The needle passes through the biopsy guide.

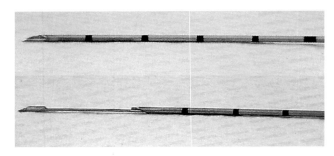

Figure 5.16

The core biopsy needle consists of two cannulas. The inner cannula is fired first, and penetrates the tissue of interest. A small core of tissue rests within the notch in this cannula. The outer cannula is fired within a split second after the inner cannula, trapping a piece of tissue inside the notch. The top image demonstrates the appearance of the needle either before or after firing. The outer cannula covers the inner cannula. The bottom image demonstrates the inner cannula as it is extended beyond the outer cannula.

small core of tissue falls into the notch. The outer cannula is then fired to cover the inner cannula and sever the tissue core from surrounding prostate tissue. A single trigger is used to initiate the automated firing sequence, which is completed within a split second. Care must be exercised to insure that the needle does not pass through the prostate and into the bladder or adjacent vessels. Most needles used for prostate biopsy have a forward throw of approximately 1.5–2 cm and obtain a core length of 1–1.5 cm.

Transrectal biopsy strategies

The sextant biopsy technique, first described in 1989, has been used widely as standard of care for the diagnosis of prostate cancer.[42] As initially described, the sextant biopsy includes three biopsy cores, which are obtained from each side of the midline – one each at the base, the mid-gland, and the apex. This sextant technique is fast and simple to perform, and is relatively well tolerated by patients. Prior to the establishment of the sextant method, various biopsy strategies were employed at different institutions, including directed biopsy limited to areas of sonographic abnormality and four-quadrant biopsy schemes. The sextant technique represented an increase in the number of biopsy specimens, but was justified as a standard technique that would improve detection of prostate cancer.

After the widespread adoption of the sextant biopsy approach, it became apparent that a significant minority of cancers were not detected on this standard biopsy. One study demonstrated a 19% positive biopsy rate in patients with an elevated PSA who were subjected to a second biopsy

after a negative sextant.[43] Another study demonstrated that if two consecutive sets of sextant biopsies were performed, the positive biopsy rate was increased by 37%.[44] A systematic five-region biopsy approach was proposed that included a sextant along with four additional lateral cores and three midline cores.[45] Approximately 35% of positive lesions detected by this approach were not found on the standard sextant. In another analysis of a PSA-screened population, 36% of cancers were missed by the standard sextant approach in glands under 30 cm^3 in volume, while 64% of cancers were missed by the standard sextant approach in larger glands.[46]

Given the number of significant cancers missed by the sextant approach, many physicians have increased the number of biopsy cores obtained in patients with an elevated PSA and a negative sextant biopsy. Several studies have suggested that adding laterally directed biopsy cores to the standard sextant protocol is useful.[47,48] Recent studies have suggested that an optimal systematic approach might require 8 or 10 biopsy cores.[49,50] In some institutions, a 'saturation biopsy' approach has been adopted.[51] A randomized trial of 6 versus 12 biopsy cores found no significant additional morbidity with the 12-biopsy approach,[52] although another study by the same group demonstrated no significant increase in the number of cancers detected with the 12-biopsy approach.[53] An analysis of the biopsy results obtained by the five-region approach suggested that the majority of additional cancers found with this technique were sampled along the lateral margin of the gland near the capsule of the prostate.[54] Furthermore, midline biopsies will increase the incidence of hematuria, but did not provide substantial additional cancer detection for the five region approach. Based upon this analysis, a modified sextant biopsy approach was proposed, with all six specimens being obtained along the lateral margins of the gland – at the base, mid-gland, and apex. The laterally directed sextant may provide superior results with fewer biopsy cores as compared with the five-region approach.[55] Needless to say, the optimal number and location of biopsy cores remains a matter of extensive research and controversy.

Although 24% of prostate cancers are thought to arise in the transition zone,[56] routine biopsy of the transition zone has a low yield of cancer and is not generally recommended.[57,58] Furthermore, anteriorly located cancers in the transition zone are rare, and biopsy of this area entails a greater risk of injury to the urethra. In the previously cited five-region biopsy approach, only 2 of 17 additional cancers not detected on the sextant approach were found in transition zone specimens. Given this relatively low yield, transition zone biopsy is recommended only for patients with an elevated PSA above 10 mg/ml and previous negative sextant biopsy.[59]

To conclude this discussion, we must address the issue of targeted biopsy. In Chapters 3 and 4, many cases were demonstrated in which sonographic abnormalities corresponded to the presence of a cancer. Unfortunately, targeted biopsy alone will miss approximately half of cancers in the prostate.[60] Nonetheless, the positive biopsy yield of targeted specimens is 1.9–3.7 times greater than that of systematic biopsy cores obtained with the sextant approach.[61] A recent analysis of Doppler evaluation in radical prostatectomy subjects suggests that the probability of a positive biopsy within a sextant that contains a cancer can be increased from 75% to 85% by directing the biopsy to the site of greatest flow velocity and volume.[62] In order to maximize biopsy yield with the smallest number of biopsy cores, the author recommends a modified systematic sextant biopsy with up to four additional directed biopsies targeted to gray-scale and Doppler abnormalities. The modified sextant cores are obtained along the capsule of the prostate in order to maximize biopsy yield along the plane of growth of prostate cancer. Additional directed biopsies are obtained to insure that all suspicious areas are sampled. In patients with a prior negative biopsy and a PSA above 10 ng/ml, additional specimens may be obtained from the transition zone.

References

1. Greenlee RT, Hill-Harmon MB, Murray T, Thun M. Cancer statistics, 2001. CA Cancer J Clin 2001; 51: 15–36.
2. Catalona WJ, Smith DS, Ratliff TL, Basler JW. Detection of organ-confined prostate cancer is increased through prostate-specific antigen-based screening. JAMA 1993; 270: 948–54.
3. Coley CM, Barry MJ, Fleming C, Mulley AG. Early detection of prostate cancer. Ann Intern Med 1997; 126: 394–406.
4. Brawer MK, Chetner MP, Beatie J et al. Screening for prostatic carcinoma with prostate specific antigen. J Urol 1992; 147: 841–5.
5. Bretton PR. Prostate-specific antigen and digital rectal examination in screening for prostate cancer: a community-based study. South Med J 1994; 87: 720–3.
6. Catalona WJ, Richie JP, Ahmann FR et al. Comparison of digital rectal examination and serum prostate specific antigen in the early detection of prostate cancer: results of a multicenter clinical trial of 6630 men. J Urol 1994; 151: 1283–90.
7. Richie JP, Catalona WJ, Ahmann FR et al. Effect of patient age on early detection of prostate cancer with serum prostate-specific antigen and digital rectal examination. Urology 1993; 42: 365–74.
8. Oesterling JE, Jacobsen SJ, Cooner WH. The use of age-specific reference ranges for serum prostate specific antigen in men 60 years old or older. J Urol 1993; 150: 1837–9.
9. Benson MC, Whang IS, Olsson CA et al. The use of prostate specific antigen density to enhance the predictive value of intermediate levels of serum prostate specific antigen. J Urol 1992; 147: 817–21.
10. Bretton PR, Evans WP, Borden JD, Castellanos RD. The use of prostate specific antigen density to improve the sensitivity of prostate specific antigen in detecting prostate carcinoma. Cancer 1994; 74: 2991–5.
11. Catalona WJ, Smith DS, Wolfert RL et al. Evaluation of percentage of free serum prostate-specific antigen to improve specificity of prostate cancer screening. JAMA 1995; 274: 1214–20.
12. Carter HB, Pearson JD, Metter EJ et al. Longitudinal evaluation of prostate-specific antigen levels in men with and without prostate disease. JAMA 1992; 267: 2215–20.
13. Brawer MK, Bigler SA, Sohlberg OE et al. Significance of prostatic intraepithelial neoplasia on prostate needle biopsy. Urology 1991; 38: 103–7.
14. Weinstein MH, Epstein JI. Significance of high grade prostatic intraepithelial neoplasia (PIN) on needle biopsy. Hum Pathol 1993; 24: 624–9.
15. Iczkowski KA, Bassler TJ, Schwob VS et al. Diagnosis of 'suspicious for malignancy' in prostate biopsies: predictive value for cancer. Urology 1998; 51: 749–57.
16. Ouyang RC, Kenwright DN, Nacey JN, Delahunt B. The presence of atypical small acinar proliferation in prostate needle biopsy is predictive of carcinoma on subsequent biopsy. BJU Int 2001; 87: 70–4.
17. Kapoor DA, Klimberg IW, Malek GH et al. Single-dose oral ciprofloxacin versus placebo for prophylaxis during transrectal prostate biopsy. Urology 1998; 52: 552–8.
18. Taylor HM, Bingham JB. Antibiotic prophylaxis for transrectal prostate biopsy. J Antimicrobial Chemother 1997; 39: 115.
19. Aron M, Rajeev TP, Gupta NP. Antibiotic prophylaxis for transrectal needle biopsy of the prostate: a randomized controlled study. BJU Int 2000; 85: 682–5.
20. Shandera KC, Thibault GP, Deshon GE Jr. Variability in patient preparation for prostate biopsy among American urologists. Urology 1998; 52: 644–6.
21. Sullivan N, Sutter V, Mims M et al. Clinical aspects of bacteremia after manipulation of the genitourinary tract. J Infect Dis 1973; 127: 49–55.
22. Dajani AS, Taubert KA, Wilson W et al. Prevention of bacterial endocarditis. Recommendations by the American Heart Association. JAMA 1997; 277: 1794–801.

23. Gatling RR. Massive retropubic hemorrhage after needle biopsy of the prostate. South Med J 1988; 81: 1188–9.

24. Brullet E, Guevara MC, Campo R et al. Massive rectal bleeding following transrectal ultrasound-guided prostate biopsy. Endoscopy 2000; 32: 792–5.

25. Collins GN, Lloyd SN, Hehir M, McKelvie GB. Multiple transrectal ultrasound-guided prostatic biopsies – true morbidity and patient acceptance. Br J Urol 1993; 71: 460–3.

26. Bastacky SS, Walsh PC, Epstein JI. Needle biopsy associated tumor tracking of adenocarcinoma of the prostate. J Urol 1991; 145: 1003–7.

27. Ryan PG, Peeling WB. Perineal prostatic tumour seedling after 'Tru-Cut' needle biopsy: case report and review of the literature. Eur Urol 1990; 17: 189–92.

28. Rietbergen JB, Kruger AE, Kranse R, Schroder FH. Complications of transrectal ultrasound-guided systematic sextant biopsies of the prostate: evaluation of complication rates and risk factors within a population-based screening program. Urology 1997; 49: 875–80.

29. Crundwell MC, Cooke PW, Wallace DM. Patients' tolerance of transrectal ultrasound-guided prostatic biopsy: an audit of 104 cases. BJU Int 1999; 83: 792–5.

30. Irani J, Fournier F, Bon D et al. Patient tolerance of transrectal ultrasound-guided biopsy of the prostate. Br J Urol 1997; 79: 608–10.

31. Renfer LG, Vaccaro JA, Kiesling V. Digital-directed transrectal core biopsy with spring-loaded biopsy device (Biopty). Urology 1991; 38: 161–2.

32. Desgrandchamps F, Meria P, Irani J et al. The rectal administration of lidocaine gel and tolerance of transrectal ultrasonography-guided biopsy of the prostate: a prospective randomized placebo-controlled study. BJU Int 1999; 83: 1007–9.

33. Nash PA, Bruce JE, Indudhara R, Shinohara K. Transrectal ultrasound guided prostatic nerve blockade eases systematic needle biopsy of the prostate. J Urol 1996; 155: 607–9.

34. Soloway MS, Obek C. Periprostatic local anesthesia before ultrasound guided prostate biopsy. J Urol 2000; 163: 172–3.

35. Wu CL, Carter HB, Naqibuddin M, Fleisher LA. Effect of local anesthetics on patient recovery after transrectal biopsy. Urology 2001; 57: 925–9.

36. Pareek G, Armenakas NA, Fracchia JA. Periprostatic nerve blockade for transrectal ultrasound guided biopsy of the prostate: a randomized, double-blind, placebo controlled study. J Urol 2001; 166: 894–7.

37. Twidwell JJ, Matthews RD, Huisam TK, Sands JP. Ultrasound evaluation of the prostate after abdominoperineal resection. J Urol 1993; 150: 902–4.

38. Renfer LG, Schow D, Thompson IM, Optenberg S. Is ultrasound guidance necessary for transrectal prostate biopsy? J Urol 1995; 154: 1390–1.

39. Fergany AF, Angermeier KW. A technique of transrectal ultrasound guided transperineal random prostate biopsy in patients with ulcerative colitis and an ileal pouch. J Urol 2000; 163: 205–6.

40. Vis AN, Boerma MO, Ciatto S et al. Detection of prostate cancer: a comparative study of the diagnostic efficacy of sextant transrectal versus sextant transperineal biopsy. Urology 2000; 56: 617–21.

41. Halpern EJ, Frauscher F, Forsberg F et al. High frequency US imaging of the prostate: impact of patient positioning. Radiology 2002; 222: 634–9.

42. Hodge KK, McNeal JE, Terris MK, Stamey TA. Random systematic versus directed ultrasound guided transrectal core biopsies of the prostate. J Urol 1989; 142: 71.

43. Keetch DW, Catalona WJ, Smith DS. Serial prostatic biopsies in men with persistently elevated serum prostate specific antigen values. J Urol 1994; 151: 1571–4.

44. Levine MA, Ittman M, Melamed J, Lepo H. Two consecutive sets of transrectal ultrasound guided sextant biopsies of the prostate for the detection of prostate cancer. J Urol 1998; 159: 471.

45. Eskew LA, Bare RL, McCullough DL. Systematic 5 region prostate biopsy is superior to sextant method for diagnosing carcinoma of the prostate. J Urol 1997; 157: 199.

46. Naughton CK, Smith DS, Humphrey PA et al. Clinical and pathologic tumor characteristics of prostate cancer as a function of the number of biopsy cores: a retrospective study. Urology 1998; 52: 808–13.

47. Chang JJ, Shinohara K, Bhargava V, Presti JC Jr. Prospective evaluation of lateral biopsy cores of the peripheral zone for prostate cancer detection. J Urol 1998; 160: 2111–14.

48. Ravery V, Goldblatt L, Royer B et al. Extensive biopsy protocol improves the detection rate of prostate cancer. J Urol 2000; 164: 393–6.

49. Presti JC Jr, Chang JJ, Bhargava V, Shinohara K. The optimal systematic prostate biopsy scheme should include 8 rather than 6 biopsy cores: results of a prospective clinical trial. J Urol 2000; 163: 163–6.

50. Gore JL, Shariat SF, Miles BJ et al. Optimal combinations of sextant and laterally directed biopsies for the detection of prostate cancer. J Urol 2001; 165: 1554–9.

51. Stewart CS, Leibovich BC, Weaver AL, Lieber MM. Prostate cancer diagnosis using a saturation needle biopsy technique after previous negative sextant biopsies. J Urol 2001; 166: 86–92.

52. Naughton CK, Ornstein DK, Smith DS, Catalona WJ. Pain and morbidity of transrectal ultrasound guided prostate biopsy: a prospective randomized trial of 6 versus 12 cores. J Urol 2000; 163: 168–71.

53. Naughton CK, Miller DC, Mager DE et al. A prospective randomized trial comparing 6 versus 12 prostate biopsy cores: impact on cancer detection. J Urol 2000; 164: 388–92.

54. Stamey TA. Editorial comment on 'Systematic 5 region prostate biopsy is superior to sextant method for diagnosing carcinoma of the prostate'. J Urol 1997; 157: 202–3.

55. Stamey TA. Making the most out of six systematic sextant biopsies. Urology 1995; 45: 2–12.

56. McNeal JE, Redwine EA, Freiha FS, Stamey TA. Zonal distribution of prostatic adenocarcinoma. Correlation with histologic pattern and direction of spread. Am J Surg Pathol 1988; 12: 897–906.

57. Lui PD, Terris MK, McNeal JE, Stamey TA. Indications for ultrasound guided transition zone biopsies in the detection of prostate cancer. J Urol 1995; 153: 1000–3.

58. Terris MK, Pham TQ, Issa MM, Kabalin JN. Routine transition zone and seminal vesicle biopsies in all patients undergoing transrectal ultrasound guided prostate biopsies are not indicated. J Urol 1997; 157: 204–6.

59. Brawer MK. Editorial: Prostate cancer. J Urol 1997; 157: 207–8.

60. Kuligowska E, Barish MA, Fenlon HM, Blake M. Predictors of prostate carcinoma: accuracy of gray-scale and color Doppler US and serum markers. Radiology 2001; 220: 757-64.

61. Halpern EJ, Strup SE. Using gray-scale and color and power Doppler sonography to detect prostatic cancer. AJR 2000; 174: 623–7.

62. Moskalik A, Carson PL, Rubin JM et al. Analysis of three-dimensional ultrasound Doppler for the detection of prostate cancer. Urology 2001; 57: 1128–32.

6

Advanced sonographic techniques for detection of prostate cancer

Ethan J Halpern

The ideal diagnostic study for prostate cancer should detect all clinically significant cancers in the prostate, and should identify patients without cancer as normal so that they need not undergo a biopsy procedure. Unfortunately, conventional sonography offers limited sensitivity and specificity for the detection of prostate cancer. A more complete review of this issue is presented in Chapters 3 and 4. Although clinical results differ among different institutions, most studies agree that conventional gray-scale and Doppler sonography are not sufficiently sensitive to exclude subjects from biopsy.[1] The author's experience suggests that gray-scale, color (frequency-shift), and power (amplitude) Doppler-directed biopsy do detect about half of cancers, but may not offer significant advantage over systematic sextant biopsy.[2]

Clinically significant cancer

Diagnostic testing for prostate cancer is further complicated by the difficulty in determining which cancers are clinically significant. Studies based upon the Connecticut Tumor Registry demonstrated no loss of life expectancy in conservatively treated men with Gleason scores of 2–4, and only a modest risk of death at Gleason scores of 5 and 6.[3,4] Initial conservative management and delayed hormone therapy may be reasonable for lower-grade localized prostate cancer.[5] A prospective study in Sweden concluded that patients with localized prostate cancer have a favorable outlook with watchful waiting, and that an aggressive approach to all patients with early disease would entail substantial overtreatment.[6]

Which features define clinically significant cancer of the prostate? An analysis of prostate cancer volumes suggests that tumors with a volume of less than 0.5 cm^3 are unlikely to be clinically significant.[7] Since serum prostate-specific antigen

(PSA) may serve as an indicator of tumor volume and stage,[8,9] the combination of a low Gleason score with a low serum PSA may be useful to identify tumors that are clinically insignificant.[10] Studies of microvessel density within the prostate demonstrate a clear association of increased microvessel density with the presence of cancer,[11] with metastases,[12] with the stage of disease,[13–15] and with disease-specific survival.[16,17] There is also evidence suggesting that quantitative assessment of microvascular density may actually provide important data to guide therapeutic decisions.[18] Thus, a diagnostic test for prostate cancer should be designed to detect all lesions with significant volume, Gleason score, and microvessel density.

Signal-processing techniques

In order to improve the diagnostic accuracy of sonography, various signal-processing techniques have been studied to improve discrimination between benign and malignant prostate tissue. For the purposes of our discussion, these techniques are grouped into three categories: application of image-processing techniques to conventional sonographic images, mathematical analysis of the reflected radiofrequency (RF) signal, and evaluation of changes in the RF signal during specific maneuvers.

The first category of image-processing techniques attempts to quantify or clarify features that are present within standard sonographic images. These features might include the shape and contour of the prostate, or its echotexture pattern. For example, one group used a computer model to measure the ratio of the lengths and areas in different parts of the prostate.[19] Others have evaluated mathematically the texture pattern of benign and malignant prostatic tissue.[20]

Several imaging features are significantly correlated with the presence of malignancy, but none of these features has proven sufficiently sensitive and specific for routine clinical application.

Spectral analysis is a quantitative approach that extracts information directly from the RF echo signal. Tissue-specific features that are not visible in the standard gray-scale presentation of an ultrasound image may be obtained by spectral analysis. A graphical plot of backscattered power versus frequency may demonstrate changes in the power spectrum related to intrinsic features of the tissue. Based upon a theoretical framework proposed by Lizzi, the intercept and midband values of this plot may be related to scatterer size and to a property called 'acoustic concentration'.[21] Both the slope and midband values obtained from malignant prostate tissue tend to be lower than those obtained from benign prostate tissue.[22] A recent study using neural networks to interpret spectral data from the prostate demonstrated substantial improvement in the discrimination of malignant and benign tissue -ROC (receiver operating characteristic) area of 0.87 for spectral analysis versus ROC area of 0.64 for conventional sonography.[23] Real-time spectral analysis may identify malignant areas that are not visible during conventional sonography, and tag these foci with color to allow for directed biopsy guidance (Figure 6.1). Such techniques are promising, but will require further development and study before they can be accepted for widespread clinical application.

Elastography represents yet another form of signal processing applied to sonographic RF data. An elastogram is a map of tissue stiffness derived from changes in the sonographic RF speckle pattern during the application of external pressure.[24] Intuitively, one would expect less displacement of the speckle pattern in stiffer tissue. In vitro examination of

prostate cancer demonstrates that malignant prostate tissue is consistently stiffer than benign tissue.[25] The elastic modulus of normal prostate tissue is lower than that of prostate tumor tissue, while the elastic modulus of tissue with benign prostatic hyperplasia is even lower than that of normal tissue.[26] Although digital rectal examination may detect malignant nodules along the posterior surface of the prostate, elastography has the potential to detect stiff tissue located deep within the gland. Elastography of prostate specimens provides precise anatomic detail throughout the gland (Figure 6.2).[27] A small study comparing conventional sonography to sono-elasticity imaging in prostatectomy specimens suggests that elastography may be more sensitive than gray-scale sonography for detection of prostate cancer in vitro.[28]

Although promising in vitro results have been reported, the in vivo application of elastography to the prostate is complicated by variability in the shape and size of the prostate. Application of a constant calibrated external pressure to all parts of the prostate is not possible in practice. Furthermore, most experimental in vitro techniques employ speckle tracking to follow the position of individual points in tissue with time. This type of analysis is not currently feasible for a real-time imaging examination. Nonetheless, initial in vivo elastography has been achieved in human subjects with simpler techniques that are feasible. The simplest of these techniques creates vibration within the prostate by 'flicking' the trans-rectal transducer against the anterior rectal wall. The resulting pattern of vibrations is then recorded with the transducer held still. A slightly more sophisticated approach applies low-frequency vibration to the perineum.

The most practical method for recording an elastographic image with current technology is by using a color Doppler technique designed to detect high-power, low-velocity

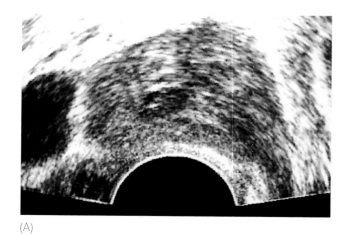

(A)

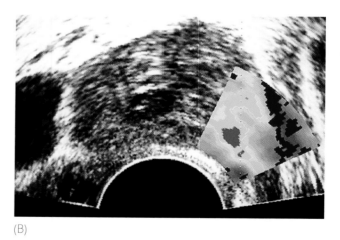

(B)

Figure 6.1

Spectral analysis technique for the identification of prostate cancer. (A) Sagittal image of the prostate. A subtle hypoechoic area is difficult to discern at the apex. (B) Color map, superimposed upon the gray-scale image. A suspicious area is highlighted at the apex for directed biopsy. The color map is based upon analysis of the radiofrequency spectrum reflected from the prostate. (Courtesy of Dr Christopher Vecchio, Spectrasonics Inc.)

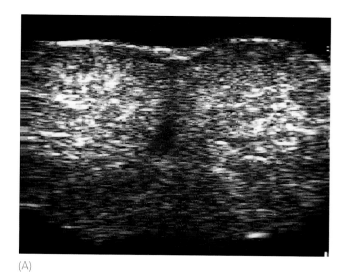

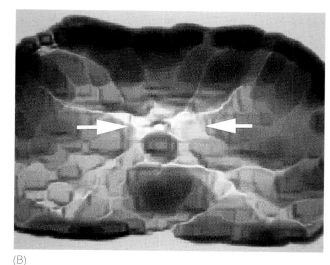

(A)　　　　　　　　　　　　　　　　　　　　　　　　(B)

Figure 6.2

Sonogram and elastogram of the canine prostate. (A) A conventional sonogram of the canine prostate demonstrates few internal architectural features of the prostate. (B) An elastogram demonstrates a radial architectural pattern, which may be related to the vascular supply of the prostate. The position of the urethra is also clearly indicated by the distinct differences in the elasticity of peri-urethral tissues from the remainder of the prostate (arrows). (Courtesy of Dr Jonathan Ophir and Dr Faouzi Kallel.)

motion. Commercially available systems for recording cardiac wall motion may be adapted for elastography of the prostate. Preliminary results with this technique have been obtained at the University Hospital of Wales.[29,30] Although elastography using this technique is not sufficiently sensitive or specific to replace systematic biopsy, it does detect some prostatic cancers that are not visible on gray-scale ultrasound imaging (Figure 6.3). The addition of targeted biopsies based upon elastography to a standard gray-scale systematic biopsy strategy results in a significant improvement in cancer detection.

Contrast-enhanced sonography

Since increased microvascular density is associated with clinically significant cancer of the prostate, selective imaging of neovasculature may provide a specific test for clinically significant disease. Unfortunately, the microvessels of interest are in the size range of 10–50 μm, which is well below the resolution of clinical ultrasound units. A recent study demonstrated a negative correlation between microvessel density count and conventional color Doppler pixel density.[31] Intravascular contrast agents, however, may provide the capability to image flow within vessels that are too small to visualize. Clinical trials of microbubble contrast agents have recently demonstrated promise for the detection of prostate cancer.[32] Furthermore two recent studies have suggested that contrast-enhanced color and power Doppler sonography

may provide selective enhancement of regions with increased microvascular density.[33,34]

Microbubble contrast agents for sonography are injectable gas-filled microbubbles that increase the echogenicity of the intravascular space, and provide a dramatic visible increase in the color Doppler signal. Modern ultrasound contrast agents have intravascular residence times of several minutes, pass through the pulmonary circulation, and may be used for parenchymal organ enhancement.[35,36] The duration of microbubble enhancement may be extended for longer periods by slow intravenous infusion of the contrast material. Some agents demonstrate only Doppler enhancement in the prostate, while others show both gray-scale and Doppler enhancement. An early study of one such agent, Echogen (Sonus Pharmaceuticals, Bothell, WA, USA), suggested that enhanced color flow with contrast may be associated with the presence of prostate cancer.[37,39] Gray-scale enhancement was not demonstrated in this early study, which was performed prior to the widespread availability of harmonic imaging techniques (see below). A dose–response relationship has been demonstrated for Doppler enhancement of the prostate with BR1 (Bracco SpA, Milan, Italy).[39] A study of men with biopsy-proven prostate cancer demonstrated that power Doppler enhancement with the contrast agent Levovist (Schering, Germany) is reduced after androgen therapy.[40]

Microbubble agents enhance the Doppler signal for both color (frequency-shift) Doppler and power (amplitude) Doppler. Focal areas of increased Doppler flow within

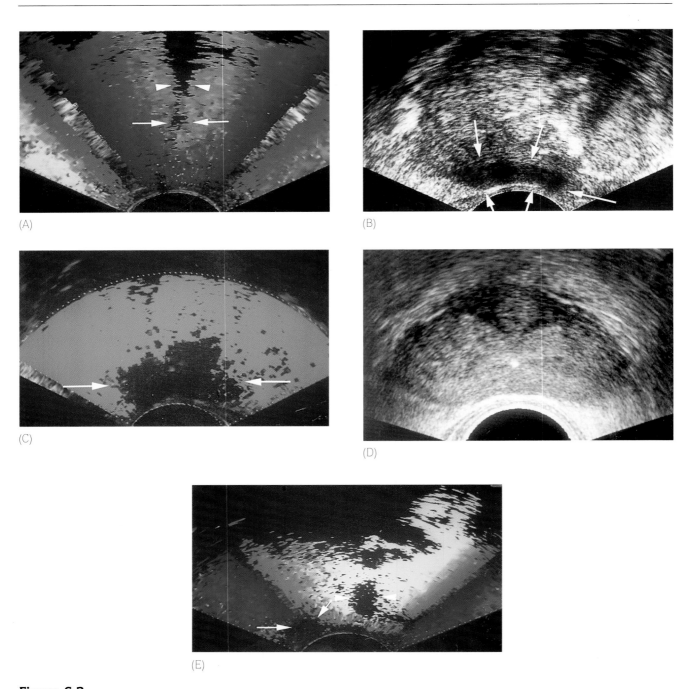

Figure 6.3
Elastography of the prostate. (A) Normal elastogram of the prostate. The periurethral area (arrows) and anterior fibromuscular stroma (arrowheads) differ in stiffness from the remainder of the prostate. (B) A hypoechoic cancer detected in a second patient with gray-scale imaging (arrows). (C) This cancer is also detected by elastography. (D) A third subject with a normal gray-scale sonogram of the prostate. (E) An elastogram obtained in the same position as (D), demonstrating the site of a cancer in the right outer gland (arrows). Arrowheads mark the periurethral zone. (Courtesy of Dr Dennis Cochlin.)

the prostate may be seen to correspond with malignancy (Figure 6.4). A study combining contrast-enhanced power Doppler with three dimensional imaging demonstrated improvement in the identification of cancer during adminis-tration of Levovist (Figure 6.5).[41] This study, however, did not demonstrate correlation of increased enhancement with positive results at individual biopsy sites. A recent study using Levovist during biopsy of the prostate demonstrated selective

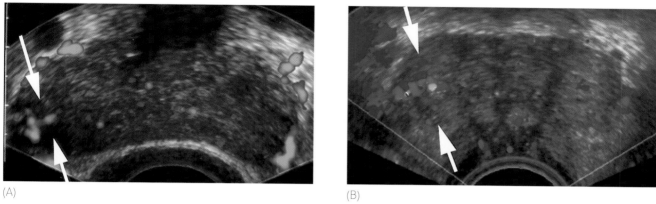

(A)   (B)

Figure 6.4
Transverse Doppler images of the prostate at the base to mid-gland level after administration of Imavist (Alliance Pharmaceutical Corp., San Diego, CA, USA). Baseline sonography without contrast infusion demonstrated no intraparenchymal Doppler signal. (A) Contrast-enhanced power Doppler demonstrates an area of flow in the right lateral aspect of the gland (arrows). A core biopsy of this site was positive for a Gleason 6 cancer. All other biopsy cores were negative. (B) Transverse sonogram at the base of the prostate in a patient with a Gleason 7 cancer extending from the right base to the mid-gland. Contrast-enhanced color Doppler after administration of Definity (DuPont Pharmaceuticals, Billerica, MA, USA) demonstrates increased flow on the side of the cancer (arrows).

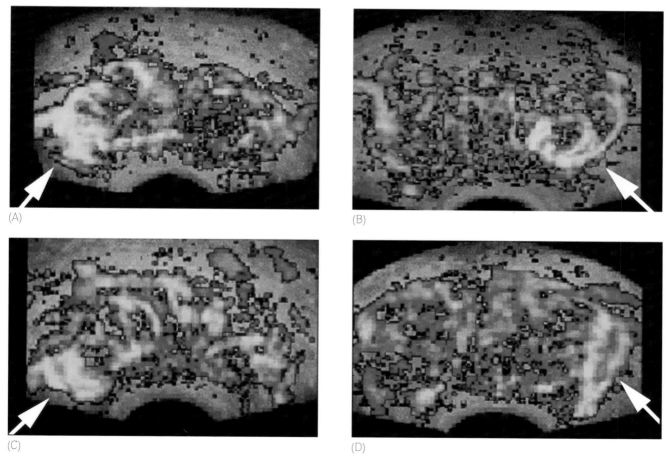

(A)   (B)

(C)   (D)

Figure 6.5
Contrast-enhanced three-dimensional power Doppler imaging of the prostate. The arrow in each image indicates the site of increased flow, corresponding to a focus of malignancy. (Courtesy of Drs JP Michiel Sedelaar, Jean JMCH de la Rosette, and Hessel Wijkstra, Department of Urology, University Medical Center Nijmegen, The Netherlands.)

Doppler enhancement of malignant foci. Prostate cancer was detected in 23 of 84 subjects (27%) with contrast-enhanced color Doppler-targeted biopsy, and in 17 of 84 patients (20%) with conventional systematic gray-scale biopsy (Figure 6.6). A significantly greater number of positive biopsy cores were obtained with fewer biopsy passes using contrast-enhanced directed biopsy of the prostate.[42]

In order to selectively enhance the neovascular bed within the prostate, contrast agents must traverse distally into the capillary bed. Unfortunately, the power levels delivered by conventional ultrasound systems destroy most microbubbles before they reach the neovasculature. One approach to this problem is the use of transient response imaging, also known as intermittent ultrasound imaging. Intermittent imaging of single image frames reduces the amount of ultrasound

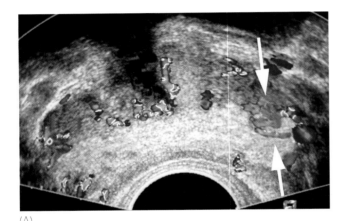

(A)

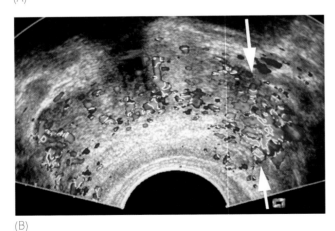

(B)

Figure 6.6

Contrast-enhanced color Doppler imaging of the prostate during infusion of Levovist (Schering, Germany). (A) Transverse color Doppler image through the mid-gland. A subtle finding of increased flow is present on the left side (arrows). (B) Contrast-enhanced color Doppler image at the same level. The area of increased flow is more obvious (arrows). Directed biopsy guided to the site of increased flow detected the presence of a Gleason 7 cancer. (Courtesy of Dr Ferdinand Frauscher.)

energy imparted to the tissue, and therefore reduces bubble destruction. Intermittent imaging has been shown to increase the enhancement provided by ultrasound contrast agents.[43–45] The observed degree of enhancement with intermittent imaging is dependent upon flow rate, acoustic power output, and frequency of insonation.[46] A conventional gray-scale ultrasound image is refreshed at approximately 30 frames per second. In the short time between frames, contrast may enter larger vessels, but will not generally reach the microcirculation. As the frame rate is reduced, more contrast material may enter the imaging plane and traverse further into the distal capillary bed between image frames. Intermittent imaging demonstrates a quantitative increase in contrast enhancement, as well as a qualitative difference in the enhancement pattern related to contrast in smaller vessels.

Harmonic gray-scale imaging represents yet another recent advance in ultrasound imaging of contrast agents.[47–51] Various harmonics of the insonating frequency are produced by resonance of the microbubbles in ultrasound contrast agents. As a result of these harmonic signals, a substantial minority of acoustic reverberations created by microbubbles differ from the frequency of insonation. Since the preponderance of reflected sound from ordinary tissue is at the fundamental frequency of insonation, most harmonic signals received during contrast infusion come from contrast material. Thus, harmonic imaging may be used to improve the imaging of contrast material, and reduce the background signal from surrounding structures. Furthermore, the spatial and temporal resolution of harmonic gray-scale imaging is far superior to the resolution achieved with conventional color and power Doppler techniques.

Although pathologic studies of prostate cancer demonstrate an increased number of small microvessels, these vessels are not selectively imaged with computed tomography, magnetic resonance, or conventional ultrasound and Doppler. Consequently, the non-selective enhancement provided with these modalities results in limited cancer detection. In contrast to these conventional forms of vascular enhancement, intermittent ultrasound combined with harmonic gray scale imaging presents a unique potential to selectively enhance different levels of the microvasculature. An early study at the Jefferson Prostate Diagnostic Center using the microbubble agent Imavist (Alliance Pharmaceutical Corp., San Diego, CA, USA) demonstrated selective gray-scale enhancement of malignant foci within the prostate (Figure 6.7).[52] The use of intermittent imaging with an inter-scan delay of 2 seconds provided a parenchymal blush, corresponding to enhancement of smaller vessels within the tumor (Figure 6.8). A larger follow-up study compared harmonic gray-scale enhancement using Definity (DuPont Pharmaceuticals, Billerica, MA, USA) with the results of sextant biopsy.[53] This study demonstrated a significant improvement of gray-scale sensitivity for cancer from 38% at baseline to 65% after infusion of the microbubble contrast

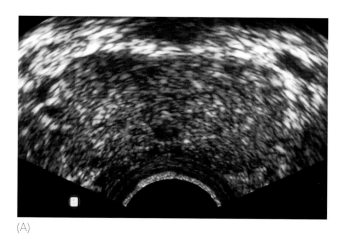

(A)

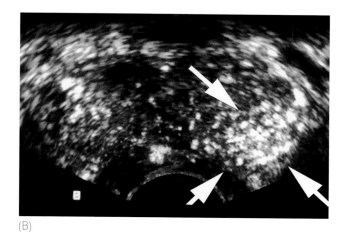

(B)

Figure 6.7

Selective gray-scale enhancement in an area of malignancy. (A) Baseline transverse sonogram at the base of the prostate. No lesion is visible. (B) Contrast-enhanced gray scale image after administration of Imavist. Focal enhancement of the left base (arrows) was observed with continuous and intermittent imaging. This area of enhancement corresponded to a Gleason 6 cancer on needle biopsy. (Reproduced with permission.[52])

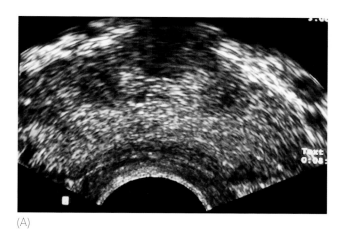

(A)

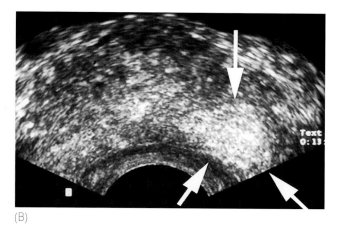

(B)

Figure 6.8

Selective gray-scale enhancement in an area of malignancy. (A) Baseline transverse sonogram at the mid-gland level. No lesion is visible. (B) Contrast-enhanced gray-scale image after administration of Imavist. A focal area of enhancement was observed (arrows), corresponding to a Gleason 9 cancer. Optimal enhancement of the cancer was obtained with intermittent imaging using an interscan delay of 2 seconds. (Reproduced with permission.[52])

agent (Figures 6.9 and 6.10). Furthermore, those lesions detected by contrast enhancement were generally larger and with a higher Gleason sum – that is, they were clinically significant cancers.

A recent study demonstrated the correlation of contrast-enhanced harmonic gray-scale sonography with whole-mount prostatectomy specimens. Infusion of the microbubble agent Sonazoid (Nycomed Amersham, Oslo, Norway) improved sensitivity for the detection of cancer in the outer portion of the prostate (Figure 6.11), but also demonstrated focal enhancement in areas of benign hyperplasia (Figure 6.12).[54] The use of a contrast agent doubled the sensitivity for detection of malignant foci in the less vascular outer portion of the prostate, but did not improve detection of inner gland cancers. The detection of enhancing malignant foci within the inner gland is complicated by heterogeneity of the gray-scale appearance and increased flow related to benign prostatic hyperplasia. The presence of prostatitis was not a major cause of false–positive diagnosis with contrast enhancement in this study.

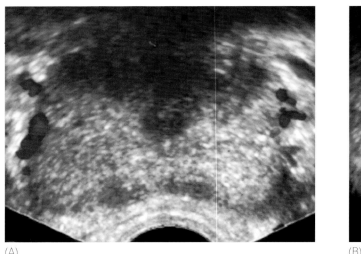

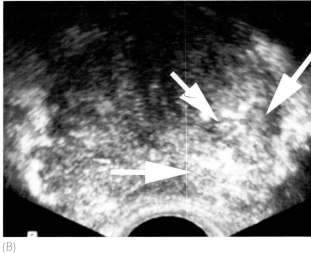

(A)

(B)

Figure 6.9

Contrast-enhanced detection of prostate cancer with harmonic imaging. (A) Transverse sonogram of the prostate with color Doppler. No focal lesion was identified, and no significant asymmetry in blood flow was observed. (B) Harmonic imaging during infusion of Definity, with intermittent imaging using an interscan delay time of 0.5 seconds. An ill-defined area of increased enhancement is identified in the left mid-gland (arrows). Biopsy cores from this area demonstrated a Gleason 7 cancer.

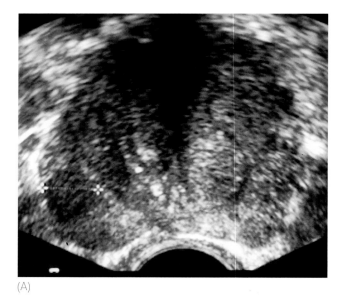

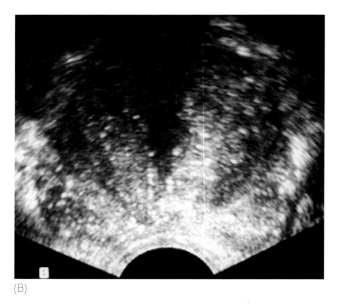

(A)

(B)

Figure 6.10

Transverse sonograms of the prostate in a patient with a Gleason 6 cancer in the right mid-gland. (A) The baseline image demonstrates a round hypoechoic lesion in the right mid-gland (calipers). (B) A harmonic gray-scale image obtained by continuous imaging during infusion of contrast demonstrates mild focal enhancement of the hypoechoic lesion. (C) A harmonic gray-scale image with intermittent imaging using an interscan delay time of 2 seconds demonstrates a clear ring of enhancement around the lesion in the right mid-gland. Directed biopsy of this lesion demonstrated a Gleason 6 cancer. (Reproduced with permission.[53])

Fig. 6.10(C), see opposite

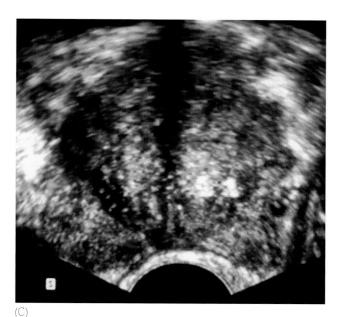

(C)

Figure 6.10
Continued.

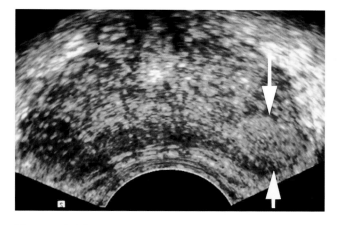

Figure 6.11
Transverse harmonic gray-scale image obtained during infusion of Sonazoid (Nycomed Amersham; Oslo, Norway). Intermittent imaging with a 2-second interscan delay demonstrates an area of focal enhancement in the left mid-gland (arrows) corresponding to a Gleason 6 cancer at radical prostatectomy. (Reproduced with permission.[54])

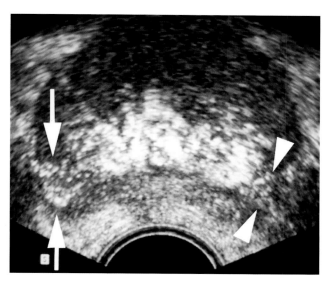

Figure 6.12
Transverse harmonic gray-scale image through the mid-portion of the prostate during infusion of Sonazoid. Transverse whole-mount prostatectomy slides were evaluated for pathology correlation with sonographic findings. Focal enhancement in the right posterolateral aspect of the prostate (arrows) corresponds to the site of a Gleason 6 cancer. Focal enhancement in the left posterolateral aspect of the prostate (arrowheads) corresponds to a focus of benign hyperplasia.

growth pattern of cancer within the prostate. Malignancy within the prostate is multifocal in 85% of cases, and often grows along the capsule. Unlike liver tumors, cancer of the prostate does not present as a large, round mass. Imaging of the prostate is further complicated by an underlying hetero-geneity of benign prostate tissue that may be secondary to benign prostatic hyperplasia or prostatitis. Nonetheless, since almost every biopsy of the prostate is performed with sono-graphic guidance, it seems prudent to explore methods that might be used to improve the diagnostic accuracy of ultra-sound for the detection of prostate cancer. Spectral analysis, elastography, and microbubble contrast agents have all demonstrated initial promising results. Future clinical studies are needed to determine whether one of these techniques might replace conventional spatially distributed, geometric biopsy schemes. Given the increasing trend toward large numbers of biopsy cores with different geometric biopsy strategies, a directed technique would be cost-effective if it could provide the diagnosis of clinically significant cancers with fewer biopsy cores.

Conclusion

In conclusion, the diagnosis of prostate cancer is complicated by the lack of sensitivity and specificity among various imaging modalities. Poor diagnostic accuracy may be related to the

References

1. Plawker MW, Fleisher JM, Vapnek EM, Macchia RJ. Current trends in prostate cancer diagnosis and staging among United States urologists. J Urol 1997; 158: 1853–8.

2. Halpern EJ, Strup SE. Using gray-scale and color and power Doppler sonography to detect prostatic cancer. AJR 2000; 174: 623–7.

3. Albertson PC, Fryback DG, Storer BE, Kolon TF, Fine J. Long-term survival among men with conservatively treated localized prostate cancer. JAMA 1995; 274: 626–31.

4. Albertsen PC, Hanley JA, Gleason DF, Barry MJ. Competing risk analysis of men aged 55 to 74 years at diagnosis managed conservatively for clinically localized prostate cancer. JAMA 1998; 280: 975–80.

5. Chodak GW, Thisted RA, Gerber GS et al. Results of conservative management of clinically localized prostate cancer. N Engl J Med 1994; 330: 242–8.

6. Johansson JE, Holmberg L, Johansson et al. Fifteen-year survival in prostate cancer. A prospective, population-based study in Sweden. JAMA 1997; 277: 467–71.

7. Stamey TA, Freiha FS, McNeal JE et al. Localized prostate cancer. Relationship of tumor volume to clinical significance for treatment of prostate cancer. Cancer 1993; 71(3 Suppl): 933–8.

8. Stamey TA, Kabalin JN, NcNeal JE et al. Prostate specific antigen in the diagnosis and treatment of adenocarcinoma of the prostate. II. Radical prostatectomy treated patients. J Urol 1989; 141: 1076–83.

9. Bluestein DL, Bostwick DG, Bergstralh EJ, Osterling JE. Eliminating the need for bilateral pelvic lymphadenectomy in select patients with prostate cancer. J Urol 1994; 151: 1315–20.

10. Epstein JI, Walsh PC, Carmichael M, Brendler CB. Pathologic and clinical findings to predict tumor extent of nonpalpable (stage T1c) prostate cancer. JAMA 1994; 271: 368–74.

11. Bigler SA, Deering RE, Brawer MK. Comparison of microscopic vascularity in benign and malignant prostate tissue. Hum Pathol 1993; 24: 220–6.

12. Weidner N, Carroll PR, Flax J et al. Tumor angiogenesis correlates with metastasis in invasive prostate carcinoma. Am J Pathol 1993; 143: 401–9.

13. Fregene TA, Khanuja PS, Noto AC et al. Tumor-associated angiogenesis in prostate cancer. Anticancer Res 1993; 13: 2377–82.

14. Brawer MK, Deering RE, Brown M et al. Predictors of pathologic stage in prostate carcinoma, the role of neovascularity. Cancer 1994; 73: 678–87.

15. Bostwick DG, Wheeler TM, Blute M et al. Optimized microvessel density analysis improves prediction of cancer stage from prostate needle biopsies. Urology 1996; 48: 47–57.

16. Lissbrant IF, Stattin P, Damber JE, Bergh A. Vascular density is a predictor of cancer-specific survival in prostatic carcinoma. Prostate 1997; 33: 38–45.

17. Borre M, Offersen BV, Nerstrom B, Overgaard J. Microvessel density predicts survival in prostate cancer patients subjected to watchful waiting. Cancer 1998; 78: 940–4.

18. Brawer MK. Quantitative microvessel density. A staging and prognostic marker for human prostatic carcinoma. Cancer 1996; 78: 345–9.

19. Craine BL, Oldani G, Engel JR et al. Computer-assisted analysis of transrectal ultrasound images. J Digital Imag 1990; 3: 219–25.

20. Basset O, Sun Z, Mestas JL, Gimenez G. Texture analysis of ultrasonic images of the prostate by means of co-occurrence matrices. Ultrason Imag 1993; 15: 218–37.

21. Lizzi FL, Greenebaum M, Feleppa EJ et al. Theoretical framework for spectrum analysis in ultrasonic tissue characterization. J Acoust Soc Am 1983; 73: 1336–73.

22. Feleppa EJ, Liu T, Kalisz A et al. Ultrasonic spectral-parameter images of the prostate. Int J Imag Syst Technol 1997; 8: 11–25.

23. Feleppa EJ, Fair WR, Liu R et al. Three-dimensional ultrasound analyses of the prostate. Mol Urol 2000; 4: 133–9.

24. Taylor LS, Porter BC, Rubens DJ, Parker KJ. Three-dimensional sonoelastography: principles and practices. Phys Med Biol 2000; 45: 1477–94.

25. Lee F, Bronson JP, Lerner RM et al. Radiology 1991; 181: 237–9.

26. Krouskop TA, Wheeler TM, Kallel F et al. Elastic moduli of breast and prostate tissues under compression. Ultrason Imag 1998; 20: 260–74.

27. Kallel F, Price RE, Konofagou E, Ophir J. Elastographic imaging of the normal canine prostate in vitro. Ultrason Imag 1999; 21: 201–15.

28. Rubens DJ, Hadley MA, Alam SK et al. Sonoelasticity imaging of prostate cancer: in vitro results. Radiology 1995; 195: 379–83.

29. Cochlin DLL, Ganatra RK, Griffiths DFS. Sonoelastography in the detection of prostatic cancer. Clin Radiol (in press).

30. Cochlin DLL, Ganatra RK. Sonoelastography of the prostate: a practical approach. Eur J Ultrasound (in press).

31. Moskalik AP, Rubin MA, Wojno KJ et al. Analysis of three-dimensional Doppler ultrasonographic quantitative measures for the discrimination of prostate cancer. J Ultrasound Med 2001; 20: 713–22.

32. Frauscher F, Klauser A, Halpern EJ. Contrast-enhanced transrectal ultrasound of the prostate: clinical utility and future applications for detection of prostate cancer. Electromedica 2000; 68: 29–34.

33. Sedelaar JP, van Leenders GJ, Hulsbergen-Van De Kaa CA, van Der Poel HG, van Der Laak JA, Debruyne FM, Wijkstra H, de La Rosette JJ. Microvessel Density: Correlation between Contrast Ultrasonography and Histology of Prostate Cancer. Eur Urol 40(3): 285–293, 2001.

34. Strohmeyer D, Frauscher F, Klauser A, Recheis W, Rogatsch H, Eibl G, Horninger W, Steiner H, Volgger H, Bartsch G. Contrast-enchanced transrectal color Doppler ultrasonography for assessment of angiogenesis in prostate cancer. Anticancer research 21: 2907–2914, 2001.

35. Goldberg BB, Liu JB, Forsberg F. Ultrasound contrast agents: a review. Ultrasound Med Biol 1994; 20: 319–33.

36. Goldberg BB. Ultrasound Contrast Agents. London: Martin Dunitz, 1997.

37. Ragde H, Kenny GM, Murphy GP, Landin K. Transrectal ultrasound microbubble contrast angiography of the prostate. Prostate 1997; 32: 279–83.

38. Rifkin MD, Tublin ME, Cheruvu SK et al. Ultrasound contrast enhanced color Doppler: initial results in the evaluation of the prostate. Radiology 1997; 205(P): 280.

39. Blomley MJ, Cosgrove DO, Jayaram V et al. Quantitation of enhanced transrectal ultrasound of the prostate: work in progress using the echo-enhancing agent Br 1. Radiology 1997; 205(P): 280–1.

40. Eckersley RJ, Butler-Barnes JA, Blomley MJ et al. Quantitative microbubble enhanced transrectal ultrasound (TRUS) as a tool for monitoring anti-androgen therapy in prostate carcinoma: work in progress. Radiology 1998; 209(P): 280.

41. Bogers HA, Sedelaar JPM, Beerlage HP et al. Contrast-enhanced three-dimensional power Doppler angiography of the human prostate: correlation with biopsy outcome. Urology 1999; 54: 97–104.

42. Frauscher F, Klauser A, Halpern EJ et al. Detection of prostate cancer with a microbubble ultrasound contrast agent. Lancet 2001; 357: 1849–50.

43. Porter TR, Xie F. Transient myocardial contrast after initial exposure to diagnostic ultrasound pressures with minute doses of intravenously injected microbubbles. Circulation 1995; 92: 239–5.

44. Colon PJ, Richards DR, Moreno CA et al. Benefits of reducing the cardiac cycle-triggering frequency of ultrasound imaging to increase myocardial opacification with FS069 during fundamental and second harmonic imaging. J Am Soc Echocardiogr 1997; 10: 602–7.

45. Broillet A, Puginier J, Ventrone R, Schneider M. Assessment of myocardial perfusion by intermittent harmonic power Doppler using SonoVue, a new ultrasound contrast agent. Invest Radiol 1998; 33: 209.

46. Porter TR, Kricsfeld D, Ceatham S, Li S. The effect of ultrasound frame rate on perfluorocarbon-exposed sonicated dextrose albumin microbubble size and concentration when insonifying at different flow rates, transducer frequencies and acoustic outputs. J Am Soc Echocardiogr 1997; 10: 593–601.

47. Schrope BA, Newhouse VL, Uhlendorf V. Simulated capillary blood flow measurement using a nonlinear ultrasonic contrast agent. Ultrason Imag 1992; 14: 134–58.

48. Schrope BA, Newhouse VL. Second harmonic ultrasound blood perfusion measurement. Ultrasound Med Biol 1993; 19: 567–79.

49. de Jong N, Cornet R, Lancee CT. Higher harmonics of vibrating gas-filled microspheres. Part one: simulations. Ultrasonics 1994; 32: 447–53.

50. de Jong N, Cornet R, Lancee CT. Higher harmonics of vibrating gas-filled microspheres. Part two: measurements. Ultrasonics 1994; 32: 455–9.

51. Forsberg F, Goldberg BB, Liu JB et al. On the feasibility of real-time, in vivo harmonic imaging with proteinaceous microspheres. J Ultrasound Med 1996; 15: 853–60.

52. Halpern EJ, Verkh L, Forsberg F et al. Initial experience with contrast-enhanced sonography of the prostate. AJR 2000; 174: 1757–80.

53. Halpern EJ, Rosenberg M, Gomella LG. Prostate cancer: contrast-enhanced US for detection. Radiology 2001; 219: 219–25.

54. Halpern EJ, McCue PA, Aksnes AK et al. Halpern EJ, McCue PA, Aksnes AK et al. Contrast-enhanced US of the prostate with Sonazoid: Comparison with whole-mount prostatectomy specimens in 12 patients. Radiology 2002; 222:361–366.

7

CT evaluation of the prostate

Ethan J Halpern

The prostate gland is imaged with computed tomography (CT) during the standard CT scan of the pelvis. In the setting of prostate cancer, CT may be obtained for radiation-therapy planning or for the purpose of staging the cancer. A CT scan is rarely obtained for primary evaluation of the prostate. Nonetheless, an understanding of the normal CT appearance of the prostate is important in order to identify abnormalities of this gland.

Normal CT anatomy

The prostate is the most caudal organ within the male pelvis, bounded posteriorly by the rectum, superiorly by the bladder, and anteriorly by the pubic symphysis (Figure 7.1). The normal prostate has an oval appearance on transaxial scans with its long axis in the transverse plane. The normal volume of the adult prostate increases with age from approximately 20 cm^3 to 40 cm^3. Typical measurements in the transaxial plane are approximately 2.5–3.0 cm in the anterior–posterior axis and 4–5 cm in the transverse axis.

The normal prostate has a smooth contour. The gland should be symmetric, with no focal bulge of the contour. Zonal anatomy of the prostate is not visualized with unenhanced imaging.[1] After the administration of intravenous contrast, however, the prostate demonstrates marked enhancement of the inner gland, related to transition zone tissue. The outer gland demonstrates less enhancement, and is often clearly demarcated from the inner gland (Figure 7.2).

The seminal vesicles are generally visible just posterior to the base of the prostate. Normal seminal vesicles are symmetric in size, and demonstrate a 'bow-tie' appearance with tapering of each seminal vesicle as it approaches the midline (Figure 7.3). Rarely, the vas deferens may be visualized as it courses into the prostate (Figure 7.4). The vas deferens courses slightly above the seminal vesicle on either side of the midline, and enters the prostate along the medial aspect of the seminal vesicle. The seminal vesicle and vas deferens on each side unite into the ejaculatory duct as they enter the prostate. The ejaculatory duct is not generally visible unless it is calcified or contains stones (Figure 7.5).

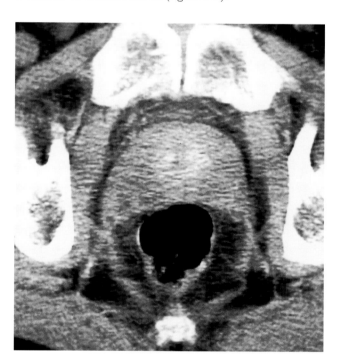

Figure 7.1
Normal CT image of the prostate. The prostate gland is located in the lowest portion of the pelvis. Anteriorly, the prostate is bounded by the symphysis pubis. Posteriorly, the prostate is bounded by the rectum. An obturator internus muscle is present on either side of the prostate.

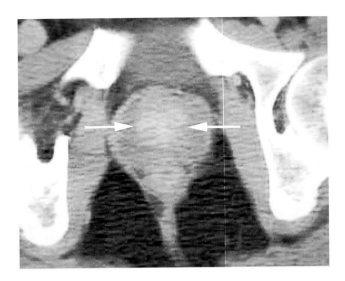

Figure 7.2
Contrast-enhanced CT scan of the prostate. The inner gland demonstrates marked enhancement (arrows). with a homogeneous low density throughout the outer gland. A thin rim of enhancement is also present along the capsule of the prostate. The floor of the bladder is seen to extend anterior to the prostate.

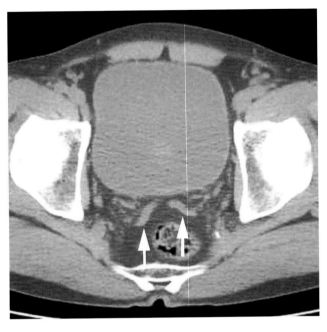

Figure 7.4
Normal vasa deferentia. The vas deferens courses above the ipsilateral ureter as the ureter enters the bladder. The vas deferens then courses medially just above the seminal vesicle, and courses caudally toward the base of the prostate on either side of midline (arrows). The ampullary portion of the vas deferens is visualized in this paramedian position.

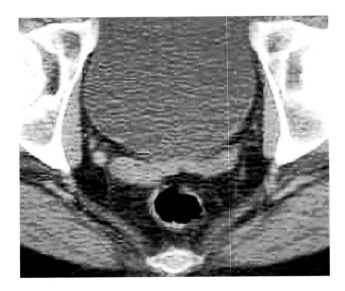

Figure 7.3
Normal seminal vesicles. The seminal vesicles are symmetric in appearance. The 'bow-tie' appearance of the seminal vesicles is seen posterior to the urinary bladder. The fat planes around the seminal vesicles, and the fat planes between the seminal vesicles and the bladder, are well defined.

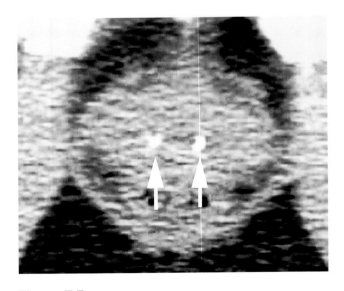

Figure 7.5
Ejaculatory duct stones. The normal ejaculatory duct is not visible on CT. Bilateral ejaculatory duct stones in this patient are visualized as calcifications within the prostate on either side of the midline (arrows).

Benign processes involving the prostate

Benign prostatic hyperplasia (BPH) is the most common pathologic process to involve the prostate, and is demonstrated with increasing frequency at increasing age. Enlargement of the prostate secondary to BPH occurs above the level of the verumontanum, and may protrude into the base of the urinary bladder (Figure 7.6). BPH may result in bladder outlet obstruction, with muscular hypertrophy of the bladder (Figure 7.7). In addition to an enlarged gland, BPH demonstrates increased heterogeneous enhancement of the inner portion of the prostate (Figure 7.8). Cystic changes within the prostate are often associated with BPH, but are generally too small to be visualized with CT. Larger cystic areas can be identified (Figure 7.9).

Inflammation of the prostate – prostatitis – is not generally visible on CT. However, when there is formation of a focal abscess, this can be identified by CT (Figure 7.10). Ductal ectasia – dilatation of tubular structures within the seminal vesicles – is commonly seen in patients with BPH. Ductal ectasia may be visible on CT as a hypodense appearance of the seminal vesicles (Figure 7.11).

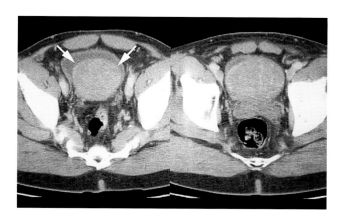

Figure 7.6
Marked enlargement of the prostate secondary to benign prostatic hyperplasia (BPH). The 'median lobe' of the prostate (which does not exist as a true lobe) protrudes into the base of the bladder (arrows).

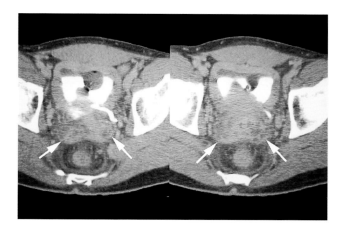

Figure 7.7
Marked prostatic enlargement resulting in bladder outlet obstruction. The bladder wall is thickened secondary to muscular hypertrophy, and the seminal vesicles demonstrate bilateral ductal ectasia (arrows). A Foley catheters is present within the bladder and a stent is present within the left ureter. The findings of BPH in this patient simulate a mass lesion at the trigone of the bladder.

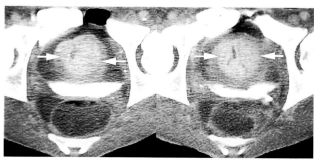

(A)

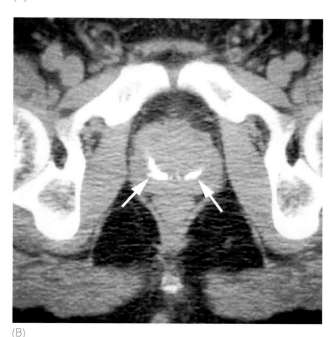

(B)

Figure 7.8
Benign prostatic hyperplasia. (A) Marked BPH with protrusion of prostate into the bladder base. The enlarged inner gland demonstrates a heterogeneous enhancement pattern (arrows). (B) Calcifications along the surgical capsule that separates the inner and outer portions of the prostate gland (arrows). Such calcifications or deposition of corpora amylacea are commonly associated with BPH.

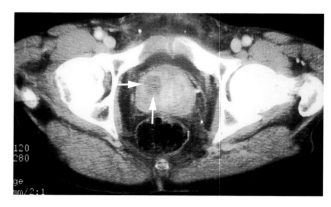

Figure 7.9

Benign prostatic hyperplasia with cystic change. The inner gland demonstrates enlargement, with a heterogeneous enhancement pattern. A cystic focus is identified on the right side of the inner gland (arrows).

CT findings of prostate cancer

Conventional CT with unenhanced imaging of the pelvis or with delayed post-contrast images is not adequate for detection of cancer within the prostate.[2] Several reports using magnetic resonance imaging, however, have demonstrated that cancer tissue within the prostate enhances earlier than normal prostate tissue on dynamic sequences.[3,4] Based upon these reports, a preliminary study was performed of arterial-phase helical CT in prostate cancer patients. This study demonstrated CT detection of outer gland cancer in 59 of 102 positive sites (58%), and overall detection of cancer in 22 of 25 patients (88%).[5] Based upon this preliminary study, the finding of a focal area of enhancement or diffuse enhancement in the outer portion of the prostate is suspicious for cancer.

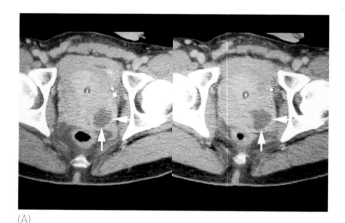

(A)

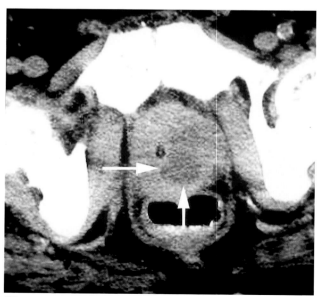

(B)

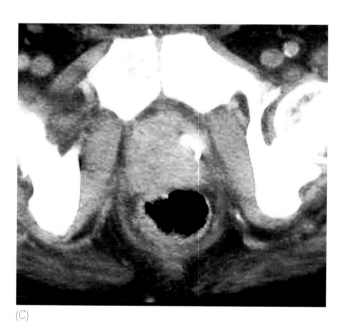

(C)

Figure 7.10

Prostate abscess. (A) An image obtained from a patient presenting with fever and pyuria. The prostate is enlarged, and demonstrates a focal abscess posteriorly and to the left of the midline (arrows). (B) A different patient with an abscess of the prostate, situated to the left of a Foley catheter (arrows). (C) The appearance of this abscess after transperineal catheter drainage.

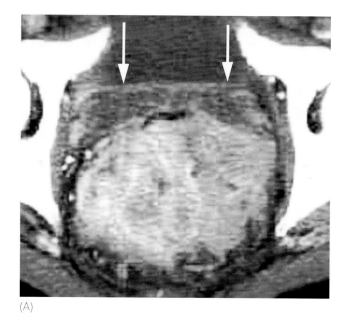

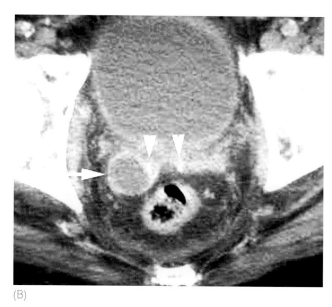

(A)   (B)

Figure 7.11
Ductal ectasia of the seminal vesicles. (A) A large mass within the rectum. There was invasion of the prostate, with obstruction of the ejaculatory ducts and ductal ectasia of the seminal vesicles. Small fluid-density dilated ducts are visualized within the seminal vesicles (arrows). (B) Unilateral dilatation of a seminal vesicle (arrows) secondary to an obstructing calculus in the ejaculatory duct. Calcification of the vasa deferentia (arrowheads) is often associated with diabetes.

Although focal enhancement within the outer gland or a focal bulge of the contour may identify the site of a cancer, the diagnostic accuracy of this technique has not been established. In an unselected population, it is likely that most abnormal areas of enhancement or a contour bulge will correspond to areas of prostatitis or BPH. In a patient with a high level of suspicion for cancer who cannot be examined with standard transrectal ultrasound, CT evaluation of the prostate may be useful if sonographically guided transperineal biopsies fail to demonstrate a cancer. CT evaluation should not be used as a standard screening examination for cancer of the prostate. Nonetheless, when a clear area of focal enhancement is identified within the outer portion of the prostate, the possibility of cancer may be raised. The findings of a bulge in the contour of the prostate together with an abnormal enhancement pattern further raises suspicion for cancer (Figure 7.12).

CT staging of prostate cancer

CT evaluation of the prostate can be used to identify macroscopic extracapsular spread of tumor (Figure 7.13) or local adenopathy (Figure 7.14). The main lymphatic drainage of the prostate drains up into pelvic nodes in the obturator area and subsequently into the iliac chains, but drainage is also present to the perineal floor and to sacral lymph nodes.[6] Lymphatic spread

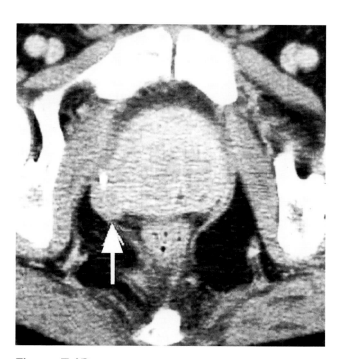

Figure 7.12
Diffusely infiltrating cancer with capsular invasion to the right of the midline. CT demonstrates a diffuse pattern of enhancement of the outer gland, with a focal bulge posterolaterally on the right side of midline (arrow). The enhancement is related to cancer in the outer gland, while the focal bulge suggests that tumor may be extending through the capsule of the prostate.

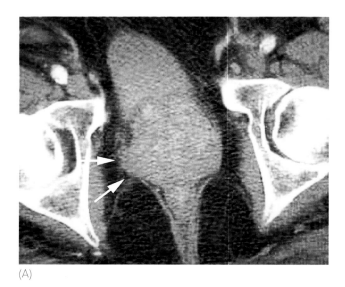

(A)

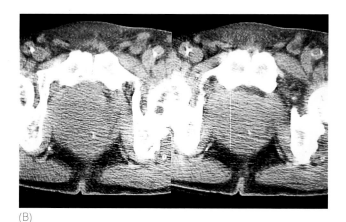

(B)

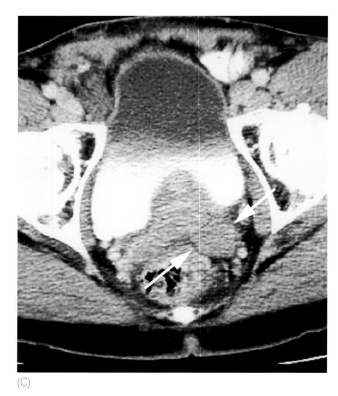

(C)

Figure 7.13

Extracapsular spread of prostate cancer. (A) A focal bulge of the right side of the prostate (arrows), corresponding to a site of capsular penetration. The fat planes around the prostate remain intact. (B) A tumor that has enlarged the prostate and spread to the pelvic side walls. The fat planes around the prostate are obliterated. (C) Tumor invasion of the left seminal vesicle. The left seminal vesicle is larger than the right seminal vesicle, and fails to demonstrate a normal tapered appearance (arrows).

of prostate cancer generally follows through contiguous nodal chains up to the para-aortic region (Figure 7.15). Pelvic lymph nodes with a short-axis measurement greater than 15 mm are suspicious for metastatic lymphadenopathy. Unfortunately, extracapsular spread may be present microscopically but not visible macroscopically. Furthermore, lymph node size may not correlate with the presence of cancer.[7]

Metastatic disease to the bones usually appears as blastic lesions on CT imaging (Figure 7.16). Although bone metastases are most commonly found within the vertebral bodies, metastatic lesions from prostate cancer may be found anywhere in the skeleton (Figure 7.17).

The staging of prostate cancer is an important step in treatment planning. Disease that is localized to the prostate should be treated differently from disease that has already spread beyond the gland. For example, most surgeons do not recommend radical prostatectomy when tumor spread outside of the prostate has been documented. CT evaluation of the abdomen and pelvis is often used for staging of prostate

cancer prior to treatment. The application of CT for staging of prostate cancer remains controversial because of the relatively poor ability of CT to identify extracapsular spread and lymphatic involvement, and because of the high costs involved in staging all prostate cancer patients with CT. Furthermore, the positive yield of CT staging studies is low among patients with a serum prostate-specific antigen (PSA) below 15 mg/ml and a Gleason score of 7 or less. A recent population-based survey of 3690 men with prostate cancer concluded that further cost-effectiveness studies are needed, but suggested that CT might be best reserved for patients with serum PSA above 20 mg/ml or a Gleason score of 8–10.[8] Another recent study of 588 patients suggested that CT is not cost-effective in patients with a clinical stage of T2b or less, Gleason score of 2–7, and PSA of 15 mg/ml or less.[9]

After treatment of prostate cancer, patients may be followed with a variety of laboratory and imaging tests for possible recurrence. Patients treated for prostate cancer are often monitored with serum PSA, prostatic acid phosphatase,

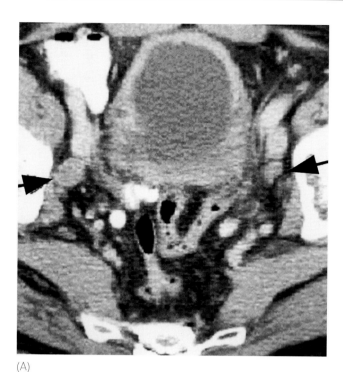

(A)

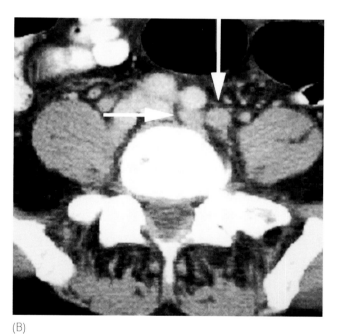

(B)

Figure 7.14
Local adenopathy secondary to prostate cancer. (A) Enlarged obturator nodes on both sides (arrows). The obturator nodes are often first to be involved by lymphatic extension of prostate cancer. (B) Several additional nodes along the iliac nodal chains in the same patient (arrows). Prostate cancer usually involves contiguous nodal levels as it extends up the nodal chains out of the pelvis.

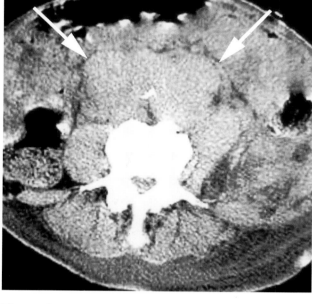

Figure 7.15
Massive para-aortic adenopathy in a patient with extensive spread of prostate cancer (arrows).

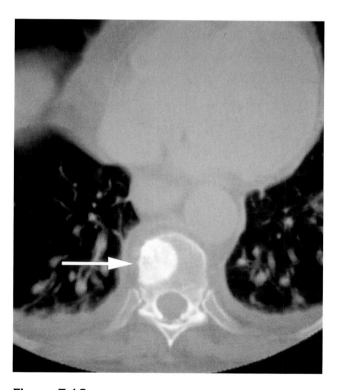

Figure 7.16
Blastic bone metastasis in a vertebral body secondary to prostate cancer (arrow).

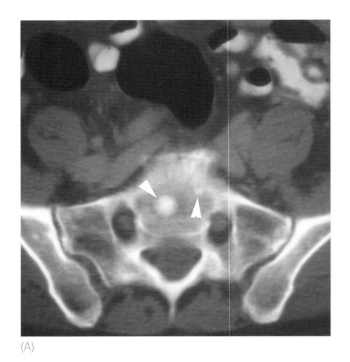

(A)

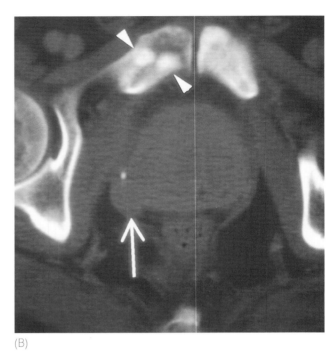

(B)

Figure 7.17
Diffuse bone metastases in patient with prostate cancer. Punctate blastic lesions (arrowheads) are seen in the sacrum (A) as well as the right pubic bone (B). There is diffuse sclerotic appearance of the left pubic bone. This is the same patient seen to have capsular invasion by cancer in Figure 7.12 (arrow).

alkaline phosphatase, digital rectal examination, bone scan, ultrasound, and CT. Among all of these tests, the serum PSA is the most sensitive tool for detection of recurrence, and is superior to follow-up CT examination.[10] Follow-up CT evaluation should be reserved for those patients in whom the serum PSA suggests a recurrence.

CT for radiation-therapy planning

CT evaluation of the prostate is often used for radiation-therapy planning. CT provides precise measurement of the three-dimensional volume of the prostate as well as visualization of surrounding organs (such as bladder and rectum). This information is critical for planning of both external-beam radiation therapy and radioactive-seed implants (brachytherapy). Furthermore, CT is used to predict whether the pubic arch will interfere with placement of seed implants into the anterior portion of the prostate.[11] In order to optimize the dose of radiation to the prostate and minimize dose to important surrounding structures, both three-dimensional conformal external-beam therapy and brachytherapy rely upon CT images to compute radiation doses to the prostate and surrounding tissues (Figure 7.18).

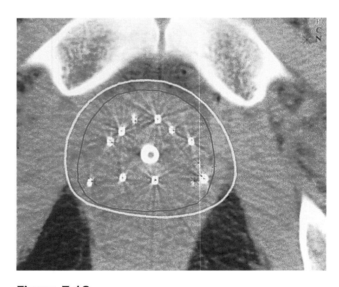

Figure 7.18
Post-implant analysis for brachytherapy. CT evaluation demonstrates the precise location of each radioactive pellet. The margin of the prostate is visualized, and an isodose line is computed to demonstrate the area that is covered with the desired level of radiation. (Courtesy of Dr Richard K Valicenti.)

The radiation-therapy planning CT is generally obtained as an unenhanced scan without intravenous contrast. However, there is little additional advantage to the performance of contrast-enhanced CT of the abdomen and pelvis in patients who have already had a CT for radiation-therapy planning.[12] Furthermore, since metastatic disease to the abdomen is uncommon in the absence of visible disease in the pelvis, a single CT scan of the pelvis may be adequate for both staging and radiation-therapy planning.[13]

References

1. Mirowitz SA, Hammerman AM. CT depiction of prostatic zonal anatomy. J Comput Assist Tomogr 1992; 16: 439–41.
2. Price JM, Davidson AJ. Computed tomography in the evaluation of the suspected carcinomatous prostate. Urol Radiol 1979; 1: 39–42.
3. Brown G, Macvicar DA, Ayton V, Husband JE. The role of intravenous contrast enhancement in magnetic resonance imaging of prostatic carcinoma. Clin Radiol 1995; 50: 601–6.
4. Jager GJ, Ruijter ET, Van de Kaa CA et al. Dynamic TurboFLASH subtraction technique for contrast-enhanced MR imaging of the prostate: correlation with histopathologic results. Radiology 1997; 203: 645–52.
5. Prando A, Wallace S. Helical CT of prostate cancer: early clinical experience. AJR 2000; 75: 343–6.
6. Brossner C, Ringhofer H, Hernady T et al. Lymphatic drainage of prostatic transition and peripheral zones visualized on a three-dimensional workstation. Urology 2001; 57: 389–93.
7. Tiguert R, Gheiler EL, Tefilli MV et al. Lymph node size does not correlate with the presence of prostate cancer metastasis. Urology 1999; 53: 367–71.
8. Albertson PC, Hanley JA, Harlan LC et al. The positive yield of imaging studies in the evaluation of men with newly diagnosed prostate cancer: a population based analysis. J Urol 2000; 163: 1138–43.
9. Lee N, Newhouse JH, Olsson CA et al. Which patients with newly diagnosed prostate cancer need a computed tomography scan of the abdomen and pelvis? An analysis based on 588 patients. Urology 1999; 54: 490–4.
10. Strohmaier WL, Keller T, Bichler KH. Follow-up in prostate cancer patients: Which parameters are necessary? Eur Urol 1999; 35: 21–5.
11. Wallner K, Chiu-Tsao ST, Roy J et al. An improved method for computerized tomography: planned transperineal[125] iodine prostate implants. J Urol 1991; 146: 90–5.
12. Miller JS, Puckett ML, Johnstone PA. Frequency of coexistent disease at CT in patients with prostate carcinoma selected for definitive radiation therapy: is limited treatment-planning CT adequate? Radiology 2000; 215: 41–4.
13. Burcombe RJ, Ostler PJ, Ayoub AW, Hoskin PJ. The role of staging CT scans in the treatment of prostate cancer: a retrospective audit. Clin Oncol 2000; 12: 32–5.

8

Magnetic resonance evaluation of the prostate

Michael Bourne

Introduction

Cross-sectional techniques such as transrectal ultrasound (TRUS), computed tomography (CT), and magnetic resonance imaging (MRI) have largely replaced the intravenous urogram (IVU) and the micturating cystogram (MCG) for imaging of the prostate. These cross-sectional techniques allow superior evaluation of the prostatic anatomy as well as direct visualization of prostatic disease processes. More recently, magnetic resonance spectroscopy (MRS) has been introduced, and now allows measurement and imaging of prostatic metabolism in both normal and disease states. As in other organ systems, MRI demonstrates significant advantages over other cross-sectional imaging techniques owing to its superior soft tissue contrast and its direct multiplanar acquisition capability. The advent of MRS techniques for the evaluation of prostate metabolism has further enhanced this diagnostic superiority.[1]

MRI examination of the prostate

Initially, MRI of the prostate was performed utilizing the body coil for both radiofrequency (RF) transmission and reception functions. However, the use of a body coil in combination with T1- and T2-weighted conventional spin echo (CSE) techniques yielded relatively low-resolution images with prolonged examination times. More recently, phased array and endoluminal surface coils have been utilized with T1- and T2-weighted fast spin echo (FSE) sequences. The combination of these hardware and software advances allows the acquisition of high-resolution images with high soft tissue contrast in acceptable examination times.

Table 8.1 Sequences and imaging planes for MRI of the prostate.

Acquisition	Sequence type[a]	Imaging plane
1	T1-weighted GRE	Multiplanar
2	T1-weighted FSE	Axial
3	T2-weighted FSE	Sagittal
4	T2-weighted FSE	Axial
5	T2-weighted FSE	Coronal

[a] GRE, gradient echo; FSE, fast spin echo.

MRI examination of the prostate should include both T1-weighted and T2-weighted acquisitions. Recommended sequences and imaging planes are outlined in Table 8.1. An endoluminal coil examination of the prostate is not routinely required for MRI of the prostate, but is required for MRS.[2,3]

Patient-related motion artefacts can be reduced by ensuring patient comfort, by placing a restraining band around the lower abdomen, and by pharmacological suppression of intestinal peristalsis.

T1-weighted imaging

On T1-weighted images, the normal prostate has a homogeneously low-signal-intensity (SI) appearance similar to that of skeletal muscle. There is therefore no useful depiction of the internal prostatic anatomy. The immediately adjacent structures such as the seminal vesicles, periprostatic veins, and the neurovascular bundles have a comparable low SI. Thus, there is no inherent soft tissue contrast between the prostate and

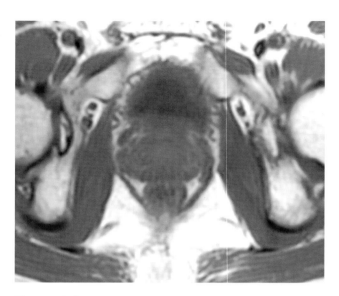

Figure 8.1
On T1 weighted sequences the signal intensity of the prostate is uniform and isointense with skeletal muscle. The anatomy of the central and peripheral zones cannot be distinguished and there is no inherent soft tissue contrast between the prostate and adjacent major anatomical structures e.g. rectum and seminal vesicles.

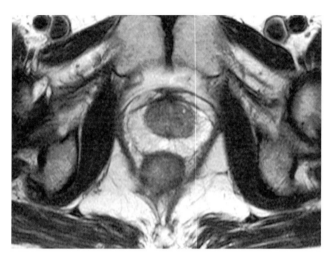

Figure 8.2
T2 weighted sequences enable the differentiation of the internal anatomy of the prostate. The normal peripheral zones exhibit uniform high signal intensity [>skeletal muscle and < fat] whilst the central zone exhibits a significantly lower signal intensity [>skeletal muscle and < fat].

these important adjacent anatomical structures. These structures, however, are surrounded by high-SI periprostatic and pelvic fat, against which they can be differentiated (Figure 8.1).

T1-weighted images should be acquired from a point just above the aortic bifurcation to the pubic symphysis. These images are principally used for the evaluation of post-biopsy changes in the prostate and the detection of lymphadenopathy and bony metastatic disease.

T2-weighted imaging

The internal anatomy of the prostate demonstrates excellent differential soft tissue contrast on T2-weighted images. The normal peripheral zone of the prostate exhibits a homogeneously high SI that is less than that of fat but greater than that of skeletal muscle. The transition and central zones have an SI that is lower than that of the peripheral zone, but still below that of fat and above that of skeletal muscle (Figure 8.2). Although the transition zone and central zone are easily distinguished by sonography, these two zones may be difficult to distinguish by MRI. The 'surgical capsule' that divides the prostate into an outer gland (peripheral and central zones) and an inner gland (transition zone and urethra) may not be visible on MRI. Conversely, the central zone and peripheral zone cannot be distinguished by sonography, but demonstrate clearly different SI on T2-weighted MRI patterns. For this reason, many MRI articles refer to the transition zone and the central zone collectively as the 'central gland'. The term

'central gland' is not used in this text in order to avoid confusion with the more anatomically accurate 'inner gland', which is removed during open prostatectomy. The reader is referred to Chapter 1 for a more complete discussion of the anatomy of the outer and inner gland.

The 'normal' MRI appearance of the central and transition zones is age-dependent, relating to the degree of benign prostatic hypertrophy (BPH). With increasing age, there is a general increase in the volume of the central and transition zones, and their SI appears more heterogeneous (Figure 8.3).

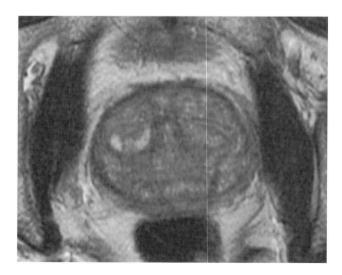

Figure 8.3
The central zone has a tendency to increase in volume [compressing the peripheral zones] and to exhibit increasingly heterogeneous signal intensity with age.

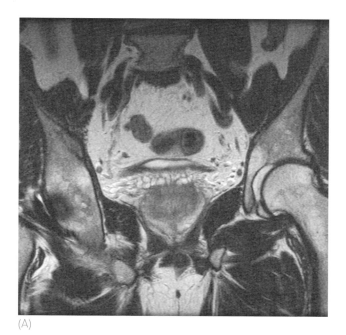
(A)

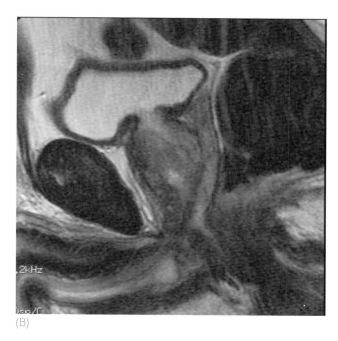
(B)

Figure 8.4

T2 weighted sequences in the coronal plane (A) complement the axial plane in the demonstration of the peripheral and central zones and in the saggital plane (B) the relationship between the prostate and the bladder base, seminal vesicle and rectum are well seen.

The T2-weighted soft tissue contrast between peripheral and central zones is thought to be due to the higher water content of the peripheral zone. Glandular elements in the peripheral zone are more numerous and less densely packed in comparison with the central zone.[4] The complex internal anatomy of the prostate is best evaluated with multiplanar T2-weighted acquisitions. The axial plane provides a good overview of all the different anatomical zones of the prostate as well as its relationship to the seminal vesicles, rectum, and levator ani. However, the evaluation of the central zone at the base of the prostate is suboptimal in the axial plane. The coronal plane is considered optimal for differentiating the peripheral and central zones (Figure 8.4a). The coronal plane complements the axial plane for the assessment of the seminal vesicles and lymphadenopathy. The sagittal plane often provides helpful information in determining the relationship of the prostate, bladder base, seminal vesicles, and rectum (Figure 8.4b).

MRS examination of the prostate

Magnetic resonance spectroscopy (MRS) and magnetic resonance spectroscopic imaging (MRSI) provide additional diagnostic information that may supplement that from MRI of the prostate alone. Advances in both hardware and software now allow the acquisition of high-resolution $^{1+}$H proton spectra

from the prostate in acceptable examination times.[5] Post-processing of these data is now essentially automated and in real time, requiring minimal user input. An MRS/MRSI acquisition can therefore be incorporated into the routine MR examination of the prostate. Metabolite overlays, utilizing pseudocolour maps, can then be overlaid on the anatomical MRI to produce an MRSI containing both anatomical and metabolic information (Figure 8.5).

Accurate imaging of cancer within the prostate is important for staging and for planning therapy. The clinical staging of prostate cancer has been demonstrated to be inaccurate, especially in the critical differentiation of T2 from T3 disease.[6–8] Up to 60% of patients thought to have stage T2 disease localized to the prostate may have extraprostatic spread. Conversely, up to 33% of patients staged clinically as T3 may have disease localized to the prostate (T2 disease). MRS is potentially more accurate, and in the future it is likely that MRI with MRS will play an important part in the planning and evaluation of therapy.

Prostate cancer

MRI appearances

The detection of prostate cancer with MRI depends upon the MRI sequence utilized and the location of the cancer within the gland. On T1-weighted images, prostate cancer may appear minimally hypointense compared with normal prostatic tissue,

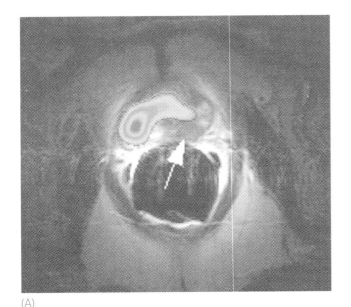

(A)

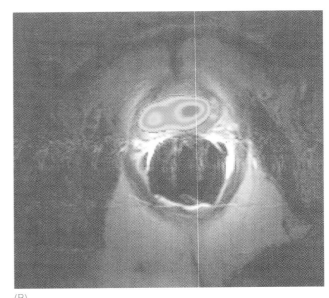

(B)

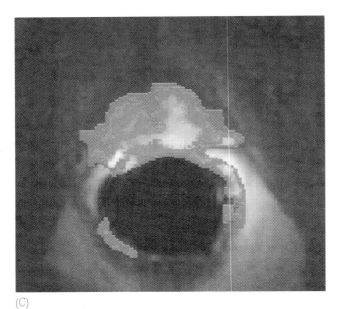

(C)

Figure 8.5

Pseudo colour overlays representing metabolite information [MRS data] can be overlaid on anatomical images [MRI data] to produce combined metabolic and anatomical image information [MRSI data]. Patient with a prostate cancer arrowed in (A). (A) T2w axial TSE image. The colour overlay represents the distribution of citrate content. (B) The colour overlay represents choline content. (C) DS time image showing enhanced intensity in the tumour region. Reproduced with permission from: Heerschap A, Jager G, van der Graaf, M, Barentz J, de la Rosette J, Oosterhof G, Ruijter E, Ruijs J. In-vivo spectroscopy reveals altered metabolite content in malignant prostate tissue. Anticancer research 1997:17, 1455–1460.

but more commonly is isointense. The lesion-to-background contrast-to-noise ratio (CNR) of T1-weighted images in this situation is generally low, and therefore lesion conspicuity is poor in the central, transition, and peripheral zones. On T2-weighted images, the normal peripheral zone appears hyperintense, with the central zone demonstrating a heterogeneous, predominantly hypointense appearance. Prostate cancer almost always appears hypointense on T2-weighted images, and therefore is most conspicuous in the normal high-SI peripheral zone (Figure 8.6). Tumour in the peripheral zone may appear as small focal abnormalities surrounded by normal tissue (Figure 8.7), as a diffusely infiltrative process within the peripheral zone (Figure 8.8), or as a large mass (Figure 8.9).

These T2-weighted appearances on MRI have a high sensitivity for the detection of prostate cancer in the peripheral zones. However, the specificity of low-SI areas in the peripheral zone is poor, since these hypointense areas may have benign or malignant aetiologies.[3,9] The sensitivity for the detection of prostate cancer in the central zone is substantially reduced owing to the inherent heterogeneous and generally hypointense SI characteristics of the central zone in comparison with the peripheral zone. A high incidence of multicentricity in prostate cancer has been demonstrated histologically.[10] This is reflected in T2-weighted MRI by multiple hypointense nodules, which may become confluent to form diffuse infiltration or mass lesions.

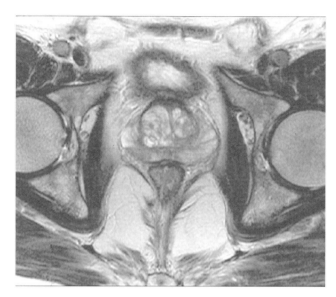

Figure 8.6
The presence of focal hypointense signal intensity within a background of normal hyperintense peripheral zone represents the typical appearance of prostate cancer on T2 weighted images.

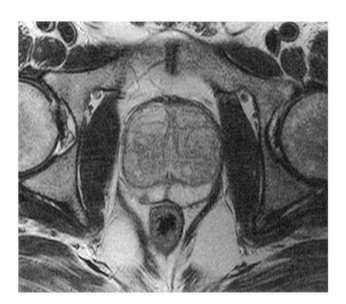

Figure 8.7
A small focus of hypointense signal intensity is seen within the right peripheral zone which TRUS guided biopsy confirmed to be a small carcinoma. There is severe central zone benign prostatic hypertrophy.

When utilizing MRI for the local staging of prostate cancer, there are some important confounding factors to be taken into account. Commonly, the patient has undergone TRUS and needle biopsy prior to the MRI examination. Intraprostatic haemorrhage and oedema are common post-biopsy findings

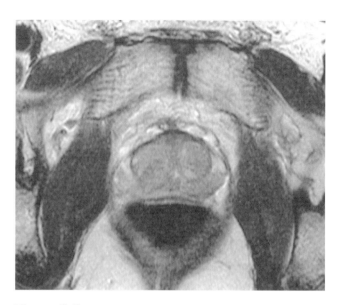

Figure 8.8
There is diffuse infiltration of both peripheral zones.

that have similar appearances to prostatic tumour on T2-weighted images. They can be differentiated on the T1-weighted images, since areas of haemorrhage demonstrate high signal intensity (Figure 8.10). The addition of MRS to MRI significantly improves the ability to determine the presence of prostate cancer and to map its spacial distribution when post-biopsy changes hinder interpretation with MRI alone.[11] The presence of BPH in the central zone may compress the peripheral zone, and this makes identification of low-signal intensity tumour within them difficult.

MRI staging of prostate cancer

The assessment of both local and distal disease by MRI can follow the standard TNM classification system (see Figure 2.6).[12,13] In this classification, local disease (≤ T2) is confined to the prostate, while more invasive disease (≥ T3) has spread into the periprostatic fat, lymph nodes, seminal vesicles, or adjacent tissues (including the bladder, rectum, and levator ani). Lymphatic spread is common, with involvement of the obturator, internal, and common iliac nodal groups. Osseous metastases via the haematogenous route are also common, and are found predominantly in the lumbar spine, pelvic bones, femora, thoracic spine, and ribs. The field of view of an MRI examination of the prostate includes a portion of the first three of these regions and provides an opportunity to detect bony metatstatic disease.

The accurate, early diagnosis of extraprostatic disease (T3 disease by the TNM classification) remains the most contentious issue in MRI of the prostate. High specificity is

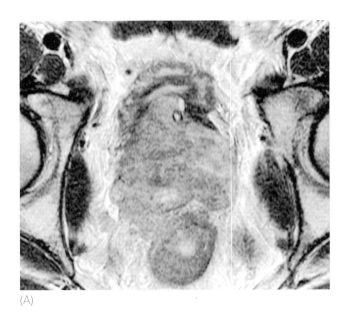

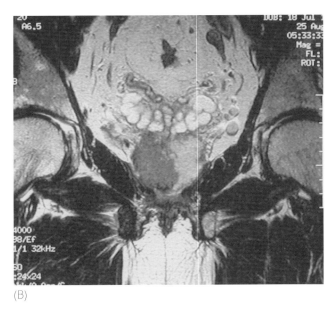

(A)   (B)

Figure 8.9
(A) There is a large mass configuration tumour occupying most of the prostate. (B) Coronal image of a mass configuration tumour.

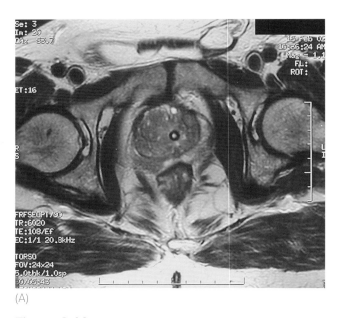

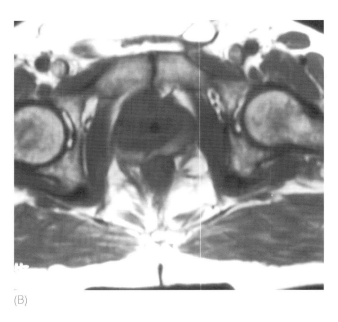

(A)   (B)

Figure 8.10
The T2W image (A) shows hypointense areas in the peripheral zone, simulating cancer. The T1W image (B) shows that these areas are hyperintense non T1. This indicates that they are due to post biopsy haemorrhage.

required so as not to deny an individual patient the chance of a potentially curative surgical procedure.[14] A number of problems exist regarding the diagnosis of extracapsular spread, not the least being the interchangeability of the terms 'capsular invasion' and 'capsular penetration'. In reality, the prostate lacks a true epithelial capsule, and infiltration of the thin fibromuscular capsule indicates spread beyond the margin of the gland. MRI cannot identify microscopic penetration of the margin of the prostate gland, and is therefore limited to the detection of macroscopic disease extension.

In the MRI determination of T2 versus T3 disease, a number of imaging appearances have been described that enable high diagnostic specificity. A tumour may be described as T2, i.e. with no capsular penetration, even if there is a broad area of contact between it and the margin of the gland, as long as the gland margins are not distorted.[9] Similarly, a tumour where there is both broad contact and smooth capsular bulging is consistent with T2 disease (Figure 8.11).[15] In comparison, irregular bulging of the prostate gland margin, asymmetry of the neurovascular bundles, or loss of the rectoprostatic angle indicate T3 disease. In T3 disease, loss of symmetry between the neurovascular bundles is caused by direct extraprostatic disease spread, with perineural and perivascular components.[16] Similarly, loss of the normal fat plane between the posterior portion of the prostate and the anterior aspect of the rectum indicates spread into the periprostatic fat. When neurovascular bundle asymmetry and obliteration of the rectoprostatic angle are both found, T3 disease can be diagnosed with a high degree of specificity (Figure 8.12).[15,16] Unfortunately, the sensitivity of this combination of imaging findings for extracapsular extension is poor.

A recent meta-analysis of studies of the accuracy of MRI in the staging of prostate cancer also examined the influence of magnetic field strength, endorectal coil usage, and pulse sequence.[17] The summary receiver operating characteristic curves (ROC) for all the studies had a maximum joint sensitivity and specificity of 74%. At a specificity of 80% on this curve, the sensitivity was 69%. The superiority of fast spin echo (FSE) techniques over conventional spin echo (CSE) techniques was confirmed. However, somewhat unexpectedly, the use of an endorectal coil and high field strengths were shown to be less accurate.

The appropriate use of MRI in the preoperative staging of prostate cancer has yet to be absolutely determined. A recent meta-analysis using a decision-analytic model compared two clinical strategies.[18] The first strategy dictated that radical prostatectomy was performed on the results of clinical staging alone, and the second that extracapsular disease detected by

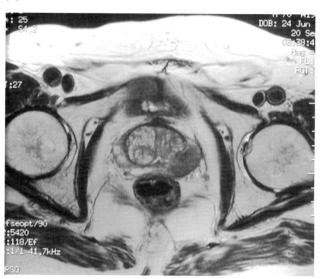

(A)

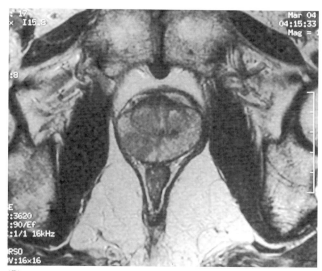

(B)

(C)

Figure 8.11

(A) (B) and (C) are all T2 stage cancers. In (A) there is a cancer in the left peripheral zone that is confined to the gland. In (B) there is a cancer in the left peripheral zone that has a broad area of contact with the pseudocapsule, but no bulging of the pseudocapsule. In (C) there is a tumour causing a large, but smooth bulge. All these patterns indicates T2 stage cancer.

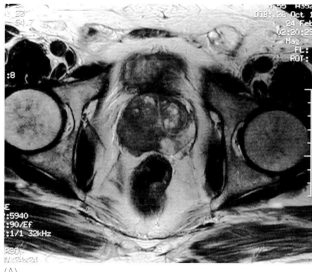

(A)

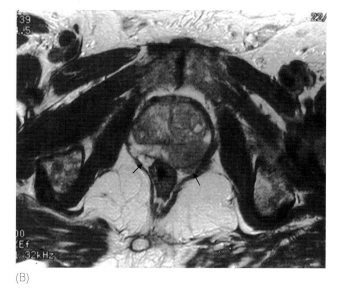

(B)

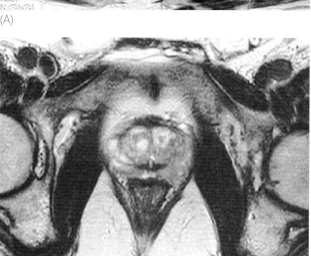

(C)

Figure 8.12

(A) There is tumour causing an irregular bulge to the prosate margin. (B) There is involvement of the left neurovascular bundle (neurovascular bundles arrowed) (C) There is irregular bulging of the prostate gland margin on the left side and asymmetry of the neurovascular bundles with loss of the rectoprostatic angle. All these patterns indicate stage T3 disease.

MRI contraindicates radical prostatectomy in patients who were considered suitable for surgery on the basis of clinical staging alone. In the absence of studies demonstrating therapeutic efficacy, the study concluded that MRI staging could not as yet be conclusively recommended. However, the sensitivity analysis indicated that the MRI-based strategy was more cost-effective when the pre-existing probability of extracapsular disease was ≥ 39% or more. The conclusion was that preoperative staging with MRI is cost-effective in men with a moderate or high prior probability of extracapsular disease.

The seminal vesicles have a variable appearance in terms of their volume, but are normally hypointense on T1-weighted and hyperintense on T2-weighted images owing to their fluid content. These SI characteristics, however, can be quite variable and are age-dependent. The peripheral portions of the seminal vesicles tend to demonstrate more serpiginous, cystic changes with age, which appear more solid as

the ducts converge towards the base of the prostate. Whilst most often there is symmetry, approximately one-third of men will exhibit some degree of asymmetry.

Involvement of the seminal vesicles by prostate cancer is suggested by the presence of focal or diffuse areas of low density around or within the seminal vesicles on T2-weighted images (Figure 8.13). Invasion of the seminal vesicles indicates stage T3 disease that is usually considered unresectable. However, a number of other disease entities can cause similar appearances, for example non-specific fibrosis, post-biopsy haemorrhage, amyloidosis, hormonal treatment, and radiation therapy. MRI detection of seminal vesicle involvement by prostate cancer is therefore sensitive but relatively non-specific. The issue of post-biopsy haemorrhage is also a factor that affects the accuracy of MRI in the detection of involvement of the seminal vesicles by prostate cancer. Post-biopsy haemorrhage and prostate cancer may both appear as

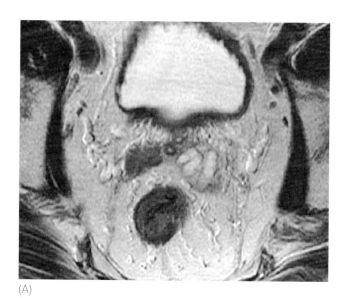

(A)

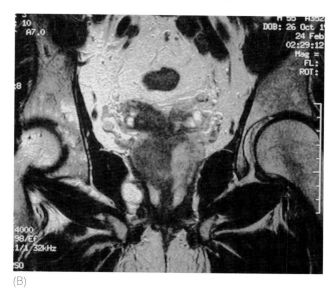

(B)

Figure 8.13

(A) Involvement of the seminal vesicles by tumour is suggested by the presence of focal or diffuse areas of low signal intensity within the seminal vesicles on T2 weighted images. (B) In this case, direct invasion of the seminal vesicle is shown. Continuity is shown between the prostatic tumour and the seminal vesicle tumour

low-SI areas on T2-weighted images. Similarly, both may be localized or diffuse in their involvement of the seminal vesicle. Fortunately, they can often be differentiated on T1-weighted images, where post-biopsy haemorrhage exhibits bright SI and tumour remains hypointense.

Local MRI staging of prostate cancer should include an evaluation of the pelvic and abdominal lymph nodes (Figure 8.14). Nodal staging is clinically relevant because of the prognostic impact of nodal metastases at the time of diagnosis. At 5 years, 80% of patients with positive nodes at diagnosis will have osseous metastases. In comparison, only 20% of patients with no nodal involvement will have osseous metastatic disease. When nodal size is used as the criterion for tumour involvement, MRI has not been shown to be superior to CT. For both CT and MRI, specificity for detection of nodal disease is high, with poor sensitivity due to their inability to detect micrometastases.

MRS of prostate cancer

Early reports of MRS/MRSI suggest that prostate cancer exhibits a different metabolic pattern in comparison with normal prostatic tissue and that this difference is statistically significant. The mean ratios of choline plus creatine to citrate in regions of histologically proven prostate cancer are significantly higher than those found in benign prostatic tissue and in the normal peripheral zones (Figure 8.15).[19] By combining the results of MRI of the prostate with MRS/MRSI of

the prostate, localization of disease within the prostate can be improved, as can the accuracy of evaluation of extraprostatic extension of tumour.[15,20,21]

The precise role of MRS in the staging and management of prostate cancer has yet to be fully defined. However, evidence is accumulating that MRS may provide information about the aggressiveness of individual tumours and the efficacy of various treatment regimens.[22,23]

Benign disease of the prostate

Benign prostatic hypertrophy (see also Chapter 11)

Although BPH is a histologically benign condition, it is responsible for considerable morbidity in men above the age of 50 years. The nodules that characterize this disease are formed from a combination of glandular and stromal proliferation. On T2-weighted images, the MRI appearances are mixed, with the glandular component contributing areas of high signal intensity and the stromal component contributing areas of low SI. The contribution of each component in individual patients is variable, but the combination results in a heterogeneous appearance (Figure 8.16). In the absence of spontaneous or post-biopsy haemorrhage, both components appear isointense with normal prostate tissue on T1-weighted images.

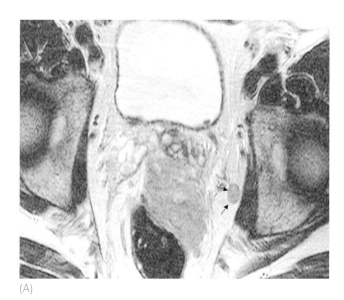

(A)

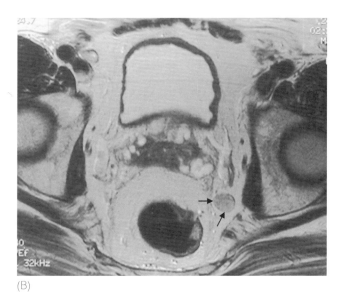

(B)

Figure 8.14

(A) and (B) show enlarged lymph nodes (arrows), strongly suggesting that they are involved by the prostate cancer This was confirmed by node excision and histology. In case (B) the seminal vesicles are also involved.

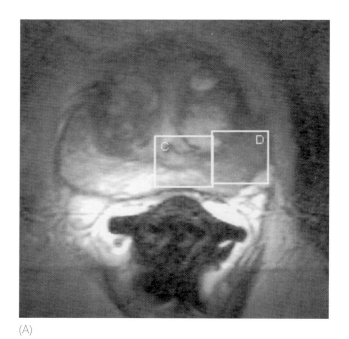

(A)

Figure 8.15

(A) shows an image of a prostate with a cancer in the left peripheral zone. (B) shows the MR spectrum from the box in the uninvolved prostate, labelled C. (C) shows the MR spectrum from the cancer defined by box D. Note the difference in the citrate and choline peaks.

Ch = (phospho) choline, Cr = creatine, Ci = citrate.

Reproduced with permission from; Heerschap A, Jager G, van der Graaf, M, Barentz J, de la Rosette J, Oosterhof G, Ruijter E, Ruijs J. In-vivo spectroscopy reveals altered metabolite content in malignant prostate tissue. Anticancer research 1997:17, 1455–1460.

The volume of nodular hyperplasia is variable, and may not be directly related to age. In the setting of extreme BPH, the peripheral zone may be severely compressed – to the extent that it is barely identifiable.

The MRI appearances of nodular hyperplasia in the central zone and transition zone cannot be differentiated reliably from those of prostate cancer. Furthermore, compression of the peripheral zone by BPH may impair the detection of prostate cancer in the peripheral zone.

Prostatitis (see also Chapter 12)

Acute and chronic prostatitis are relatively common clinical entities, but are rarely imaged with MRI. Coliform bacteria are most often the cause of acute prostatitis, and may give rise to a suppurative episode. When prostatitis is generalized, the prostate demonstrates diffusely increased signal intensity on T2-weighted images and a slightly reduced SI on T1-weighted images. When prostatitis progresses to the formation of a

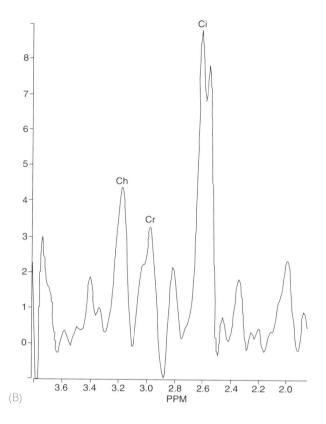

(B)

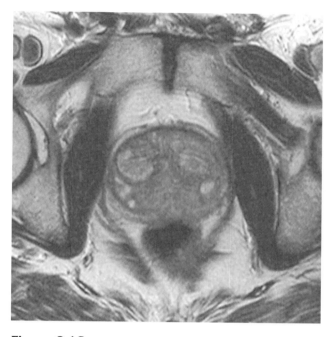

Figure 8.16

The central zone has been expanded by nodules of varying size that characterise this disease. On T2 weighted acquisitions the high signal component is caused by change in the glandular element and the low signal by the stromal element.

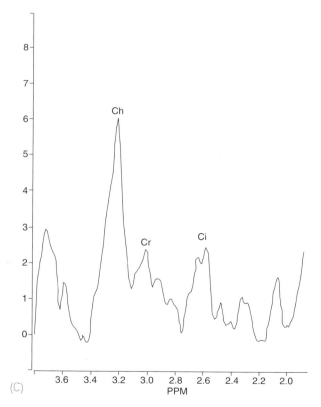

(C)

Figure 8.15

Continued.

prostatic abscess, these SI characteristics become localized. Chronic prostatitis has a non-specific appearance, and may present as an area of low SI in the peripheral zone on T2-weighted images.

Post-therapy evaluation

Evaluation of the prostate with MRI after local therapy (cryotherapy) or systemic (hormonal or radiation) therapies is often difficult owing to therapy-induced anatomical and signal intensity disturbances.[24] In general, the response of prostate cancer to both localized and systemic therapies is similar. The treated area becomes generally hypointense on T2-weighted images. Treated tumuor can be very difficult to differentiate from residual or recurrent disease. After treatment, the peripheral zone may regain its relatively hyperintense signal intensity on T2-weighted images in comparison with the central zone.

MRI should not be used as a primary screening modality to detect preclinical recurrent disease after radical prostatectomy. These patients should be monitored for recurrence with serial prostatic specific antigen (PSA) measurements. When recurrent disease is suspected because of a rising PSA level, MRI may be useful for evaluation of the prostatic bed and the vesicoureteric anastomosis. The obturator, internal iliac, and common iliac nodal groups as well as the bone marrow can also be evaluated.

It is in this post-therapy scenario that MRS may prove to have a most significant role to play in the management of prostate cancer. Evidence from early studies suggest that residual and recurrent tumour can be distinguished from both normal and treated normal prostate tissue by MRS. Sequential evaluation with MRS may provide a non-invasive method for monitoring of response to treatment (localized and systemic) and for early detection of recurrent disease.[25,26]

Conclusions

When MRI was first applied to the prostate, results were inconsistent owing to both software and hardware defficiencies as well as reader inexperience. More recently, there has been a trend towards improved consistency and accuracy in the MRI staging of prostate cancer. Nonetheless, MRI staging of all patients with a new diagnosis of prostate cancer is unlikely to prove cost-effective. Definitive guidelines for the performance of an MRI examination for prostate cancer have not been determined.[27,28]

However, the patients who are most likely to benefit from MRI examination are those whose clinical, biochemical, and histological indicators combined indicate a significant risk for possible T3 disease. The accurate determination of T2 versus T3 disease in this patient group may have a significant effect on their management and prognosis. The clinical impact of MRS is most likely to be seen in the area of post-therapy evaluation owing to the poor results from MRI alone.

References

1. Wefer AE, Hricak H, Vigneron DB et al. Sextant localization of prostate cancer: comparison of sextant biopsy, magnetic resonance imaging and magnetic resonance spectroscopic imaging with step section histology. J Urol 2000; 164: 400–4.

2. Hricak H. Given the improvement in pelvic coils for MR, is an endorectal coil necessary to evaluate prostate carcinoma? AJR 1995; 165: 733–4.

3. Hricak H, White S, Vigneron D et al. Carcinoma of the prostate gland: MR imaging with pelvic phased-array coils versus integrated endorectal–pelvic phased-array coils. Radiology 1994; 193: 703–9.

4. Maio A, Rifkin MD. Magnetic resonance imaging of prostate cancer: update. Top Magn Reson Imag 1995; 7: 54–68.

5. Kurhanewicz J, Vigneron DB, Hricak H et al. Three-dimensional H-1 MR spectroscopic imaging of the in situ human prostate with high (0.24–0.7-cm^3) spatial resolution. Radiology 1996; 198: 795–805.

6. Partin AW, Kattan MW, Subong EN et al. Combination of prostate-specific antigen, clinical stage, and Gleason score to predict pathological stage of localized prostate cancer. A multi-institutional update. JAMA 1997; 277: 1445–51.

7. Reckwitz T, Potter SR, Partin AW. Prediction of locoregional extension and metastatic disease in prostate cancer: a review. World J Urol 2000; 18: 165–72.

8. Ravery V, Boccon-Gibod L. T3 prostate cancer: How reliable is clinical staging? Semin Urol Oncol 1997; 15: 202–6.

9. Outwater EK, Petersen RO, Siegelman ES et al. Prostate carcinoma: assessment of diagnostic criteria for capsular penetration on endorectal coil MR images. Radiology 1994; 193: 333–9.

10. Miller GJ, Cygan JM. Morphology of prostate cancer: the effects of multifocality on histological grade, tumor volume and capsule penetration. J Urol 1994; 152: 1709–13.

11. Kaji Y, Kurhanewicz J, Hricak H et al. Localizing prostate cancer in the presence of postbiopsy changes on MR images: role of proton MR spectroscopic imaging. Radiology 1998; 206: 785–90.

12. Schroder FH, Hermanek P, Denis L et al. The TNM classification of prostate cancer. Prostate Suppl 1992; 4: 129–38.

13. Iyer RV, Hanlon AL, Pinover WH, Hanks GE. Outcome evaluation of the 1997 American Joint Committee on Cancer staging system for prostate carcinoma treated by radiation therapy. Cancer 1999; 85: 1816–21.

14. Rifkin MD, Zerhouni EA, Gatsonis CA. Comparison of magnetic resonance imaging and ultrasonography in staging early prostate cancer: results of a multi institutional cooperative trial. N Engl J Med 323: 621–6.

15. Yu KK, Hricak H, Alagappan R et al. Detection of extra-capsular extension of prostate carcinoma with endorectal and phased-array coil MR imaging: multivariate feature analysis. Radiology 1997; 202: 697–702.

16. Villers A, McNeal JE, Redwine EA et al. The role of perineural space invasion in the local spread of prostatic adenocarcinoma. J Urol 1989; 142: 763–8.

17. Sonnad SS, Langlotz CP, Schwartz JS. Accuracy of MR imaging for staging prostate cancer: a meta-analysis to examine the effect of technologic change. Acad Radiol 2001; 8: 149–57.

18. Jager GJ, Severens JL, Thornbury JR et al. Prostate cancer staging: should MR imaging be used? A decision analytic approach. Radiology 2000; 215: 445–51.

19. Kurhanewicz J, Vigneron DB, Nelson SJ. Three-dimensional magnetic resonance spectroscopic imaging of brain and prostate cancer. Neoplasia 2000; 2: 166–89.

20. Yu KK, Scheidler J, Hricak H et al. Prostate cancer: prediction of extracapsular extension with endorectal MR imaging and three-dimensional proton MR spectroscopic imaging. Radiology 1999; 213: 481–8.

21. Scheidler J, Hricak H, Vigneron DB et al. Prostate cancer: localization with three-dimensional proton MR spectroscopic imaging – clinicopathologic study. Radiology 1999; 213: 473–80.

22. Kurhanewicz J, Swanson MG, Wood PJ, Vigneron DB. Magnetic resonance imaging and spectroscopic imaging: improved patient selection and potential for metabolic intermediate endpoints in prostate cancer chemoprevention trials. Urology 2001; 57: 124–8.

23. Kurhanewicz J, Vigneron DB, Hricak H et al. Prostate cancer: metabolic response to cryosurgery as detected with 3D H-1 MR spectroscopic imaging. Radiology 1996; 200: 489–96.

24. Kalbhen CL, Hricak H, Shinohara K et al. Prostate carcinoma: MR imaging findings after cryosurgery. Radiology 1996; 198: 807–11.

25. Kurhanewicz J, Vigneron DB, Males RG et al. The prostate: MR imaging and spectroscopy. Present and future. Radiol Clin North Am 2000; 38: 115–19

26. Kurhanewicz J, Swanson MG, Wood PJ, Vigneron DB. Magnetic resonance imaging and spectroscopic imaging: Improved patient selection and potential for metabolic intermediate endpoints in prostate cancer chemoprevention trials. Urology 2001; 57: 124–8.

27. Garnick MB. Prostate cancer: screening, diagnosis, and management. Ann Intern Med 1993; 118: 804–18.

28. Yu KK, Hricak H. Imaging prostate cancer. Radiol Clin North Am 2000; 38: 59–85.

9

Nuclear medicine evaluation and therapy of the prostate

Rakesh H Ganatra

Introduction

The assessment of metastatic disease is vital for both treatment planning and prognostic evaluation of prostate cancer. The success of definitive local surgical and radiation therapy is limited by extraprostatic spread of tumour. Historically, nuclear medicine has played a significant role in the management of prostate cancer, with the conventional isotope bone scan being used as a primary technique to assess extraprostatic spread throughout the skeleton. More recently, the role of nuclear medicine has expanded, not only in its imaging contribution, but also in a therapeutic role. Advances in immunoscintigraphy and positron emission tomography (PET) demonstrate potential to contribute to the future management of patients with prostate cancer. In the field of therapeutics, the role of nuclear medicine is twofold. Palliation of bone pain from prostate metastases may be achieved with intravenously administered isotopes such as strontium, rhenium and samarium. Curative approaches to treatment of organ-confined tumour include brachytherapy, immunotherapy, and external-beam radiotherapy. Intratumoral injection of isotope is currently being pioneered for a variety of tumours, including prostate cancer. This delivers a high radiation dose locally and shows promise for definitive treatment of prostate cancer. This chapter will address both the current role and the future potential of these nuclear medicine techniques.

IMAGING

Bone scintigraphy

History

The idea of isotope bone imaging was conceptualized from the observation that luminous watch dial painters accumu-

lated radioactive isotope in bone. Metabolic studies with radionuclides were commenced in 1935 by Chiewitz and Hevesy[1] with [^{32}P]orthophosphate, and continued in the early 1940s with the use of flourine-18 (^{18}F), calcium-45 (^{45}Ca) and strontium-89 (^{89}Sr). Successful bone imaging, however, was not achieved until 1961, when Fleming et al[2] used strontium-85 (^{85}Sr). The search for an 'ideal' isotope has continued since that time and technetium-99m methylene diphosphonate (^{99m}Tc-MDP) is now the standard agent used, fulfilling the majority of the criteria for an 'ideal' imaging agent.

Instrumentation

Standard static images can be acquired using a static camera and a moving table that acquires whole-body views. Alternatively, spot views can be acquired using a static camera. Single- or multiple-head cameras are now available, the main advantage of the latter being increased speed of acquisition. Advances in instrumentation have also led to the optimization of image acquisition and the capability of single-photon emission tomography (SPECT), with more accurate localization of lesions. SPECT has significant advantages over conventional imaging, particularly in spinal imaging, where the localization of abnormal activity to the body or posterior elements may help differentiate benign from malignant causes of abnormal uptake.

Bone scan staging of prostate cancer

The skeleton is a relatively common site for metastatic spread of prostate cancer, possibly as a result of the production by bone cells of growth factors that stimulate proliferation of malignant cells.[3] Prostate cancer cells that metastasize to bone produce additional growth factors that stimulate bone formation. The propensity for spread of prostate cancer to the vertebral column may be related to a network of venous connections around the lumbar spine first described by Batson[4] in 1940.

Isotope uptake by bone is related to bone turnover from the complex interaction of osteoblastic and osteoclastic activity. This interaction is controlled by a variety of stimulatory and inhibitory factors. Abnormal bone uptake is associated with a disruption in the normal balance of bone turnover. Owing to the profound effect of metastatic prostate cancer upon metabolism within bone tissue, the isotope bone scan is an excellent test for the assessment of skeletal spread of disease.

The presence of bone metastases affects staging, alters treatment options, and has prognostic implications. Furthermore, the localization of skeletal metastases guides radiation therapy for bone pain and is essential prior to systemic isotope therapy. Approximately 50% of patients with metastatic carcinoma of the prostate die within 30 months and 80% die within 5 years of diagnosis. Bone metastases occur in 85% of patients dying of carcinoma of the prostate[5] and are present in about 8% at presentation.[6] Lund et al[7] showed that patients with an abnormal bone scan at presentation have a mortality rate of 45% at 2 years, compared with 20% for those with a normal scan.

Various studies have shown that the bone scan is the most sensitive method for the early detection of metastatic disease.[8,9] Although a strong case can be made for all patients to have a staging bone scan at presentation, routine use of the bone scan in all patients diagnosed with prostate cancer may not be cost-effective. Many centres limit the bone scan to patients with a serum prostate-specific antigen (PSA) above a specified level (see the section below on indications for a bone scan). Serial bone scans may be of value in therapeutic decision-making, particularly when used in combination with clinical and biochemical data.

Plain radiography provides excellent anatomical detail of bones. Often, it is possible to diagnose bony metastatic disease from carcinoma of the prostate on a skeletal survey. However, bone scanning provides additional functional information and is more easily adapted to whole-body imaging. Furthermore, the bone scan demonstrates metastatic deposits earlier than plain radiographs.[10,11] In four series comparing scintigraphy with X-ray in 1430 cases, 28% more abnormalities were detected by scintigraphy and only 1.5% of X-ray abnormalities were not detected by scintigraphy. This excellent sensitivity of bone scanning is largely due to the fact that the bone scan is able to identify as little as a 5–15% change in bone turnover.[12] In some circumstances, it may be necessary to perform plain radiography to help differentiate benign from malignant causes of abnormal uptake on bone scan. In this regard, both imaging modalities may be complementary in the assessment of metastatic disease.

Bone scan appearance of prostate metastases

The classical pattern of metastatic disease from prostate to bone is of multiple, randomly distributed areas of increased uptake in the axial skeleton (Figure 9.1). This appearance rarely poses a diagnostic challenge. However, a haematogenously disseminated condition such as infection or mast cell disease can give a similar pattern, and clinical correlation should always be made. Lobo et al[13] showed that the most frequently involved sites with metastatic deposits from prostate cancer were the pelvis (86%), rib cage (67%), and spine (57%). Krishnamurthy et al[14] demonstrated that 60% of metastases occurred in the axial skeleton, while 40% occurred in the appendicular skeleton.

The distribution of bone metastases on the initial bone scan should be considered as a variable for the prognostic stratification of patients with metastatic prostate cancer. A study by Yamashita et al[15] assessed the survival rates of patients on hormonal treatment according to the distribution of the metastasis. They showed that the presence of bone metastases outside the pelvis and lumbar spine is predictive of a shorter survival time.

Only about 15% of patients with proven metastatic disease from prostate cancer have a single osseous lesion (usually in the spine) (Figures 9.2 and 9.3). A solitary metastasis is more difficult to diagnose with certainty. However, certain features of solitary metastases may be useful. Bony metastases from prostate cancer characteristically show intense uptake. Although benign conditions such as degenerative disease and Paget's disease may demonstrate intense uptake, they can easily be differentiated with a plain radiograph. Furthermore, SPECT may be used to demonstrate the characteristic involvement of the vertebral body and posterior elements in Paget's disease. The posterior part of the vertebral body is the most common site of involvement by metastatic deposits. Uptake in the posterolateral elements or the anterolateral aspect of the vertebral body is generally due to benign disease.[16]

Solitary rib metastases demonstrate linear uptake that spreads along a rib and can be distinguished from rib fractures, which show more focal uptake (Figures 9.2 and 9.4). Lesions that line up in adjacent ribs are more likely to represent fractures while lesions in non-contiguous ribs are more likely to be metastases. Exceptions do occur and alternative imaging methods or follow-up scanning is sometimes necessary. Solitary rib metastases are uncommon; Tumeh et al[17] reported only 10% of solitary rib lesions were due to metastases.

A significant proportion of solitary lesions on the bone scan are due to benign causes, even in the presence of a known extraosseous primary cancer. Corcoran et al[18] found that solitary abnormalities occurred in 15% of a series of 1129 patients with an extraskeletal primary carcinoma. In two-thirds of these 15%, the cause was metastatic, while in one-

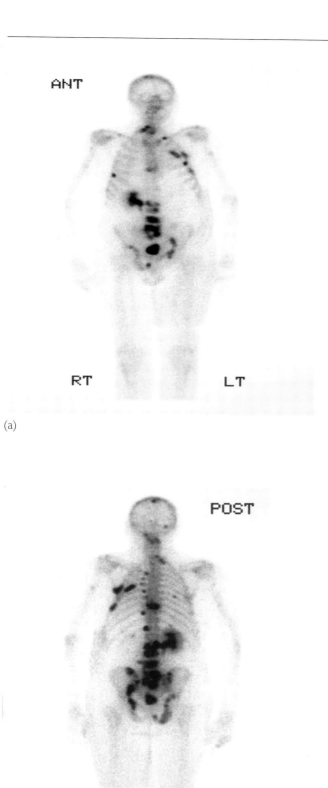

(a)

(b)

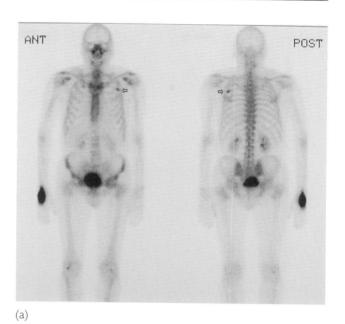

(a)

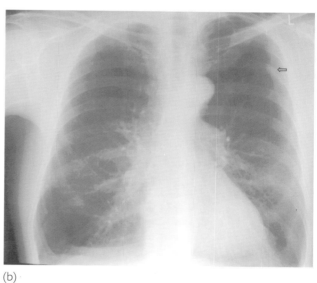

(b)

Figure 9.2

(a) This bone scan shows a solitary rib metastasis in the left 5th rib posteriorly (arrow). (b) A chest X-ray of the same patient shows a sclerotic lesion in the corresponding rib (arrow).

Figure 9.1

This bone scan shows the typical appearance of bone metastases from carcinoma of the prostate with multiple, randomly distributed areas of increased uptake throughout the axial skeleton. There is also a right hydronephrosis and a non-functioning left kidney as a result of chronic bladder outflow obstruction.

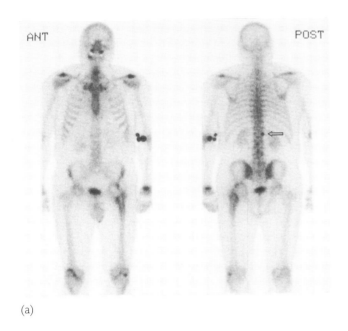

(a)

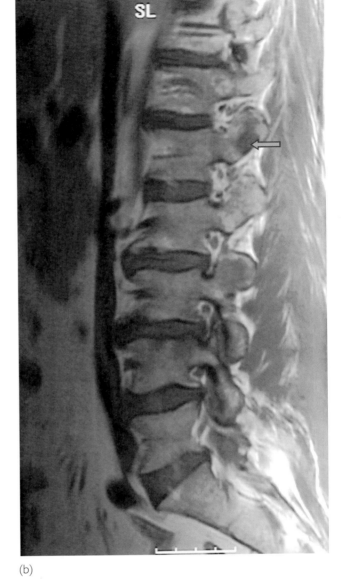

(b)

Figure 9.3

(a) This bone scan shows a solitary metastasis in the L1 vertebra on the right (arrow). There is also increased activity surrounding the femoral component of the left total hip replacement due to loosening. (b) T1-weighted MRI on the same patient shows a low-signal lesion in the posterior element of L1 (arrow), confirming the presence of the metastasis.

third, the cause was a benign lesion. Plain radiographic correlation is particularly important in solitary lesions. However, if doubt still remains, computed tomography (CT), magnetic resonance imaging (MRI), or even a bone biopsy can be employed (Figure 9.5). MRI of a vertebral metastasis may demonstrate an epidural mass and paravertebral extension of the tumour.

A variety of less common appearances are seen in metastatic bone disease from carcinoma of the prostate. A photopenic area with peripheral enhancement may be due to a peripheral reparative response, for example, following hormonal therapy. Cold metastases have also been described, but these are much more common in renal and breast carcinoma.

A feature that is not uncommonly seen in prostate cancer is the metastatic superscan. This is readily recognized by intense bone uptake, with a paucity of renal or soft tissue uptake (Figure 9.6). Superscans are seen in a variety of malignant and benign conditions. Malignant causes include prostate cancer, breast cancer, and lymphoma. In the absence of a known primary tumour, a superscan involving bones throughout the axial and peripheral skeleton should raise the suspicion of a metabolic superscan, which may be seen with primary or secondary hyperparathyroidism. A normal bone scan may be seen in the early stage of metastatic disease when malignant cells are confined to bone marrow and are not inciting an osteoblastic/osteoclastic response.

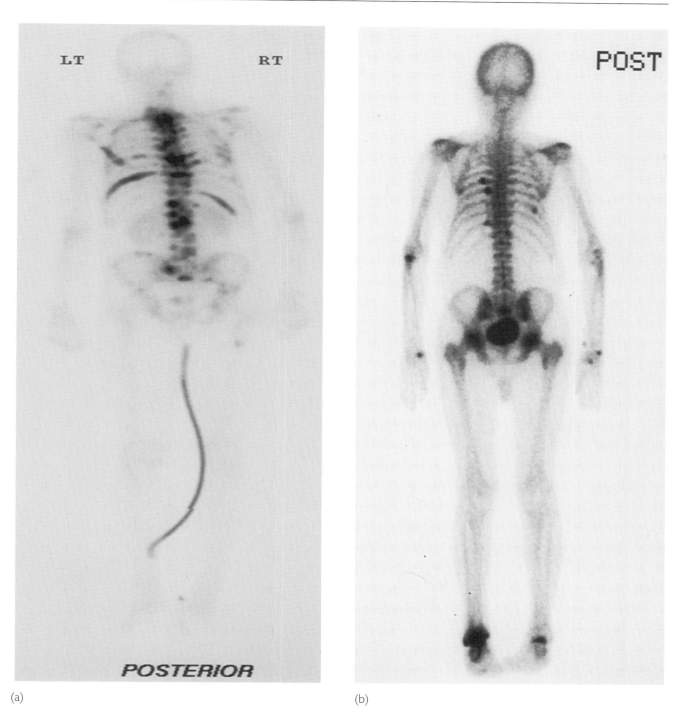

(a) (b)

Figure 9.4

(a) This bone scan shows multiple bone metastases from carcinoma of the prostate. Note the spread of the metastatic deposits along the line of the ribs. (b) Typical appearance of rib fractures, which show more focal uptake and involve adjacent ribs.

The 'flare' phenomenon

The 'flare' phenomenon, first described by Greenberg et al,[19] is the finding of increased activity on bone scan that typically occurs following chemotherapy and is due to an increase in bone turnover. It is a particular problem in bone metastases from lung and breast cancer (where it is reported to occur in up to 20% of cases) but occurs much less commonly in prostate cancer. It accounted for only 6% of positive bone scans in prostate cancer patients in a study

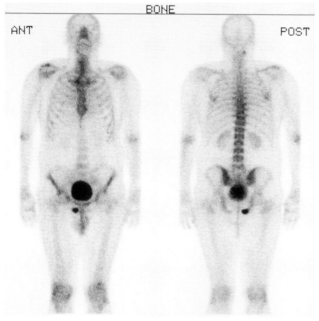

(a)

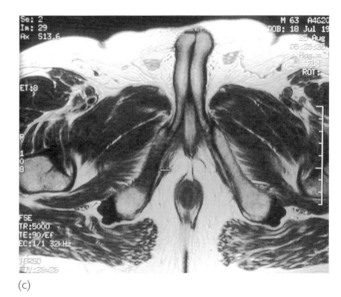

(c)

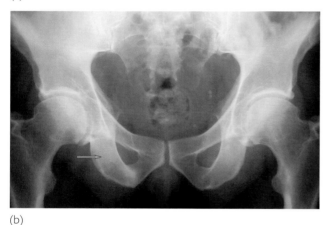

(b)

Figure 9.5

(a) This bone scan shows a solitary metastasis in the right inferior pubic ramus. A plain X-ray (b) shows subtle sclerosis at the corresponding site (arrow) and T2-weighted MRI (c) shows low signal at this site, confirming the presence of a metastasis.

by Pollen et al,[20] but was seen in 23% of cases in a study by Levenson et al.[21]

The flare phenomenon can cause confusion when trying to decide whether increased uptake following the start of chemotherapy is due to residual disease. Increased activity within the first 3 months of chemotherapy is likely to be due to the flare phenomenon. Bone lesions that appear 6 months or later after treatment almost always indicate disease progression.

Indications for a bone scan in prostate cancer

Staging

Bone is the only extraprostatic site of disease in 65% of patients with metastatic prostate cancer, and about 80–85% of patients who die of prostate cancer have skeletal involvement.[22] Between 30% and 51% of initial staging scans in proven carcinoma of the prostate are abnormal. The frequency of skeletal metastases, however, is related to the clinical stage, the Gleason histological grade, and the PSA value. The frequency of skeletal metastases increases from 5% for clinical stage 1 to 10% for clinical stage 2, and 20% for clinical stage 3.[23,24] Prior to the introduction of PSA in the early 1990s, the bone scan was routinely performed for staging of patients with prostate cancer. More recently, it has been accepted that PSA levels may be used to predict metastatic disease to the skeleton. A more cost-effective approach to the staging of prostate cancer will apply the bone scan only to those patients who have an elevated PSA, but the cutoff point for this decision is not universally agreed and ranges from 8 to 20 ng/ml.[25,26] Various studies have demonstrated good correlation between PSA and the presence of a positive bone scan.[27,28]

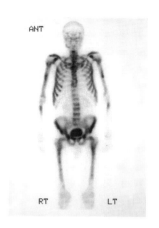
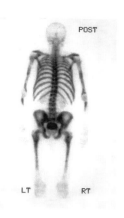

Figure 9.6

Typical appearance of a superscan, showing intense bone uptake and a paucity of renal and soft tissue uptake.

With a serum PSA of less than 10 ng/ml, the chance of the bone scan being negative is greater than 96% (providing the patient is not on hormonal therapy). Freitas et al[29] demonstrated a negative predictive value of 98.5% for a bone scan with a PSA of less than 8 ng/ml. However, in the setting of hormonal therapy, the PSA level is suppressed even in the presence of bone metastases. One-third of patients on hormonal therapy have a normal PSA level despite the presence of bone metastases.[30] Lin et al[31] also showed that a PSA cutoff level of less than 10 ng/ml had a high negative predictive value for bone metastasis, but concluded that this criterion did not exclude bone metastasis, and that a baseline bone scan should be routinely obtained. Similar conclusions were reached in studies by Wolff et al[32] and Bruwer et al.[33]

Lorente et al[34] have suggested that the combined utility of serum alkaline phosphatase (<20 ng/ml) and PSA obviated the need to perform a bone scan in patients with a PSA level between 10 and 20 ng/ml, hence reducing cost in the management of patients with prostate cancer. The American Urological Association has recently recommended that routine use of skeletal scintigraphy is not indicated when the PSA level is less than 20 ng/ml.

Re-staging and evaluation of therapy

Between 10% and 25% of patients with newly diagnosed prostate cancer without bone metastases at the time of diagnosis will develop metastases during follow-up. However, it is generally accepted that the routine use of bone scans in the follow-up of prostate cancer patients treated for localized disease is not indicated.[35,36] The routine use of follow-up bone scans adds significant cost and burden to the already stretched health system. Follow-up is simpler and cheaper with serial serum PSA levels and monitoring of clinical symptoms. A study by Stokkel et al[37] demonstrated that in patients with prostate cancer but without bone metastases at the time

of diagnosis, PSA could be used for the assessment of risk of metastases during follow-up. However, there do remain some advocates of the routine use of bone scanning for follow-up.[38] Furthermore, follow-up scans are useful where the initial bone scan is inconclusive, for symptomatic patients with pain that may be related to the skeleton, to plan further therapy in the setting of metastatic disease, and for research purposes to assess the benefits of therapy. The presence of pain shows positive correlation with the presence of metastases. The absence of this symptom should not, however, be used as an exclusion criteria for metastases. In a study by Palmer et al,[39] 82% of 64 consecutive prostate cancer patients who had bone pain had bone metastases, while only 34% of patients without pain had metastases.

Systemic treatment for bone pain

A bone scan is an essential part of the workup prior to isotope treatment for palliation of bone pain. It aids in deciding which patients are suitable for such treatment and which isotope to use. This topic is discussed more fully in the section below on isotope therapy.

Single-photon emission computed tomography (SPECT)

The posterior portion of the vertebral body is the most frequent site for the spread of prostate cancer to bone. This may be related to the better vascular supply at this site and the propensity of haematogenous spread of metastasis from prostate cancer.

Although it is difficult to locate the position of abnormal uptake within a vertebra on planar imaging (Figure 9.4), SPECT imaging has improved the assessment of vertebral metastases with increased sensitivity (87–100%) and specificity (91–95%) for detection of metastatic deposits compared with planar imaging.[40–42]

Bone scan index (BSI)

The bone scan index (BSI) estimates the fraction of the skeleton that is involved by tumour, and assesses the regional distribution of skeletal metastases. Quantitative or semiquantitative measures of skeletal uptake can be used. Semi-automated image segmentation programs are available to reduce the processing time. Practical applications of the BSI might include the assessment of response to treatment and prognostication for survival. However, even with the use of semi-automated programs, the calculation of the BSI is time-consuming and currently has limited clinical use.[43,44] As a research tool, the BSI is useful in predicting treatment response and allowing objective comparison of different therapies.

Bone marrow scintigraphy

Marrow scintigraphy has little use in the routine management of patients with prostate cancer. A study by Bourgeois et al[45] demonstrated that bone marrow scintigraphy was less sensitive than the conventional bone scan in diagnosing skeletal metastasis (94% for marrow scintigraphy versus 100% for bone scanning). However, marrow scintigraphy may be useful in cases of dubious bone scans and for evaluating the response of skeletal metastasis to treatment.

Positron emission tomography (PET)

Although PET has been available since the 1960s, it is only recently that it has been accepted as the optimal method for staging a variety of tumours, including lung cancer, melanoma and lymphoma. PET presents a unique ability to image biochemical processes with high-resolution, whole-body images. The technique utilizes a positron-emitting isotope. The positron combines with an electron to produce two photons (gamma rays) of 511 keV, which are emitted at 180° to each other. Coincident detection of these photons by two oppositely positioned photomultiplier tubes allows the scanner to determine the anatomical location of the radiotracer in the body. Three-dimensional images are produced using sophisticated computer software.

The agent used most commonly for PET imaging is ^{18}F-labelled deoxyglucose ([^{18}F]-2-fluoro-2-deoxyglucose, ^{18}F-FDG), which is utilized by tissue as a glucose analogue. The tracer is preferentially metabolized in malignant tissue because of increased glycolytic metabolism in that tissue. A number of studies have evaluated the use of ^{18}F-FDG PET in the management of prostate cancer. Most such studies have concluded that it was not useful in differentiating benign from malignant prostate pathology or in the evaluation of metastatic disease.[46–48] Unlike other malignancies, such as lung cancer, melanoma and lymphoma, prostate cancer demonstrates poor glucose metabolism and does not demonstrate preferential uptake of ^{18}F-FDG. In addition, since ^{18}F-FDG is excreted in the urine, it is difficult to differentiate pelvic pathology from urinary activity in the bladder. Furthermore, PET is not as sensitive as bone scintigraphy for the detection of osseous metastases. With the use of PET, Shreve et al[49] found a sensitivity of 65% for the detection of bone metastases, while Yeh et al[50] found a sensitivity of only 20%.

A few studies have suggested that ^{18}F-FDG PET can be useful in prostate cancer. Oyama et al[51] found that a higher ^{18}F-FDG uptake correlated well with high Gleason grade, advanced clinical stage, and higher PSA level. Based upon these findings, it is possible that PET may be helpful in evaluating the malignant potential of tumours. Saltzer et al[52] suggested that PET was better than CT and monoclonal antibody scanning in detecting PSA relapse following treatment for localized prostate cancer. Schirrmeister et al[53] found PET to be better than planar bone scans at detecting bone metastases.

Quantitative studies have evaluated prostatic blood flow to differentiate benign from malignant prostatic lesions. These studies demonstrate a significant difference in prostatic vascularity in benign prostatic hypertrophy (BPH) and tumour.[54] However, it is generally accepted that ^{18}F-FDG PET has no useful role to play in the routine management of prostate cancer. Other PET tracers relying on protein synthesis rather than glucose metabolism may have greater potential for future clinical use.

Immunoscintigraphy

The two main clinical applications of immunoscintigraphy are:

- accurate local staging of apparent organ confined tumour prior to radical treatment;
- localization of soft tissue recurrence in a patient who has a rising PSA level following radical treatment.

Local staging with immunoscintigraphy may be most useful for high-risk patients.

Goldberg et al[55] first described immunoscintigraphy of the prostate using iodine-131 (^{131}I)-labelled polyclonal antibody to prostatic acid phosphatase in 1983. Dillman et al[56] later described indium-111 (^{111}In)-labelled monoclonal antibody to PSA. These tracers were of limited clinical utility owing to the binding of antibodies with enzymes in the circulation. More recently, a monoclonal antibody against prostate-specific membrane antigen (PSMA) has been described.[57] This antibody appears to be more specific for imaging of prostate cancer. A radioimmunoconjugate based on PSMA, capromab pendetide (ProstaScint), is now available for clinical use in newly diagnosed cancer patients and in patients with biochemical failure after radical treatment. Studies have shown its usefulness in predicting lymph node involvement in high-risk patients prior to radical treatment, hence avoiding unnecessary morbidity.[58] This radioimmunoconjugate is also useful in finding occult recurrences after primary treatment failure of prostate cancer.[59] Immunoscintigraphy has been shown to outperform CT, MRI, and ultrasound in detecting lymph node metastases, with a sensitivity of 75%, a specificity of 86%, an accuracy of 81%, and a positive predictive value of 79%.[60,61] Other studies suggest that PET and CT may be better than monoclonal antibody scans at detecting nodal metastases.[62] The different findings in these studies may reflect differences in the amount of nodal involvement and the PSA levels in these studies. The detection threshold for this antibody appears to be disease foci of at least 5 mm.[63] This 5 mm threshold is smaller than the 1 cm threshold level for defining pathological nodes in most lymph node regions on CT.

The technique of immunoscintigraphy involves labelling a suitable monoclonal antibody with an isotope. The best isotopes currently available are ^{111}In and ^{99m}Tc. The main contraindication to this procedure is an allergy to foreign proteins as demonstrated by an adverse reaction to a previous inoculation. SPECT is essential for imaging with this technique. Following intravenous administration of the labelled antibody, planar anterior and posterior images are obtained, followed by squat views (to eliminate genital uptake from the field of view) and SPECT of the pelvis. Images are acquired during the first hour after injection and repeated at 24 and 48 hours for ^{111}In-labelled antibody, and at 24 hours for ^{99m}Tc-labelled antibody. Figure 9.5 shows typical immunoscintigraphy images. The main pitfalls in the interpretation of these images are the presence of vascular activity and urinary activity when using ^{99m}Tc-labelled antibody, and rectal and marrow activity with ^{111}In-labelled antibody. These other sources of activity can usually be identified by comparing images acquired at different times. Activity in vascular, urinary, bowel, and marrow structures should decrease with time, while activity in malignant tissue increases with time. Dual-isotope imaging, using ^{111}In-labelled antibody and ^{99m}Tc-labelled red cells can be used with a subtraction technique to eliminate activity from the vascular component.[64]

Although immunoscintigraphy is now an established technique, it is costly and its availability is limited to specialist centres.[65] Its clinical applications are already helping management decisions, but larger studies are needed to define its role in the routine management of prostate cancer.

Therapy

Nuclear medicine plays a significant role in the management of prostate cancer, both as a curative form of treatment as well as for the palliation of bone pain. Details of the imaging strategy from the viewpoint of the radiation oncologist are discussed in Chapter 18.

Prostate brachytherapy

Prostate brachytherapy has come in and out of fashion since the early 1900s. Brachytherapy was first used for the treatment of prostate and bladder cancer by implantation of radium needles.[66,67] In the 1970s, the technique experienced a revival with the use of ^{125}I-seed implantation via an open retropubic approach.[68] The main problem with the retropubic approach was the difficulty in accurately placing the activity at the tumour site. Poorly positioned implants resulted in local morbidity from radiation effects and a significant recurrence rate. In 1983, Holme et al[69] described the use of transrectal ultrasound and the use of a template to guide the accurate placement of the radioactivity. This technique is now accepted as the method of choice for inserting radioactive 'seeds' into the prostate.

The main advantage of brachytherapy over external-beam therapy is the ability to deliver a higher, focused radiation dose at the treatment site, with reduced adverse radiation effects on surrounding tissues. The technique involves performing a transrectal ultrasound scan or CT to assess the prostate volume and plan the number and position of radioactive sources needed to deliver a homogenous dose to the prostate. The sources are then inserted via the perineal skin into preplanned positions within the prostate using ultrasound guidance. The dose delivered to the prostate is calculated using computer software.

The procedure is performed under spinal or general anaesthesia, usually as a day case. Patients are routinely given antibiotics before and after the procedure. Brachytherapy is suitable for organ-confined disease. Patients with a PSA level greater than 25 ng/ml should undergo lymph node sampling prior to the procedure. Previous transurethral resection of the prostate (TURP) is a relative contraindication because of the potential for seed loss, which causes underdosing and subsequent local radiation morbidity.

Patients who are deemed at high risk for local extraprostatic spread of disease because of a high Gleason grade or high PSA level may have external-beam radiation combined with seed implantation. Several studies have reported good survival rates using this technique.[70, 71]

Using transrectal ultrasound guidance, the complication rate of the procedure is low. Proctitis, urinary incontinence, and urethral strictures have been reported. As already mentioned, these rates are higher in patients who have undergone a TURP.

Intratumoral injection of isotope

The direct intratumoral injection of isotope is not a new idea, but work is currently being done to evaluate its use in the treatment of prostate cancer. Very high doses can be administered with this technique, using ultrasound or CT to target the activity into the tumour. Several agents are being evaluated, but rhenium currently shows the most promise.

Systemic treatment for bone pain

The management of bone pain in patients with multiple osseous metastases poses a significant clinical problem. Phosphorus-32 has been used as systemic radioisotope therapy for the management of bone pain for over 40 years. However, its use is limited by the side-effect of bone marrow suppression. More recently, the bone-seeking radiopharmaceuticals ^{89}Sr, samarium-153 (^{153}Sm) and rhenium-186 (^{186}Re) have all been used as palliative treatment for patients with clinically significant bone pain. ^{89}Sr (Metastron) is the most widely used. It is a calcium analogue that is selectively absorbed by bone at sites of increased osteoblastic activity. It is a pure beta-emitter, with a bone penetration of 0.8 cm, and it has been used in multiple trials with response rates of up to 80%. Like ^{186}Re and ^{153}Sm, it is administered intravenously. Patients should have a bone scan prior to administration to assess the sites and extent of osseous deposits. Excess tumour load, particularly in the spine, is a relative contraindication because of the risk of spinal cord compression and significant myelosuppression. The risks appear to be less with ^{186}Re and ^{153}Sm.[72]

The most common side-effect of the bone-seeking radiopharmaceuticals is mild thrombocytopenia that typically recovers in 3 or 4 months. Subclinical disseminated intravascular coagulation is reported to be present in approximately 10–20% of patients with advanced prostate cancer.[73]

Treatment with bone-seeking radiopharmaceuticals has been shown to improve quality of life in 65% of patients.[74,75]

Radioimmunotherapy

Radioimmunotherapy (RIT) uses a tumour-specific monoclonal antibody to deliver systemic, targeted radiation to cancer cells. A number of agents are currently in clinical trials and show promise for the future. For further details, the reader is referred to oncology texts.

External-beam radiation

Two forms of external beam radiation are in use: three-dimensional conformal radiation therapy (3DCRT) and intensity-modulated radiation therapy (IMRT). These are described in more detail in Chapter 18.

Acknowledgement

I am grateful to Dr John Rees, Consultant Radiologist, University Hospital of Wales, Cardiff for his contribution to this chapter.

References

1. Chiewitz O, Hevesy G. Radioactive indicators in the study of phosphorus metabolism in rats. Nature 1935: 754–5.

2. Fleming WH, McIlradith JD, King ER. Photoscanning of bone lesions utilising strontium 85. Radiology 1961; 77: 635–6.

3. Gleave M, Hsieh JT, Gao CA et al. Acceleration of human prostate cancer growth in vivo by factors produced by prostate and bone fibroblasts. Cancer Res 1991; 51: 3753–61.

4. Batson OV. Function of vertebral veins and their role in spread and metastasis. Ann Surg 1940; 112: 138–49.

5. Murray IPC. The evaluation of malignancy: primary bone tumours. In: Nuclear Medicine in Clinical Diagnosis and Treatment (Murray IPC, Ell PJ, eds). Edingburgh: Churchill Livingstone, 1998: 1176.

6. American Cancer Society. Cancer Facts and Figures 1997. Atlanta: ACS, 1997: 4.

7. Lund F, Smith PH, Suciu S. Do bone scans predict the prognosis in prostate cancer? A report of the ERCOT Protocol 30762. Br J Urol 1984; 26: 58–63.

8. Schaffer DL and Pendergrass HP. Comparison of enzyme, clinical, radiographic and radionuclide methods of detecting bone metastasis from carcinoma of the prostate. Radiology 1976; 121: 431–4.

9. Letaief B, Boughattas S, Hassine H et al. Bone scan and prostate cancer. Ann Urol 2000; 34: 256–65.

10. Tofe AJ, Francis MA, Harvey WJ. Correlation of neoplasms with incidence and localisation of skeletal metastasis: an analysis of 1355 diphosphonate bone scans. J Nucl Med 1975; 16: 896.

11. Pistenman DA, McDougall IR, Kriss JP. Screening for bone metastasis: Are only scans necessary? JAMA 1975; 231: 46–50.

12. Murray IPC. The evaluation of malignancy: primary bone tumours. In: Nuclear medicine in clinical diagnosis and treatment (Murray IPC, Ell PJ, eds). Edinburgh: Churchill Livingstone, 1998: 1169.

13. Lobo G, Ladron de Guevara D, Salgado G et al. Bone scintigraphy in prostatic cancer. Correlation with clinical and laboratory features and with survival. Rev Med Chil 1999; 127: 181–8.

14. Krishnamurthy GT, Tubbis M, Hiss J et al. Distribution pattern of metastatic bone disease: a need for total body skeletal image. JAMA 1997; 237: 2504–6.

15. Yamashita K, Denno K, Ueda T et al. Prognostic significance of bone metastases in patients with metastatic prostate cancer. Cancer 1993; 71: 1297–302.

16. Algra PR, Heimans JJ, Valk J et al. Do metastases in vertebrae begin in the pedicles? AJR 1992; 158: 1275–9.

17. Tumeh SS, Beadle G, Kaplan WD. Clinical significance of solitary rib lesions in patients with excess skeletal malignancy. J Nucl Med 1985; 26: 1140–3.

18. Corcoran RJ, Thrall JH Kyle RW et al. Solitary abnormalities in bone scans in patients with extra osseous malignancies. Radiology 1976; 121: 663–5.

19. Greenberg EJ, Chu FCH, Dwyer AJ et al. Effects of radiation therapy on bone lesions as measured by ^{47}Ca and ^{85}Sr local kinetics. J Nucl Med 1972; 13: 747–9.

20. Pollen JJ, Witztum KF, Ashburn WL. The flare phenomenon on radionuclide bone scans in metastatic prostate cancer. AJR 1984; 142: 773–6.

21. Levenson RM, Sauerbraunn BJL, Bates HR et al. Comparative value of bone scintigraphy in radiography in tumour response in systemically treated prostate cancer. Radiology 1983; 146: 513–17.

22. Jacobs SC. Spread of metastatic cancer to bone. Urology 1983; 21: 337–44.

23. Shih WJ, Mitchell B, Wierzbinski B et al. Prediction of radionuclide bone imaging findings by Gleason histological grading of prostate carcinoma. Clin Nucl Med 1991; 16: 763–6.

24. McKillop JH. Bone scanning in clinical practice. In: Bone Scanning in Clinical Practice (Fogelman I, ed). London: Springer-Verlag, 1987: 41–60.

25. Haukaas S, Roervik J, Halvorsen OJ et al. When is bone scintigraphy necessary in the assessment of newly diagnosed, untreated prostate cancer? Br J Urol 1997; 79: 770–6.

26. Hunchereck H, Muscat J. Serum prostate specific antigen as a marker of bone metastasis in patients with prostate cancer. Urol Int 1996; 156: 169.

27. Lee N, Fawaaz R, Olsson CA et al. Which patients with newly diagnosed prostate cancer need a radionuclide bone scan? An analysis based on 631 patients. Int J Radiat Oncol Biol Phys 2000; 48: 1443–6.

28. Gleave ME, Coupland D, Drachenberg D et al. Ability of serum prostate specific antigen levels to predict normal bone scans in patients with newly diagnosed prostate cancer. Urology 1996; 47: 708–12.

29. Freitas JE, Gilvydas R, Ferry DJ et al. The clinical utility of PSA and bone scintigraphy in prostate cancer follow-up. J Nucl Med 1991; 32: 1387–90.

30. Leo ME, Bilhartz DL, Bergstralh EJ et al. Prostate-specific antigen in hormonally treated stage D2 prostate cancer: is it always an accurate indicator of disease status? J Urol 1991; 145: 802–6.

30. Lin K, Szabo Z, Chin et al. The value of baseline bone scans in patients with newly diagnosed prostate cancer. Clin Nucl Med 1999; 24: 579–82.

32. Wolff JM, Zimny M, Borchers H et al. Is prostate-specific antigen a reliable marker of bone metastasis in patients with newly diagnosed cancer of the prostate? Eur Urol 1998; 33: 376–81.

33. Bruwer G, Heyns CF and Allen FJ. Influence of local tumour stage and grade on reliability of serum prostate specific antigen in predicting skeletal metastases in patients with adenocarcinoma of the prostate. Eur Urol 1999; 35: 223–7.

34. Lorente JA, Valenzuela H, Morote J et al. Serum bone alkaline phosphatase levels enhance the clinical utility of prostate specific antigen in the staging of newly diagnosed prostate cancer patients. Eur J Nucl Med 1999; 26: 625–32.

35. Ercole CJ, Lange PH, Mathisen M et al. Prostatic specific antigen and prostatic acid phosphatase in monitoring and staging of patients with prostatic cancer. J Urol 1987; 138: 1181–4.

36. Smith PH, Bono A, Calais da Silva F et al. Some limitations of the radioisotope bone scan in patients with metastatic prostatic cancer. A subanalysis of EORTC trial 30853. The EORTC Urological Group. Cancer 1990; 66(5 Suppl): 1009–16.

37. Stokkel M, Zwinderman A, Zwartendijk J et al. The value of pre-treatment clinical and biochemical parameters in patients with newly diagnosed, untreated prostate carcinoma and no

indications for bone metastasis on bone scintigraphy. Eur J Nucl Med 1997; 24: 1215–20.

38. Hetherington JW, Siddall JK and Cooper EH. Contribution of bone scintigraphy, prostatic acid phosphatase and prostate specific antigen to the monitoring of prostate cancer. Eur Urol 1988; 14: 1–5.

39. Palmer E, Henrickson K, McKusick K et al. Pain as an indicator of bone metastasis. Acta Radiol 1988; 29: 445–9.

40. Kodusa S, Kaji T, Yokoyama H et al. Does bone SPECT actually have lower sensitivity for detecting vertebral metastasis than MRI? J Nucl Med 1996; 37: 975–8.

41. Han LJ, Au-Yong, Tong WC et al. Comparison of bone single-photon emission tomography and planar imaging in the detection of vertebral metastasis in patients with back pain. Eur J Nucl Med 1998; 25: 635–8.

42. Savelli G, Maffioli M, Maccauro E et al. Bone scintigraphy and the added value of SPECT in detecting skeletal lesions Q J Nucl Med 2001; 45: 27–37.

43. Erdi YE, Humm JL, Imbriaco M et al. Quantitative bone metastases analysis based on image segmentation. J Nucl Med 1997; 38: 1401–6.

44. Imbriaco M, Larson SM, Yeung HW et al. A new parameter for measuring metastatic bone involvement by prostate cancer: the Bone Scan Index. Clin Cancer Res 1998; 4: 1765–72.

45. Bourgeois P, Malarme M. Van Franck R et al. Bone scintigraphy in prostatic carcinomas. Nucl Med Commun 1991; 12: 35–45.

46. Effert PJ, Bares R, Handt S et al. Metabolic imaging of untreated prostate cancer by positron emission tomography with 18 fluorine-labelled deoxyglucose. J Urol 1996; 155: 994–8.

47. Sanz G, Robles JE, Gimenez M et al. Positron emission tomography with 18 fluorine-labelled deoxyglucose: utility in localised and advanced prostate cancer. BJU International 1999; 84: 1028–31.

48. Ricchiuti VS, Hass C, Resnick MI et al. The accuracy of PET scanning in detecting prostatic fossa recurrence after radical prostatectomy. J Urol 1999; 161:393.

49. Shreve PD, Grossman HB, Gross MD, Wahl RL. Metastatic prostate cancer: initial findings of PET with 2-deoxy-2-[F-18]fluoro-D-glucose. Radiology 1996: 751.

50. Yeh SDJ, Imbriaco M, Garza D et al. Twenty percent of bony metastases of hormone resistant prostate cancer are detected by PET FDG whole body scanning. J Nucl Med 1995; 36(Suppl): 198.

51. Oyama N, Akino H, Kanamaru H et al. Fluorodeoxyglucose positron emission tomography in the diagnosis of untreated prostate cancer. Nippon Rinsho 1998; 56: 2052–5.

52. Saltzer M, Nerth J, Cangiano T et al. Comparison of computer tomography (CT), positron emission tomography (PET) and monoclonal antibody scan (MAB) for evaluation lymph node metastases in patients with PSA relapse after treatment for localised prostate cancer (CAP). In: Proceedings of the American Urological Association Congress, 1998.

53. Schirrmeister H, Guhlmann A, Elsner K et al. Sensitivity in detecting osseous lesions depends on anatomical localisation: planar bone scintigraphy versus 18F PET. J Nucl Med 1999; 40: 1623–9.

54. Inaba T. Quantitative measurements of prostatic blood flow and blood volume by positron emission tomography. J Urol 1992; 148: 1457–60.

55. Goldberg DM, DeLand FH, Bennett SJ et al. Radioimmuno-detection of prostatic cancer: in vivo use of radioactive antibodies against prostatic acid phosphatase for diagnosis and detection of prostatic cancer by nuclear imaging. JAMA 1983; 250: 630–5.

56. Dillman RO, Beauregard J, Ryan KP et al. Radioimmuno-detection of cancer with the use of [111]I labelled monoclonal antibody. J Natl Cancer Inst Monogr 1987; 3: 33–6.

57. Wynant GE, Murphy GP, Horoszewicz JS et al. Immunoscintigraphy of prostate cancer: preliminary results with [111]I labelled monoclonal antibody 7E11C5.3 CYT-356. Prostate 1991; 18: 229–41.

58. Polascik TJ, Manyak MJ, Haseman MK et al. Comparison of clinical staging algorithms and 111 indium–capromab pendetide immunoscintigraphy in the prediction of lymph node involvement in high risk prostate carcinoma patients. Cancer 1999; 85: 1586–92.

59. Murphy GP, Elgamal AA, Troychak MJ et al. Follow-up ProstaScint scans verify detection of occult soft-tissue recurrence after failure of primary prostate cancer therapy. Prostate 2000; 42: 315–17.

60. Hinkle GH, Burgers JK, Neal CE et al. Multicenter radioimmunoscintigraphic evaluation of patients with prostate carcinoma using [111]I capromab pendetide. Cancer 1998; 83: 739–47.

61. Haseman MK, Reed NL and Rosenthal SA. Monoclonal antibody imaging of occult prostate cancer in patients with elevated PSA. PET and biopsy correlation. Clin Nucl Med 1996; 21: 704–13.

62. Saltzer MA, Barbaric Z, Belldegrum A et al. Comparison of helical CT, PET and monoclonal antibody scans for evaluation of lymph node metastases in patients with PSA relapse after treatment for localised prostate cancer. J Urol 1999; 162: 1322–8.

63. Babaian RJ, Sayer J, Podoloff D et al. Radioimmunoscintigraphy of pelvic lymph nodes with [111]I labelled monoclonal antibody CYT-356. J Urol 1994; 153: 1952–5.

64. Quintana JC and Blend MJ. The dual-isotope ProstaScint imaging procedure: clinical experience and staging results in 145 patients. Clin Nucl Med 2000; 25: 33–40.

65. Britton KE, Feneley H, Jan VU et al. Prostate cancer: the contribution of nuclear medicine. BJU Int 2000; 86(Suppl 1): 135–42.

66. Pasteau O, Degrais P. De L'emploi du radium dans le traitement des cancer de la prostate. J Urol Med Chir 1913; 4: 314–66.

67. Barringer BS. Radium in the treatment of carcinoma of the bladder and prostate. JAMA 1917; 68: 1227.

68. Whitmore WF, Hilaris BS, Grabstald H. Retropubic implantation of iodine 125 in the treatment of prostate cancer. J Urol 1972; 108: 918–20.

69. Holm HH, Jul N, Pedersen JF et al. Transperineal 125-iodine seed implantation in prostatic cancer guided by trans-rectal ultrasonography. J Urol 1983; 130: 283–6.

70. Blasko JC, Wallner K and Grimm PD. PSA based disease control following ultrasound-guided I-125 implantation for stage T1/T2 prostate carcinoma. J Urol 1995; 154: 1096–9.

71. Ragde H, Balasko JC, Grimm PD et al. Interstitial iodine 125 radiation without adjuvant therapy in the treatment of clinically localised prostate carcinoma. Cancer 1997; 80: 442–53.

72. Li S, Liu J, Zhang et al. Rhenium-188 help to treat painful bone metastases. Clin Nucl Med 2001; 26: 919–22.

73. Paszkowski AL, Hewitt DJ, Taylor A Jr. Disseminated intravascular coagulation in a patient treated with strontium-89 for metastatic carcinoma of the prostate. Clin Nucl Med 1999; 24: 852–4.

74. Turner SL, Gruenewald S, Spry N, Gebski V. Less pain does equal better quality of life following strontium-89 therapy for metastatic prostate cancer. Br J Cancer 2001; 84: 297–302.

75. Kraeber-Bodere F, Campion L, Rousseau C et al. Treatment of bone metastases of prostate cancer with strontium-89 chloride: efficacy in relation to the degree of bone involvement. Eur J Nucl Med 2000; 27: 1487–93.

Section III

Benign disease of the prostate

10

Cysts and congenital anomalies of the prostate and ejaculatory ducts

Dennis Ll Cochlin

General considerations

Cysts in the prostate occur commonly in middle-aged and elderly men, in whom most are acquired and of little significance. Prostatic cysts are less common in young men, in whom most are congenital. Some of these (although only a minority) are clinically significant. Certain types of cyst are significant because they are associated with other urogenital anomalies, while others are important because they may be associated with infertility. A minority of cysts develop complications, principally infection, calculi, and (very rarely) malignancy. The largest proportion of congenital cysts that are detected are found incidentally in men being examined for suspected prostatic cancer. Most of these men have no associated anomalies or complications, and have been fertile. It must therefore be assumed that only a minority of congenital cysts are clinically significant.

Acquired prostatic cysts

Acquired cysts are the most common type of prostatic cysts in middle-aged and elderly men. They are small, typically less than 5 mm and rarely more than 1 cm in diameter. They are common in the hyperplastic inner gland of benign prostatic hypertrophy (BPH), although they may also occur in the outer gland. Those found in the hyperplastic inner gland of BPH have been shown to be caused by haemorrhagic degeneration.[1] The aetiology of those not associated with BPH, particularly those occurring in the outer gland, is unproven. There is a theory that these cysts may result from chronic outlet obstruction.[2] There is evidence that they may be more common in patients who have had repeated urinary tract

infections.[3] It is also possible that, like renal cysts, they simply become more common with increasing age.

Acquired prostatic cysts have the same ultrasonic characteristics as simple cysts anywhere in the body. They are thin-walled with anechoic contents. The larger ones exhibit posterior acoustic enhancement, although this may not be appreciated in small cysts (Figure 10.1). They are often multiple. A frequent pattern is a group of closely packed very small cysts (Figure 10.2). Some cysts have an irregular shape, perhaps reflecting their origin from areas of haemorrhagic necrosis (Figure 10.3). Irregularity is not a cause for concern, since the vast majority of prostatic parenchymal cysts are benign.[1]

Acquired cysts are of little clinical significance. Large tense cysts in the posterior part of the gland may sometimes be

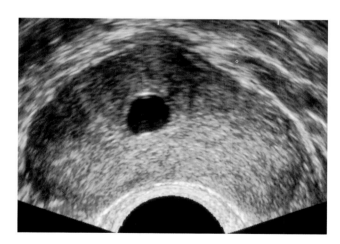

Figure 10.1
Simple acquired cyst. A typical simple prostatic cyst is seen in the inner gland.

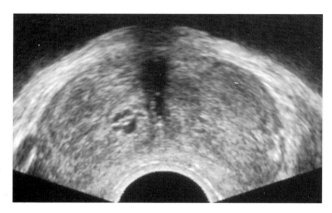

Figure 10.2
Simple acquired cysts. A group of closely packed simple cysts are seen in the inner gland.

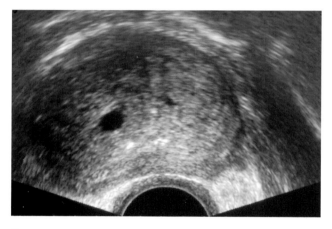

Figure 10.3
Simple acquired cyst. This cyst is irregular in outline. Irregularity in prostatic cysts is of no clinical importance.

palpable on digital rectal examination and may mimic prostatic cancer. Some cysts seen on a transrectal ultrasound study may be difficult to distinguish from hypoechoic tumours, although this is becoming less of a problem as the resolution of ultrasound systems improves. If this dilemma occurs during a study of suspected prostatic cancer, it is best to biopsy the suspected area. A lesion that is a cyst will visibly deflate during the biopsy. If the lesion is solid, the histology of the biopsy core will establish the nature of the lesion (Figure 10.4).

Congenital prostatic cysts

Three types of lesions are commonly termed congenital prostatic cysts, although two of them are not true cysts. A Müllerian duct cyst is a true cyst. A congenitally enlarged

prostatic utricle and an ejaculatory duct cyst are diverticulae. In addition, some prostatic parenchymal cysts, particularly those in the outer gland, may be congenital.

A congenitally enlarged prostatic utricle (often termed a utricular cyst) and Müllerian duct cysts both occur in essentially the same embryonic anlage, although their aetiology and significance are different. In order to facilitate an understanding of these cysts, a brief review of the embryology is given here.

Basic embryology

The Müllerian ducts (also termed the paramesonephric ducts) are paired structures present in the early embryo in both sexes. In the female, they develop into the uterus and possibly also a portion of the vagina. In the male, they largely atrophy owing to the effect of testosterone, but a small portion remains in the form of the testicular appendices and the fused caudal parts that form the prostatic utricle. The prostatic utricle is therefore a homologue of the female uterus – hence its name. The Müllerian ducts and prostatic utricle are derived from the same embryonic structure. Congenitally enlarged prostatic utricles and Müllerian duct cysts differ in their anatomic location and in their communication with the urethra. The prostatic utricle always communicates with the urethra at the level of the verumontanum.

The ejaculatory ducts are formed from the Wolffian ducts. In response to hormonal stimulation by testosterone, various Wolffian structures develop, including the epididymes, vasa deferentia, seminal vesicles, and ejaculatory ducts.[5–8]

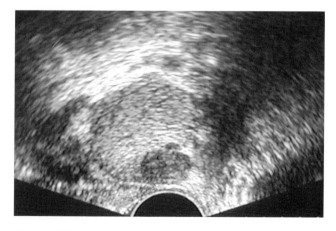

Figure 10.4
Cyst simulating tumour. The medium-echodensity rounded lesion in the outer gland was thought to be a cancer. On biopsy, it partly deflated. The biopsy core showed some solid tissue and some debris, with no malignant change. The medium-echodensity contents may be due to a previous bleed into the cyst.

Congenitally enlarged prostatic utricle

The terminology of this condition may be misleading. Congenital enlargement of the prostatic utricle is termed a utricular cyst, although the lesion is not a true cyst. To add to the confusion, Müllerian duct cysts are sometimes called utricular cysts. In the interests of clarity and anatomic accuracy, the terms 'congenitally enlarged prostatic utricle' and 'Müllerian duct cyst' should be used for the two separate conditions, and the term 'utricle cyst' should be dropped.

The prostatic utricle is derived from the Müllerian and Wolffian ducts as well as the urogenital sinus. During the standard embryonic development of the prostate, the utricle atrophies to a small, insignificant structure. Failure of this atrophy results in a congenitally enlarged prostatic utricle.

Development of the prostate and penis depends upon 5α reductase, a hormone secreted by the urogenital sinus that converts testosterone to dihydrotestosterone. It is probable that a variable deficiency of this enzyme causes an enlarged prostatic utricle.[9,10] This biochemical deficiency may also account for the association of congenitally enlarged utricle with congenital anomalies of the penis.

A congenitally enlarged prostatic utricle is a diverticular projection from the posterior wall of the prostatic urethra. There are always associated genital anomalies. Hypospadias is by far the most common. Ambiguous genitalia, undescended testes and congenital urethral polyps are less common associations (Table 10.1).[11] The size of the utricle varies, as does the position of the neck. They have been graded by Ikama et al[12] according to their appearance at urethrography (Figure 10.5). About 15–40% of boys with hypospadias have a congenitally enlarged utricle, whose size is approximately related to the severity of the hypospadias (Table 10.2).[13]

Congenitally enlarged utricles are usually found when performing urethrography as part of the workup of hypospadias or ambiguous genitalia. The enlarged diverticular projection fills with contrast, although sometimes only on descending urethrography and not on ascending urethrography (Figure 10.5).[14,15] An enlarged utricle may be found incidentally on transabdominal pelvic ultrasound studies as an ovoid anechoic

or low-echodensity structure lying posterior to the bladder (Figure 10.6). The history of associated genital anomalies helps to clarify the diagnosis in these cases. A congenitally enlarged prostatic utricle is rarely found in adults undergoing transrectal ultrasound. The appearance of an enlarged utricle may be identical to that of a Müllerian duct cyst (Figure 10.7). However, a history of hypospadias or another genital anomaly suggests the diagnosis of a congenitally enlarged utricle.

Table 10.1 Congenitally enlarged prostatic utricle: associated anomalies

- Hypospadias
- Ambiguous genitalia
- Undescended testes
- Congenital urethral polyps

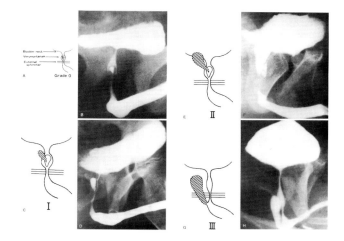

Figure 10.5
Congenitally enlarged prostatic utricle. Classification of congenitally enlarged prostatic utricles by urethrography. Reproduced with permission from Ikoma F, Shima H, Yabumoto H. Classification of enlarged prostatic utricle in patients with hypospadias. Br J Urol 1985; 57: 334–7.

Table 10.2 Relation between degree of enlargement of congenitally enlarged utricle and severity of hypospadias

	Percentage associated with congenitally enlarged utricle	Grade of hypospadias
Glandular hypospadias	10	0–I
Penile hypospadias	20	0–I
Penoscrotal hypospadias	30	0–II, occasionally III
Perineal and scrotal hypospadias	40	Usually III

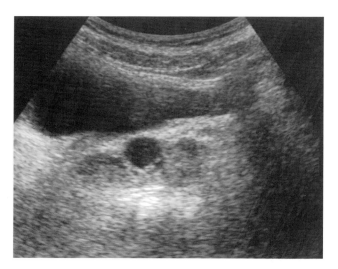

Figure 10.6
Congenitally enlarged prostatic utricle seen on a transabdominal scan through the full bladder in a teenage boy with a history of hypospadias.

A congenitally enlarged prostatic utricle is present in all cases of prune-belly syndrome. These utricles are invariably small and asymptomatic.[16]

Complications of a congenitally enlarged utricle are uncommon. They include chronic infection, with symptoms similar to prostatitis, and formation of calculi within the utricle. Calculi within the utricle cause no symptoms unless they become infected.

Müllerian duct cysts

Müllerian duct cysts occur when the Müllerian ducts fail to develop a communication with the urethra. Glands of Müllerian origin from the medial portion of the prostate become distended when prostatic secretions develop at the time of puberty. A midline cyst then develops in the prostate.[17–21] Rarely, the embryologically twin Müllerian ducts fail to fuse at their lower end as well as failing to communicate with the urethra. In this case, paired Müllerian duct cysts occur. This anomaly is usually associated with unilateral renal atrophy.[22]

Appearance

A Müllerian duct cyst is typically shaped like an inverted pear, although sometimes ovoid cysts occur. The neck of the cyst lies at the verumontanum, sometimes with a small dimple at its tip. The body extends for a variable distance cranially into

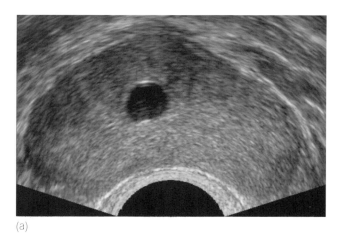

(a)

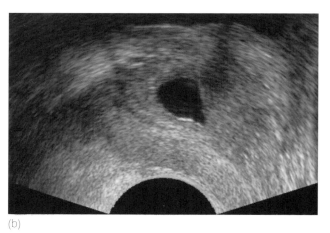

(b)

Figure 10.7
Congenitally enlarged prostatic utricle. A transrectal ultrasound scan performed for infertility in a 22-year-old man shows a midline enlarged utricle: (a) axial scan; (b) sagittal scan. The patient gave a history of repaired hypospadias. This is therefore a congenitally enlarged utricle.

and sometimes beyond the prostatic parenchyma (Figure 10.8). Cysts vary from a few millimetres in diameter to very large cysts with a volume of over a litre (Figure 10.9). The smaller ones are only visible on transrectal ultrasound or magnetic resonance imaging (MRI). The larger ones are visible on transabdominal pelvic ultrasound.

The contents of the cyst may be clear fluid, which is anechoic on ultrasound, low signal on T1-weighted and high signal on T2-weighted MRI. When cyst contents are mucoid they appear as medium echodensity on ultrasound (Figure 10.10),[23] and of medium signal on both T1- and T2-weighted MRI.[24–26] Infected cysts also have medium-echodensity contents and occasionally a fluid/fluid level (Figure 10.11). The wall of the cyst is usually thin. Infection, particularly chronic infection, however, causes thickening of the wall (Figure 10.12). Rings of small calculi are sometimes seen surrounding the cyst, lying in the openings of the prostatic ducts (Figure 10.13).

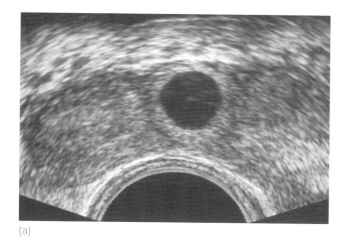

(a)

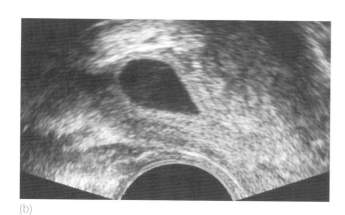

(b)

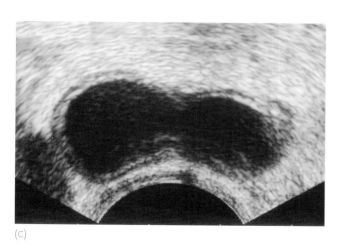

(c)

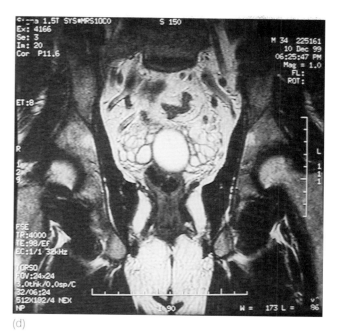

(d)

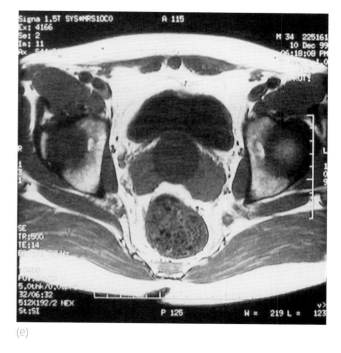

(e)

Figure 10.8

Müllerian duct cyst. (a,b) A typical pear-shaped Müllerian duct cyst is seen in the midline of the prostate: (a) axial view; (b) sagittal view. (c) A bilateral Müllerian duct cyst. (d,e) Magnetic resonance imaging (MRI) studies: (d) T2-weighted, with TR = 4000 and TE = 98. (e) T1-weighted, with TR = 500 and TE = 14. There is a midline Müllerian duct cyst with dilatation of the seminal vesicles secondary to ejaculatory duct obstruction.

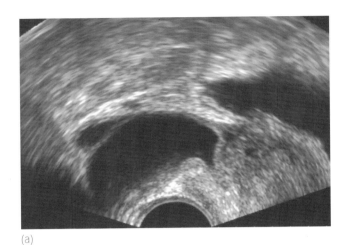

(a)

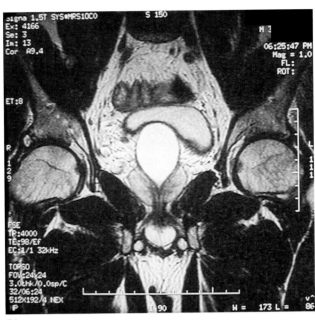

(b)

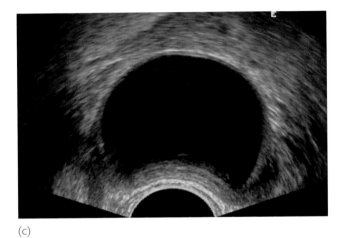

(c)

Figure 10.9

Large Müllerian duct cyst. (a) Transrectal ultrasound study. (b) T2-weighted MRI study, with TR = 4000 and TE = 98. These show a large Müllerian duct cyst. (c) A very large Müllerian duct cyst.

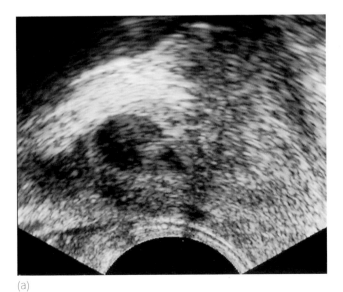

(a)

Figure 10.10

Mucinous Müllerian duct cyst. Sagittal (a) and (b) transrectal scans of a cyst with medium-echodensity contents, indicating a mucinous cyst. (c) Axial view of a cyst with very echodense contents. Because of the unusual appearance, the cyst was aspirated through a wide-bore needle and mucin was obtained.

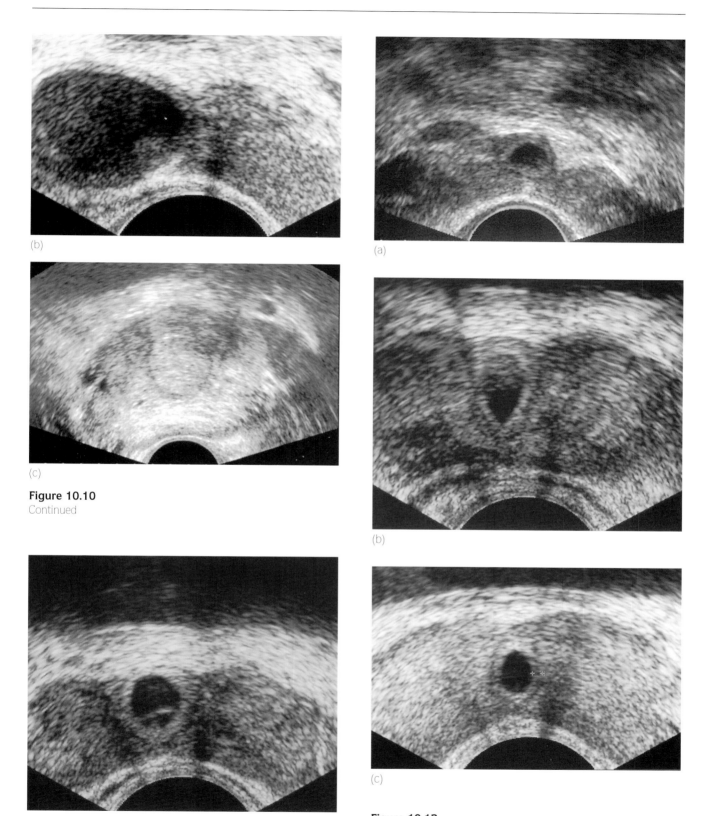

(b)

(a)

(c)

(b)

Figure 10.10
Continued

(c)

Figure 10.11
Infected Müllerian duct cyst. Layering is seen in this cyst. The patient had clinical symptoms of prostatitis. Aspiration revealed pus.

Figure 10.12
Chronically infected Müllerian duct cyst. (a–c) Thick-walled cysts in different patients with symptoms of prostatitis. These cysts are presumably chronically infected, although proof was not obtained.

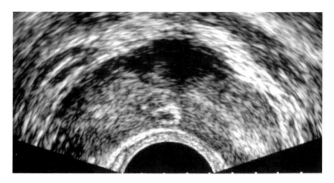

Figure 10.13
Calculi around a Müllerian duct cyst. A ring of calcifications is seen in the prostatic ducts around this small cyst.

Complications (Table 10.3)

Small Müllerian duct cysts are not infrequently found incidentally during transrectal ultrasound examinations in men who have never had any symptoms related to them. It is indeed likely that the majority of Müllerian duct cysts are asymptomatic and never develop any complications. Most men in whom these cysts are found incidentally have fathered children. Large Müllerian duct cysts may present in teenagers with symptoms of bladder outlet obstruction similar to those of BPH.[27] The symptoms are due to a pressure effect on the urethra. Large cysts may displace the verumontanum and cause angulation of the urethra. They may also push the bladder base upwards.[28,29] Very large cysts have been reported as causing erosion of the pubic bones.[28]

Müllerian duct cysts may cause infertility in one of two ways. The presence of a Müllerian duct cyst may be associated with embryonic failure of the Wolffian ducts to communicate with the urethra. In this case, the blind-ending ejaculatory ducts do not deliver sperm into the urethra. In other cases, the cyst itself may obstruct otherwise normal ejaculatory ducts by a pressure effect. Aspiration of the cyst may relieve the obstruction and result in fertility.[23,25,30,31]

However, these cysts may recur after simple aspiration, and may require surgical deroofing.[32] The fact that many small Müllerian duct cysts are found incidentally in fertile men suggests that a small cyst may also be an incidental finding in a patient with infertility due to other causes.

Müllerian duct cysts may become infected. In these cases, symptoms are those of prostatitis. Diagnosis is important, since aspiration of the cyst aids treatment. Infected cysts may have echogenic contents, sometimes with layering. In other cases, however, the contents remain anechoic. Chronically infected cysts may develop a thick wall (Figure 10.11).[32,33]

Calculi may develop in some cysts. Simple calculi are asymptomatic, but may predispose the prostate to infection. Calculi within the utricle may present on imaging studies as a diagnostic puzzle of a highly echogenic calcification with posterior acoustic shadowing lying posterior to the urethra (Figure 10.14).[13]

Malignant change has been reported in Müllerian duct cysts. Published studies have reported malignant change in up to 3%.[7,34,35] The author's experience, however, suggests a lower risk. Excision of a Müllerian duct cyst is, in any case, technically very difficult because of its location. It is therefore not normal practice to excise an uncomplicated Müllerian duct cyst.

Ejaculatory duct cysts

The ejaculatory ducts and vasa deferentia are derived from the Wolffian ducts in response to testosterone. Cysts of the ejaculatory ducts are congenital and may be associated with other congenital anomalies of the ejaculatory ducts. These anomalies include discontinuity of the ejaculatory duct, which may cause azoospermia.[5–8]

Table 10.3 Müllerian duct cysts: complications (the majority are asymptomatic)

- Large cysts cause bladder outlet obstruction in teenagers
- Infertility due to pressure
- Infertility due to ejaculatory duct agenesis
- Bilateral cysts can be associated with unilateral renal agenesis
- Infection, giving symptoms of prostatitis
- Calculus, causing predisposition to infection
- Malignancy: up to 3% (possibly rarer)

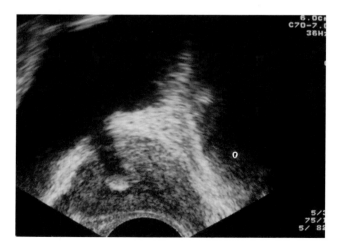

Figure 10.14
Calculus in a Müllerian duct cyst. This calculus lying posterior to the urethra was removed because of chronic infection. It lay in a Müllerian duct cyst.

Ejaculatory duct cysts are actually diverticula of the ducts that retain a communication with the ducts. They may be bilateral or unilateral. They tend to lie slightly to the side of the midline, along the course of the ejaculatory ducts. Occasionally, however, they lie in the midline with both ducts opening into the cyst. They are usually small, rarely more than 1 cm. However, larger cysts, particularly those lying in the midline, may occur.

Imaging appearances

The ultrasonic and MRI appearances of ejaculatory duct cysts are rounded, thin-walled cysts with fluid contents that are anechoic on ultrasound and of low signal on T1-weighted and high signal on T2-weighted MRI (Figure 10.15). Infected or haemorrhagic cysts have contents of mixed echogenicity and variable MRI signal (Figure 10.16). Infected cysts may have a thick wall (Figure 10.17).[23,25,26]

The ejaculatory ducts from which the cysts arise may be dilated, in which case the ducts are seen as tubular structures adjacent to the cyst. Normal-sized ejaculatory ducts are inconsistently demonstrated on transrectal ultrasound or MRI as very fine tubular structures, 0.4–0.8 mm in diameter.[36] With high-resolution ultrasound systems, however, the ducts are seen in most young men. Even when the ducts are shown, however, communication with the cyst is not visualized (Figure 10.18). The diagnosis of ejaculatory duct cysts is therefore assumed when cysts are seen bilaterally, or when they are unilateral but lie in the appropriate location, particularly in young men. Dilated ejaculatory ducts and a history of infertility make the diagnosis even more likely. Midline cysts are more problematic. Based upon the appearance of midline prostatic cysts, both on ultrasound and MRI, it is often not possible to distinguish between ejaculatory and Müllerian duct cysts. The definitive distinction may only be made by vasography.[37]

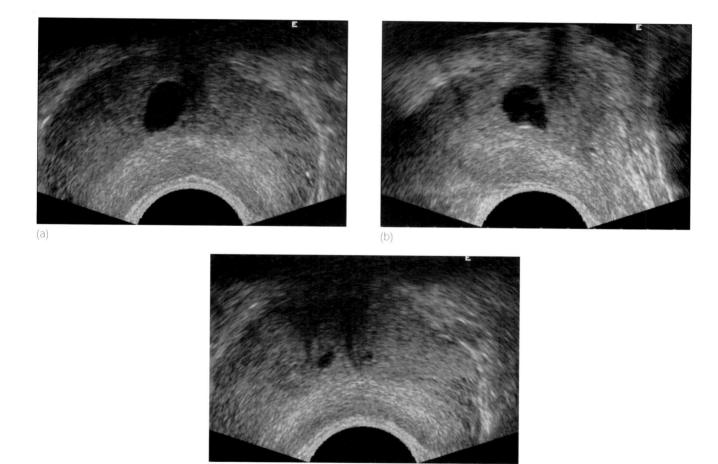

(a)

(b)

(c)

Figure 10.15
Ejaculatory duct cyst: (a) axial view; (b) sagittal view. These show a cyst just to the right of the midline. (c) The ejaculatory duct above the cyst is dilated. (There is also borderline dilation of the left duct.)

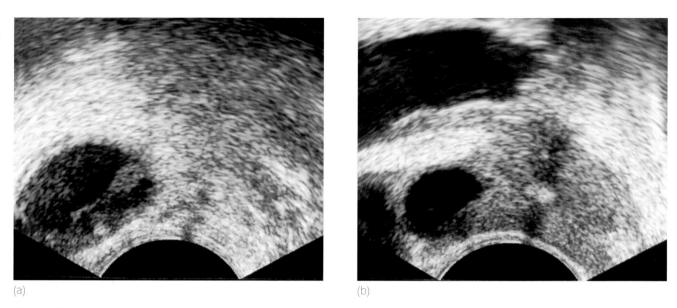

(a)

(b)

Figure 10.16
Echogenic ejaculatory duct cyst. (a) A large, echogenic infected cyst. (b) An infected cyst with layered contents.

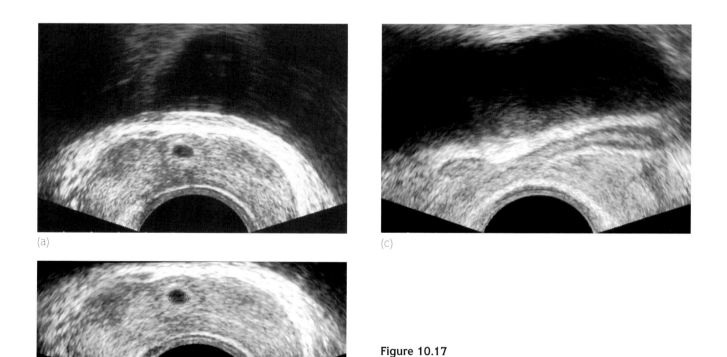

(a)

(c)

(b)

Figure 10.17
Thick-walled ejaculatory duct cyst. (a,b) A thick-walled ejaculatory duct cyst, probably infected. (c) Debris in the lumina of the proximal vasa deferentia.

Symptoms

Ejaculatory duct cysts are often, although probably not invariably, associated with infertility. In many cases, this is caused by obstructive azoospermia due to associated obstruction of the ducts, resulting from either congenital anomalies of the duct or, less often, pressure from the cysts. Haematospermia, a symptom traditionally regarded as being most often

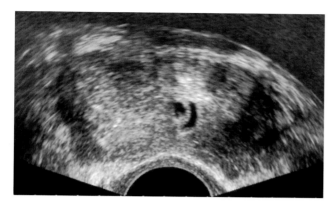

Figure 10.18
Ejaculatory duct cyst. A small cyst is seen adjacent to the dilated left ejaculatory duct, but no communication can be demonstrated between the cyst and the duct.

idiopathic, is often found in patients with ejaculatory duct cysts. Painful ejaculation is another symptom described. If infected, the symptoms are those of prostatitis.[23,25,26]

Other congenital anomalies of the ejaculatory ducts

The other important congenital anomalies are congenital obstruction (often associated with cysts), agenesis, and ectopic insertion of a ureter into a dysplastic seminal vesicle–ejaculatory duct complex.

The normal ejaculatory ducts are very fine tubular structures about 0.4–0.8 mm in diameter,[36] lying just to each side of the midline, slightly posterior to the plane of the urethra. As already mentioned they are difficult to visualize on transrectal ultrasound, but with high-resolution equipment can usually be seen in young men (Figure 14.2). In the setting of BPH, they are difficult or impossible to see. As they are not detectable in all normal patients, total aplasia may only be truly diagnosed by vasography. Dilatation of the ducts to more than 1 mm in diameter makes it highly likely that they are obstructed – either from congenital obstruction or acquired obstruction. The latter can be secondary to urethritis,[45] it can be due to pressure from a Müllerian duct or ejaculatory duct cyst, or it can be caused by a calculus. Calculi are easily detectable on the transrectal ultrasound study. Confirmation of atrophy or obstruction may be obtained from vasography. MRI may also demonstrate the normal and abnormal ejaculatory ducts, but has little or no benefit over good-quality transrectal ultrasound. An ectopic ureter may enter an abnormal, dysplastic seminal vesicle–ejaculatory duct complex (this complex has been

termed the common duct[39]) (Figure 10.19). Symptoms include recurrent episodes of epididymo-orchitis. The diagnosis is made by intravenous urogram[19] or computed tomography urogram (CTU). The ectopic ureter, which is usually single, is seen to drain via the common sinus, because the seminal vesicles fill with contrast.

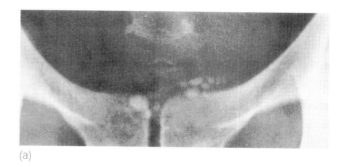

(a)

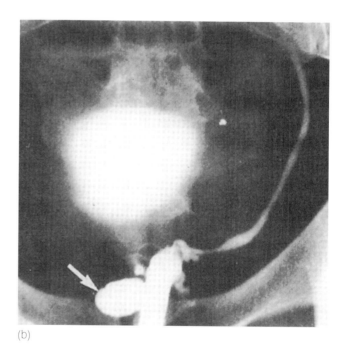

(b)

Figure 10.19
Ectopic ureter inserted into the vas deferens. An ectopic left ureter terminates in a left common duct with the seminal vesicle. (a) A preliminary radiograph of the pelvis shows calculi in the left common duct and the left seminal vesicle extending over to the right. (b) Transurethral injection of contrast into the left common duct outlines the left seminal vesicle, which extends over to the right (arrow), as well as the distal end of the left ectopic ureter. Reproduced with permission from Nino-Murcia M, Friedland WG, de Vries PA. Congenital anomalies of the male genitalia. In: Clinical Urography. Vol 1 (Pollack HM, McClennan BL, eds). Philadelphia: WB Saunders, 2000: 872.

Congenital parenchymal cysts

Congenital cysts of the prostatic parenchyma also occur. They are usually small and asymptomatic, although it is reported that they may cause outlet obstruction by pressure on the urethra. They may be palpated on digital rectal examination if they lie posteriorly, and they may displace the urethra. When these cysts are hard to palpation, they may simulate prostatic cancer. They are assumed to result from dilatation of blind-ending prostatic ducts. When aspirated, they do not contain sperm. It is impossible on imaging to distinguish congenital prostatic parenchymal cysts from acquired cysts, although they are probably separate entities. The occasional occurrence of parenchymal cysts in young men without prostatic hypertrophy or the presence of cysts in the outer gland does suggest that they are congenital (Figure 10.20).[24,40]

Urethral diverticula and peri-urethral cysts

Urethral diverticula and cysts in the prostatic urethra cause cystic lesions within the prostatic parenchyma that are difficult to distinguish from prostatic cysts.

Acquired urethral diverticula are uncommon in the male. They may occur following repeated catheterization.[41] Some may occur when a prostatic abscess ruptures into the urethra.[42,43]

Appearances are extremely variable. Both cysts and diverticula may have smooth or irregular walls, they may be unilocular or multilocular, and they may have wide or narrow necks (Figure 10.21). Their lumina sometimes contain calculi.[42]

Benign periurethral cysts may also occur in the prostatic urethra. Transrectal ultrasound will show a cyst close to the urethra, but will not demonstrate its communication with the urethra (Figure 10.22). Puncture of the cysts during transrectal ultrasound with aspiration of the contents and injection of contrast under fluoroscopic control will demonstrate a connection with the urethra if one exists.[3] Other diagnostic procedures that may be used are urethrography and sono-urethrography.[44,45]

Congenital hypoplasia of the prostate

Congenital hypoplasia is a condition in which the prostate is apparently absent. In reality, a very small volume of prostatic

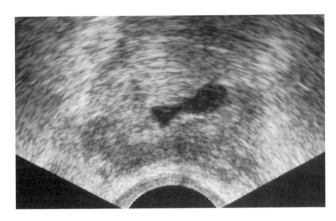

Figure 10.21
Urethral diverticulum. The diverticulum is seen to extend from the urethra in this micturating transrectal ultrasound study.

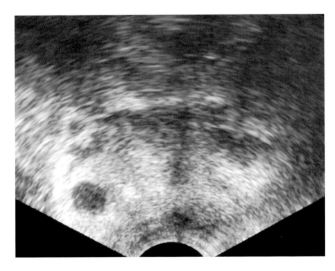

Figure 10.20
Congenital prostatic cyst. This cyst lies in the outer gland in a young man, suggesting that it is congenital.

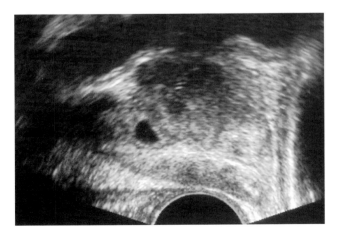

Figure 10.22
Periurethral cyst. A cyst is seen adjacent to the urethra. Urethrography revealed that this was a periurethral cyst.

tissue is always present in the posterior part of the gland (Figure 10.23). The verumontanum is small or absent and the prostatic urethra is dilated and elongated, often with a diverticular projection from its posterior wall. This condition is most commonly, although not invariably, found in patients with prune-belly syndrome.

The most commonly used imaging modality is urethrography, which demonstrates the associated urethral abnormalities.[46-51]

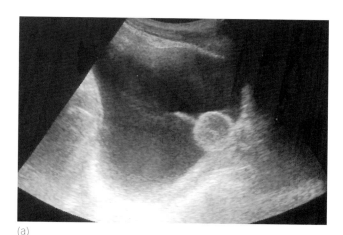

(a)

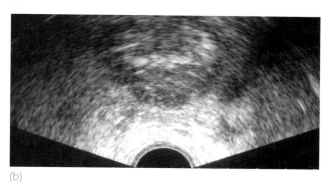

(b)

Figure 10.23
Congenital hypoplasia of the prostate: (a) transabdominal scan through the catheterized bladder; (b) transrectal scan. These show no discernible prostatic tissue

References

1. Hamper UM, Epstein JI, Sheth S et al. Cystic lesions of the prostate gland: a sonographic–pathologic correlation. J Ultrasound Med 1990; 9: 395–402.

2. Alexander AA. The prostate and seminal vescicles. In: Cochlin D LL et al, Urogenital Ultrasound: A Text Atlas. London: Martin Dunitz, 1994.

3. Rickards D. Interventional radiology in the lower urinary and genital tract. In: Pollack HM, Clinical Urography, 2nd edn. Philadelphia: WB Saunders, 2000.

4. hesbat PA. Urological Pathology. Philadelphia: Lea & Febiger, 1952. 886–988.

5. Johnson FP. The later development of the urethra in the male. J Urol 1920; 4: 447–501.

6. Lowsley OS. The development of the human prostate gland with reference to the development of other structures at the neck of the urinary bladder. Am J Anat 1912; 13: 299–349.

7. Cunha GR. Epithelial stromal interactions in the development of the urogenital tract. Int Rev Cytol 1976; 47: 137–94.

8. Glenister TW. The development of the utricle and the so-called 'middle' or 'median' lobe of the human prostate. J Anat (Lond) 1962; 96: 443–55.

9. Wilson JD, Lasnitzki I. Dihydrotestosterone formation in fetal tissues of the rabbit and rat. Endocrinology 1971; 89: 659.

10. Lasnitzki I, Mezuno T. Role of mesenchyma in the induction of the rat prostate by androgens in organ culture. J Endocrinol 1979; 82: 171–8.

11. Gregg DC, Sty JR. Sonographic diagnosis of enlarged prostatic utricle. J Ultrasound Med 1989; 8: 51–2.

12. Ikoma F, Shima H, Yabumoto H. Classification of enlarged prostatic utricle in patients with hypospadias. Br J Urol 1985; 57: 334–7.

13. Nino-Murcia M, Friedland GW, deVries PA. Congenital anomalies of the male genitalia. In: Clinical Urography, 2nd edn (Pollack HM, McClellan BL, eds). Philadelphia: WB Saunders, 2000: 872.

14. Myers GH Jr, Lynn HB, Kelalis PP. Giant cyst of the utricle. J Urol 1969; 101: 369–73.

15. Schuhrke TD, Caplan GW. Prostatic utricle cysts (Müllerian duct cysts). J Urol 1978; 119: 765–7.

16. Morgan RJ, Williams DI, Pryor JP. Müllerian duct remnants in the male. Br J Urol 1979; 51: 488–92.

17. Culbertson LR. Müllerian duct cysts. J Urol 1947; 58: 134–6.

18. Deming CL, Bernecke RR. Müllerian duct cysts. J Urol 1944; 51: 563–8.

19. Landes RR, Ransom CL. Müllerian duct cysts. J Urol 1949; 61: 1089–93.

20. Lloyd FA, Bennet D. Müllerian duct cysts. J Urol 1950; 64: 777–82.

21. Rusche C, Butler OW. Müllerian duct cysts. J Urol 1948; 59: 962–65.

22. McDermott V, Orr JD, Wild SR. Duplicated Müllerian duct remnants associated with unilateral renal agenesis. Abdom Imag 1993; 15: 193–5.

23. Kuligowska E, Fenlon HM. Transrectal US in male infertility: spectrum of findings and role in patient care. Radiology 1998; 207: 173–81.

24. McDermott VG, Meakem TG 3rd, Stolpen AH et al. Prostatic and periprostatic cysts: findings on MR imaging. AJR 1995; 164: 123–7.

25. Parsons RB, Fisher AM, Bar-Chama N, Mitty HA. MR imaging in male infertility. Radiographics 1997; 17: 627–37.

26. Choi IR, Lee MS, Rha KH et al. Magnetic resonance imaging in hemospermia. J Urol 1997; 157: 258–62.

27. Zhu JP, Mayhoff HH. Prostatic cyst. An unusual but important finding in male urogenital dysfunction. Scand J Urol Nephrol 1995; 29: 345–9.

28. Sanchez-Chapado M, Angulo JT. Giant Müllerian duct cyst mimicking prostatic malignancy. Scand J Urol Nephrol 1985; 29: 229–31.

29. Thambi Dorai CR, Couper RT, Smith AJ, Duwan PA. Müllerian duct cyst associated with posteriorly prolapsing verumontanum. Aust NZ J Surg 1997; 67: 63–5.

30. Hendry WF, Pryor JP. Müllerian duct (prostatic utricle) cyst: diagnosis and treatment in subfertile males. Br J Urol 1992; 69: 79–82.

31. Stricker HJ, Kunin JR, Foerber GJ. Congenital prostatic cyst causing ejaculatory duct obstruction: management by transrectal cyst aspiration. J Urol 1993; 149: 1141–3.

32. Halpern EJ, Hirsch IH. Sonographically guided transurethral laser incision of a Müllerian duct cyst for treatment of ejaculatory duct obstruction. AJR 2000; 175: 777–8.

33. Miglaeri R, Scarpa RM, Campus G, Usai E. Percutaneous drainage of utricular cyst under ultrasound guidance. Br J Urol 1988; 62: 385.

34. Ngheim HT, Kellman GM, Sandberg SA, Craig MM. Cystic lesions of the prostate. Radiographics 1990; 10: 635.

35. Carter SSC, Shinohara K, Lipshultz LI. Transrectal ultrasonography in disorders of the seminal vesicles and ejaculatory ducts. Urol Clin North Am 1989; 16: 773.

36. Jarrow JP. Transrectal ultrasound in infertile men. Fertil Steril 1993; 60: 1035–9.

37. Ford K, Carson CL III, Dunnick NR, et al. The role of seminal vesiculography in the evaluation of male infertility. Fertil Steril 1982; 37: 552–6.

38. Greenberg SH. Male reproductive tract sequelae of gonococcal and non-gonococcal urethritis. Arch Androl 1979; 3: 317.

39. Williams DI. Urology in childhood. Springer: New York, 1974: 139–143 and 195–212.

40. Siegel A, Snyder H, Duckett JW. Epididymitis in infants and boys: underlying urogenital anomalies and efficacy of imaging modalities. J Urol 1987; 138: 1100–3.

41. Seidman E, Hanno P (eds). Current Urologic Therapy. Philadelphia: WB Saunders, 1994:145.

42. Maged A. Urethral diverticula in males. Br J Urol 1965; 37: 566.

43. Marya S, Kumar S, Swanatar S. Acquired male urethral diverticulum. J Urol 1977; 118: 765.

44. Berman LH, Bearcroft PW. The urethra. In: Rifkin M, Cochlin D, Imaging of the Scrotum and Penis. London: Martin Dunitz, 2002.

45. Gluck CD, Bundy AL, Fine C et al. Sonographic urethrogram: comparison to roentgenographic techniques in 22 patients. J Urol 1988; 140: 1404–8.

46. Nunn IN, Stephens FD. The triad syndrome: a composite anomaly of the abdominal wall, urinary tract and testes. J Urol 1961; 86: 782.

47. Woodward JR. The prune-belly syndrome. Urol Clin North Am 1978; 5: 75–93.

48. Berdon WE, Baker DH, Wigger HJ, Blanc WA. The radiologic and pathologic spectrum of prune-belly syndrome. The importance of urethral obstruction in prognosis. Radiol Clin North Am 1977; 15: 83–92.

49. Kroovand RL, Al-Ansari RM, Perlmutter AD. Urethral and genital malformations in prune-belly syndrome. J Urol 1982; 127: 94–6.

50. Cremin BJ. The urinary tract anomalies associated with agenesis of the abdominal walls. Br J Radiol 1971; 44: 767.

51. Greskovich FJ III, Nyberg LM Jr. The prune-belly syndrome: a review of its etiology, defects, treatment and prognosis. J Urol 1988; 140: 707–12.

11

Benign prostatic hypertrophy

Dennis Ll Cochlin

General considerations

Benign prostatic hypertrophy (benign prostatic hyperplasia) is a condition that occurs to a greater or lesser extent in all men from middle age onwards, and causes progressive enlargement of the prostate. Histologically, it is a true hyperplasia, with an increase in the number of glandular elements associated with a degree of hypertrophy.[1] Hyperplasia and hypertrophy are both acceptable terms to describe the condition. In this chapter, the term benign prostatic hypertrophy is used, abbreviated to BPH. The prevalence of BPH at a given age appears to be similar in all countries, and has notably been studied in Scotland, UK,[2-3] Michigan, USA,[4] and Minnesota, USA.[5] Many studies demonstrate a similar prevalence of under 20% for men below age 50, rising to 50% between ages 50 and 80 years, and 80% for men in their eighties. A study of autopsy findings in Chinese men from Beijing showed a similar prevalence,[6] as did a comparative study comparing Japanese, American, and Scottish men[2] (Table 11.1). It appears from these studies that there is no significant racial difference in the prevalence of BPH. The actual cause of BPH is not known, although the condition is hormonally driven. Smoking has been suggested as a protective factor, as has beer

Table 11.1 Prevalence of benign prostatic hypertrophy (BPH), according to age

Age group (years)	Prevalence per 1000 men
0–49	138
50–59	237
60–69	430
70–79	400

drinking. Heavier men tend to have larger prostates. These factors, however, demonstrate only a weak association with the degree of hypertrophy.[7-10]

Benign prostatic hypertrophy occurs mainly in the transition zone, causing bilateral lobar enlargement, and, to a lesser degree, in the periurethral zone, causing central enlargement (Figure 11.1). The peripheral zone is affected to a far lesser degree, so that the outer gland is usually stretched and thinned by the inner gland BPH. In advanced cases, the outer gland may be thinned to a barely discernible rim.[1]

Symptoms

Symptoms related to BPH, loosely termed prostatism, are only weakly related to the degree of enlargement of the prostate or the pattern of enlargement.[11,12] The symptoms are those of bladder outlet obstruction. However, the mechanism is more complicated than simple mechanical obstruction. There is certainly an element of obstruction due to the prostatic enlargement, but additional factors, including changes in smooth muscle tone in the adenoma capsule and in the bladder neck, contribute to the obstruction.[13] Bladder outlet obstruction may take two forms. When obstructive symptoms predominate, there is difficulty passing urine, difficulty and slowness in initiating micturition, a poor stream, and dribbling at the end of the stream. When irritative symptoms predominate, the presentation includes urinary urgency and frequency. Although one form or the other may be predominant, symptoms of both usually coexist. Symptoms depend not only on the effect of the enlarged prostate but also on the response of the bladder. In an aging population, a proportion of men will develop bladder dysfunction unrelated to prostatic enlargement. Some elderly women will develop bladder

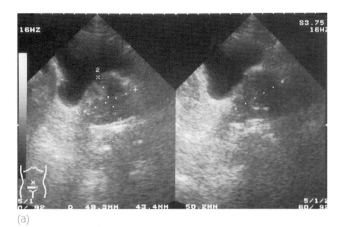

(a)

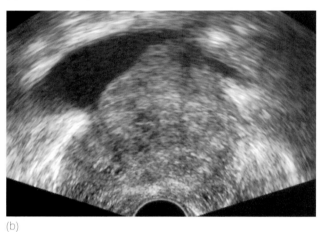

(b)

Figure 11.1

Benign prostatic hypertrophy (BPH) with median lobe hypertrophy: (a) transabdominal view; (b) transrectal scan. The median lobe of the prostate is enlarged and is bulging into the bladder.

outlet obstruction with the same symptoms as those found in elderly men.[14] The bladder outlet obstruction in these elderly men and women must be related to additional factors other than prostatic enlargement. These factors include obstruction, impaired detrussor contractibility, and detrussor instability.[15,16] Given the complexity of the situation and the variability of factors involved, it is not surprising that prostatism is poorly related to simple prostatic volume and that response to treatment is variable.

Symptoms of prostatism are common in older men, but may also be seen in middle-aged men. These symptoms are distressing and usually lead the patient to seek medical advice. Untreated bladder outlet obstruction due to BPH may lead to progressive hydronephrosis, with a reduction of renal function and ultimately renal failure. About 3% of patients with BPH will present with renal failure and its related symptoms, the earlier symptoms of disordered bladder emptying being absent or not sufficiently distressing for the patient to seek advice.[17,18]

Imaging

In the majority of patients with BPH, the diagnosis is made from the clinical history and a digital rectal examination of the prostate. Serum urea and creatinine levels are measured to assess whether the condition has affected renal functions. A diagnosis of BPH is made on clinical grounds. It is arguable that no imaging studies are necessary in these patients, and indeed this is the situation in some centres. Most centres, however, assess residual bladder volume as a further aid to deciding on treatment and as a baseline for further assessment of the patient.

Post-micturition bladder volume

Post-micturition bladder volume is determined by transabdominal ultrasound of the bladder. It is customary to first examine the full bladder and then to examine the bladder after voiding. It is not usually necessary to measure the volume of the filled bladder. However, if the patient feels full when there is only a small volume within the bladder, then it is worth measuring the maximum full volume. The post-voiding (post-micturition) residual volume is assessed with three orthogonal linear measurements (a, b, and c) of the bladder. Assuming an ellipsoidal shape (Figure 11.2), the volume is then calculated from the formula: $a \times b \times c \times \pi/6$ ($\approx a \times b \times c \times 0.52$). Accuracies of $\pm 15\%$ have been quoted for bladder volumes of less than 150 cm^3. The normal bladder empties completely. In practice, however, a small post-micturition residue is often found. It is important to remember that a short delay between micturition and measurement of the post-micturition volume can result in some refilling of the bladder. In practice, therefore, a post-micturition residue of less than 10 cm^3 is regarded as normal, and in older men, less than 20 cm^3 may be regarded as not clinically significant.[19–24] When a patient is asked to micturate before the bladder is reasonably full, a falsely high residual volume may remain. It is important to wait until the bladder holds at least 200 cm^3 of urine before the patient is asked to micturate.

In many clinics residual bladder volume is measured using a simple B-mode ultrasound device. These devices have the advantage that they are cheap, easy to use and eminently suitable for a clinic environment. However, only the bladder volume may be assessed. Prostatic volume cannot be measured nor can the upper tracts be assessed. Furthermore, any coincidental bladder tumours that may be present are not seen. For this reason, any patient with haematuria or raised urea or creatinine should have a full ultrasound study and, in the case of haematuria, cystoscopy. Perhaps the most worrying aspect of this method of measuring post-micturition residue is that any fluid-filled structures within

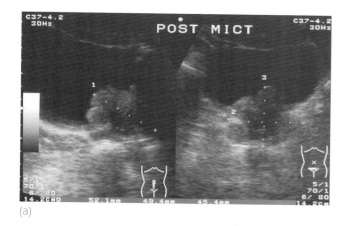
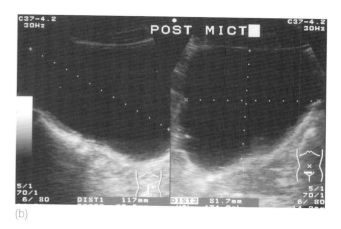

(a)

(b)

Figure 11.2

Prostate volume and post-micturition bladder volume. (a) The enlarged prostate is seen at the bladder base and its volume has been measured. (b) The post-micturition bladder volume has been measured. Both methods use three orthogonal measurements multiplied by 0.52 (formula for the volume of an ellipsoid).

the pelvis are measured as bladder. Errors have therefore occurred due to the presence of large ovarian cysts and bladder diverticulae.

Urine flow rate

Ultrasound assessment of post-micturition residue may be combined with measurements of urinary flow. The flow study produces a graphical representation of the rate of flow against time that reflects bladder function. A low peak flow rate is related to bladder outlet obstruction. A rate of less than 10 ml/s suggests obstruction; a rate of more than 15 ml/s is probably normal; a rate of between 10 and 15 ml/s is equivocal and requires further study by urodynamics. Unfortunately, there is a significant overlap among the flow rates of these patient groups (Table 11.2).[25] The shape of the flow curve may contribute additional information. The normal pattern demonstrates a prompt rise to maximum flow of more than 20 ml/s, a relatively smooth curve, and a rapid fall to zero at the end of micturition. Outlet obstruction with a high pressure but otherwise normally functioning bladder gives a slower rise and a low flat prolonged peak. An underactive detrussor muscle gives a

slow rise and an irregular peak, although the maximum flow rate may be normal. The anxious bladder, in which the muscle is oversensitive, gives a similar pattern but with slower contractions, while an atonic bladder gives more rapid intermittent contractions with low peaks. A painful bladder will give a similar pattern (Figure 11.3).

While the majority of patients with BPH will give a pattern ranging from normal to severe outlet obstruction, any of the other patterns may be superimposed. If this is the case, then treatment may be modified to reflect the bladder pathology as well as the prostatic enlargement.[26–34]

Urodynamic studies

Urodynamic studies combine urinary flow rate estimation with pressure recordings of the intravesicular pressure and the intrarectal pressure. This is achieved by using catheters connected to external pressure devices or pressure transducers within the bladder and rectum. The intrarectal pressure is a barometer of the intra-abdominal pressure. Subtraction of the intrarectal pressure from the intravesicular pressure gives the detrussor pressure. A normal bladder

Table 11.2   Numbers of patients with or without bladder outlet obstruction, according to peak urinary flow rate (total number of patients = 134). Reproduced with permission.[25]

	Maximum flow rate (ml/s)		
	>10	10–15	>15
Obstructed	106	41	10
Unobstructed	15	21	21

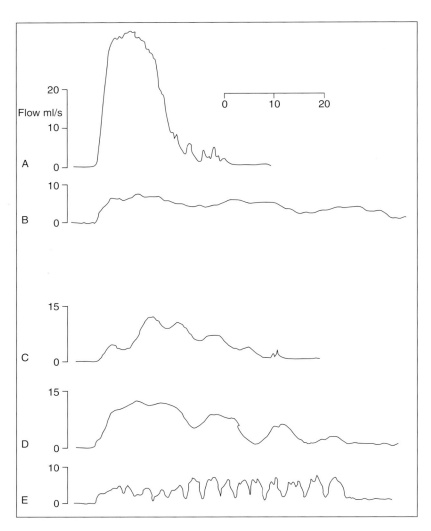

Figure 11.3
Typical urinary flow studies. (a) Normal.
(b) Obstructed. (c) Underactive detrussor muscle.
(d) Anxious bladder syndrome. (e) Atonic
bladder.

and bladder outlet will demonstrate a high flow rate and low detrussor pressure on micturition. Bladder outlet obstruction results in a low flow rate with high pressure. Poor detrussor function gives a low flow rate with low pressure (Figure 11.4). Flow and pressure studies may be combined with fluoroscopic studies of the contrast-filled bladder and urethra during bladder emptying. More detailed studies may incorporate urethral pressures and sphincter electromyography if neurogenic disease is suspected. A detailed discussion of urodynamics is outside the scope of this book, but can be found in the literature.[35–43]

Prostate size

When imaging the full bladder, the prostate size may be estimated. An estimate of prostate size is obtained by angling the transducer into a plane that extends behind the symphysis pubis to the bladder base and obtaining three orthogonal measurements of the prostate (Figure 11.2). The volume cal-

culation is the same as for bladder volume. It is customary to express the size of the prostate in terms of weight in grams. As the prostate is very nearly of water density (average specific gravity 1.05), the volume in cubic centimetres is the same as the weight in grams. Assessment of prostate size by this method is approximate but is sufficiently accurate for clinical purposes and more accurate that digital rectal examination.[44–48] In obese men, however, adequate visualization by this means may not be possible. It must be emphasized that transabdominal imaging of the prostate, while adequate for gross assessment of prostate size and patterns of enlargement, i.e. median or lateral lobe,[48] is inadequate for the detection of prostatic cancer.

Appearances of the bladder in BPH

Chronic bladder outlet obstruction leads to thickening of the bladder wall. When thickened, the loosely woven muscle

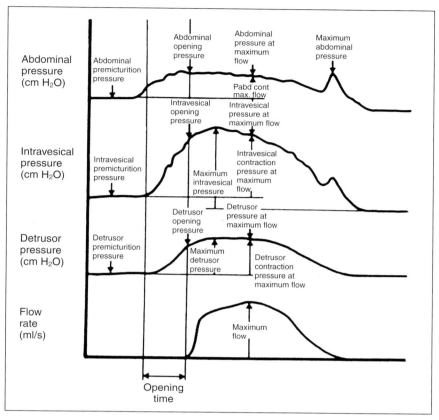

Figure 11.4
Urodynamic studies. (a) The parameters that should be measured according to the International Continence Society. (b) Patterns found in abnormal studies.

(a)

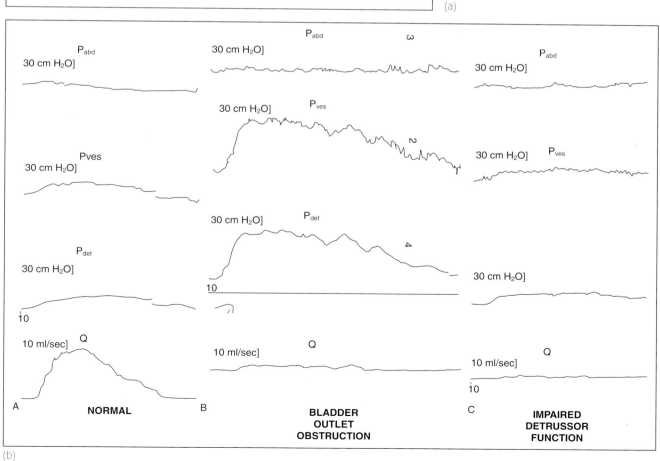

(b)

bundles of the bladder wall cause an irregular outline to the inner bladder wall known as trabeculation (Figure 11.5). This appearance is commonly called hypertrophy, although the thickening may be due to infiltration by collagen.[49] The thickness of the bladder wall may be measured. Normal bladder wall thickness varies with the degree of bladder filling. It has been suggested[52] that this variability may be overcome by measuring bladder wall thickness at a constant volume of 150 cm^3. In practice, the bladder volume is not critical, and, provided the bladder is neither over-full nor nearly empty, diagnostically useful measurements may be achieved (Figure 11.6). Furthermore, for management of patients with BPH, bladder wall measurement is rarely necessary, although a qualitative assessment is appropriate if the bladder wall is thick and trabeculated.[49,52]

Bladder diverticula may occur in cases of BPH, and should be recorded on the ultrasound examination as they may be missed on cystoscopy if narrow-necked (Figure 11.7).

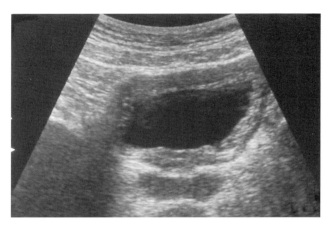

Figure 11.6
Thickened bladder wall. In this case the muscle is more hypertrophied than in Figure 11.5, giving a thick, slightly irregular bladder wall.

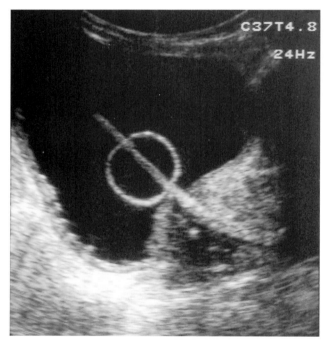

Figure 11.5
Trabeculated bladder. Thickening of the muscle is visible in the posterior wall of the bladder. The bladder is catheterized. The prostate is enlarged.

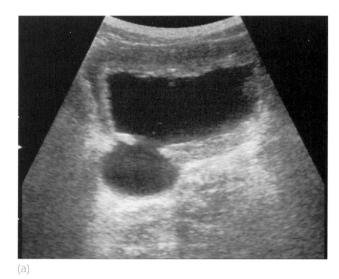

(a)

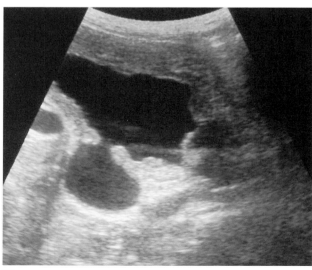

(b)

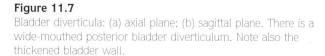

Figure 11.7
Bladder diverticula: (a) axial plane; (b) sagittal plane. There is a wide-mouthed posterior bladder diverticulum. Note also the thickened bladder wall.

The upper urinary tract in BPH

The upper tracts were traditionally examined in patients with BPH by intravenous urography (IVU) and more recently by ultrasound. The argument for these tests was they may detect hydonephrosis or renal tumours. The presence of hydronephrosis, however, does not affect management of BPH, and renal tumours are no more common in patients with BPH than those without. It is therefore no longer routine practice to examine the upper tracts in patients with BPH. An elevated serum creatinine, however, does indicate a need to examine the upper tracts, since renal failure may be related to outlet obstruction or due to other causes. Renal size, cortical echogenicity, and vascularity are important to assess. Haematuria in the setting of BPH is another legitimate reason for examination of the upper tract. Although BPH is a common cause of haematuria in older men, evaluation of the upper tracts should be performed to detect coexisting upper urinary tract tumours. Cystoscopy and bladder ultrasound are useful in such cases to further evaluate the urinary bladder.

The appearance of the prostate in BPH

Pathological descriptions of the development of BPH as briefly outlined earlier in the chapter are based on the classical description by O'Neil of the zonal anatomy of the prostate. While this description is embryologically accurate, the simpler pragmatic anatomy that divides the prostate into inner and outer glands is more appropriate for most clinical use. In the case of BPH, however, it is descriptively helpful to use the concept of medial and lateral lobes. These lobes do not exist anatomically, but may be used to describe areas of hyperplasia in BPH.

BPH primarily affects the inner gland, where it causes hypertrophy of the gland in the transitional zone and, to a lesser degree, in the periurethral area. Transition zone hypertrophy classically causes bilateral rounded nodules, descriptively termed lateral lobes. These nodules displace the outer gland outwards and thin it. The lateral lobes also compress the urethra, thus causing outlet obstruction (Figure 11.8). Hypertrophy of the periurethral glands is associated with so-called median lobe enlargement that bulges upwards into the bladder base and compresses the urethra from its posterior aspect (Figure 11.9). Both types of inner gland hypertrophy usually coexist, although one often predominates.

BPH may affect the outer gland histologically. In practice, however, inner gland hypertrophy predominates. Even when there is histologic evidence of hypertrophy in the peripheral and central zones, the outer gland is displaced outwards,

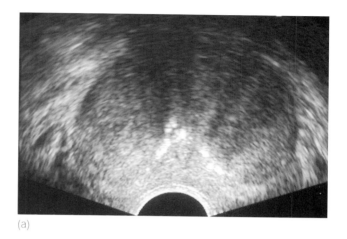

(a)

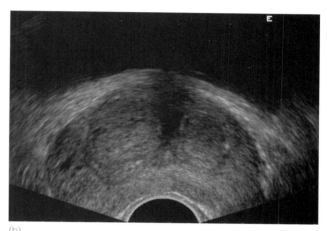

(b)

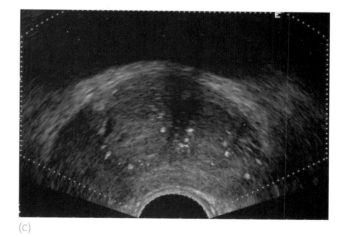

(c)

Figure 11.8

BPH: lateral lobe hypertrophy. (a) There is symmetrical enlargement of both lateral lobes causing thinning of the outer gland (although in this case the thinning was not marked). There is calcification in the surgical capsule. (b) This shows a hypoechoic rim around the BPH nodule representing a capsule. (c) There is displacement of normal prostatic vessels around the hypertrophied lobes.

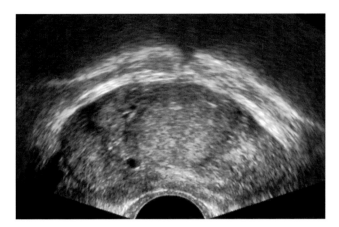

Figure 11.9
BPH: median lobe hypertrophy. In this case, most of the hypertrophy has occurred in the median lobe. Note the dilatation of the right ejaculatory duct due to obstruction by the BPH.

stretched, and thinned by macroscopic enlargement of the inner gland (Figure 11.10). Macroscopic nodules are uncommon in the outer gland.

Lateral lobe hyperplasia is usually symmetrical (Figure 11.8), although marked asymmetry does sometimes occur (Figure 11.11). Median lobe enlargement is also usually symmetrical about the midline, although asymmetry is not uncommon (Figure 11.12). The median lobe is well seen on transabdominal ultrasound of the bladder and on IVU. It should not be mistaken for a bladder tumour (Figure 11.13). It must be remembered, however, that BPH and bladder tumours are both common and often coexist (Figure 11.14). Any doubt warrants cystoscopy. The hypertrophied median

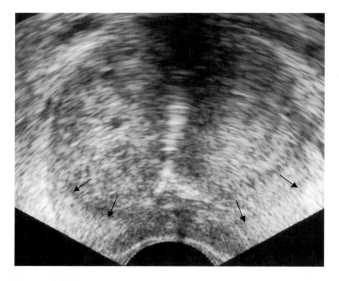

Figure 11.10
BPH: thinning of the outer gland. The hypertrophied central gland has caused marked thinning of the outer gland (arrows).

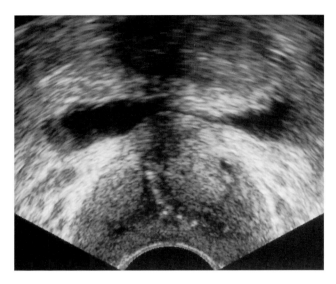

Figure 11.11
BPH: asymmetrical enlargement of the lateral lobes. Both lateral lobes and the median lobe are hypertrophied, but the left lateral lobe is significantly larger than the right.

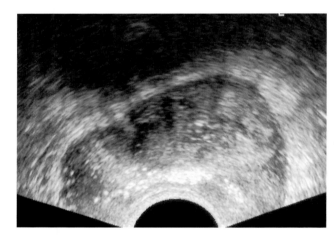

Figure 11.12
BPH: asymmetrical median lobe enlargement. The hypertrophied median lobe is very asymmetrical.

lobe may be rounded, ovoid, heart-shaped, or asymmetrical. On some views – both on ultrasound and on IVU – it has the curious appearance of seeming to lie free within the bladder (Figure 11.15).

The echotexture of BPH is very variable. The uncomplicated hypertrophied and hyperplastic tissues are similar in texture to the normal prostate, but are prone to cystic change, necrosis, and calcification. This gives rise to a very mixed echoic pattern, with mostly medium echodensity but with other areas of high and low echodensity, anechoic areas, and highly echoic shadowing areas of calcification (Figure 11.16). Hypertrophied nodules are sometimes dis-

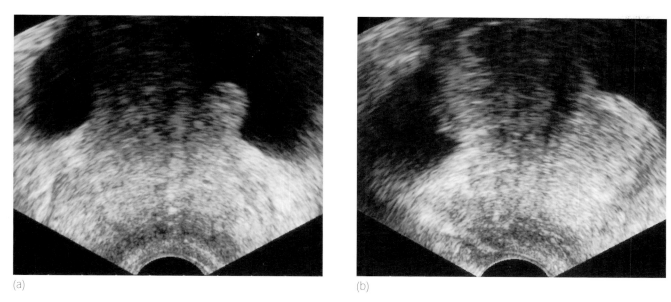

(a)   (b)

Figure 11.13
BPH: hypertrophied median lobe bulging into the bladder: (a) axial plane; (b) sagittal plane. The large median lobe is seen bulging well into the bladder.

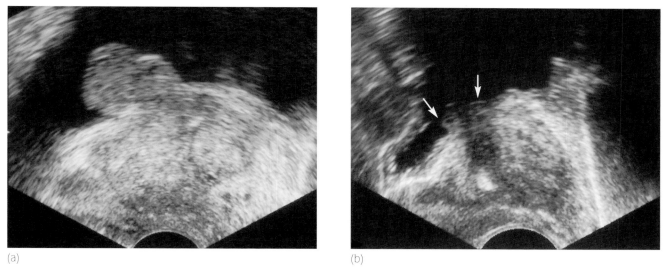

(a)   (b)

Figure 11.14
Median lobe hypertrophy simulating a bladder tumour. (a) In this case, the enlarged median lobe is very asymmetrical, making it difficult to distinguish from a bladder tumour. In some cases, the bladder mucosa and the layers of the bladder wall may be identified, helping to make the distinction. In this case, the prostate is large and the bladder wall is outside the best focal plane for the transducer. (b) In this case, there is an enlarged prostate indenting the bladder, but there is also a bladder tumour adjacent to it (arrows).

crete, but often several nodules merge into one. The nodules have a thin fibrous capsule, which may sometimes be seen on ultrasound as a hypoechoic rim, although the capsule is often not visible (Figure 11.17). Magnetic resonance imaging (MRI) appearances parallel the ultrasound appearances, with the hypertrophied tissue itself being similar in signal to normal prostatic tissue on both T1- and T2-weighted images, but with areas of high and low signal and signal voids particularly marked on T2-weighted images. The fibrous capsule is often better seen on MRI (Figure 11.18).

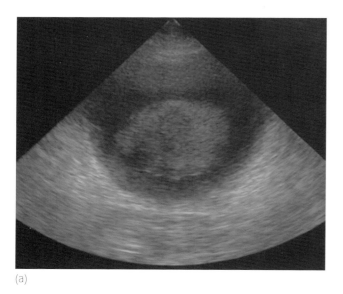

(a)

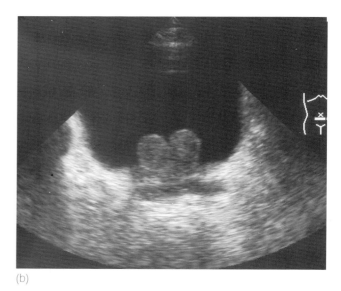

(b)

Figure 11.15
BPH: hypertrophied median lobe appearing to lie within the bladder. (a) An asymmetrical hypertrophied median lobe appears to lie within the bladder. (b) This symmetrical heart shape is often seen in median lobe hypertrophy.

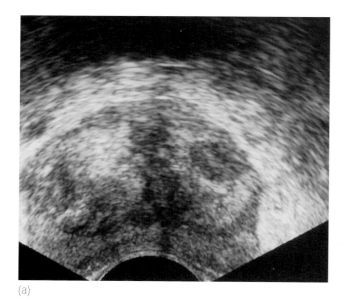

(a)

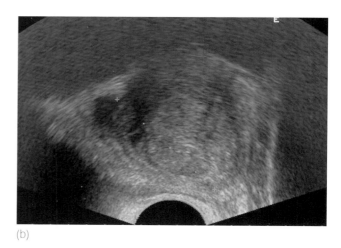

(b)

(c)

Figure 11.16
BPH: different parenchymal patterns on ultrasound study.
(a)–(d) show different common ultrasound patterns. (a) Mixed echodensity, predominantly hyperechoic. (b) The BPH nodule on the left is homogeneously hyperechoic. (c) The lateral lobe nodule on the left is hypoechoic. (d) Calcified lateral lobe nodules. (e) A nodule with cystic change.

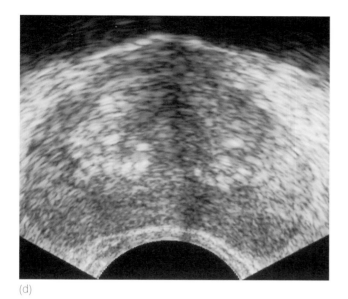

(d)

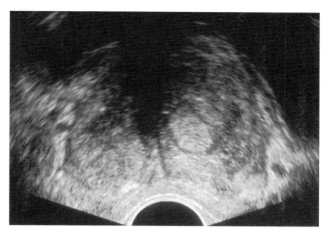

Figure 11.17
BPH nodule with visible capsule. The nodule on the left has a clearly defined hypoechoic rim representing the capsule.

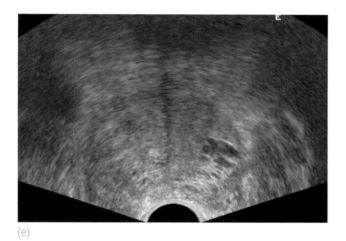

(e)

Figure 11.16
Continued

Imaging in the treatment of BPH

Once a diagnosis has been made, the majority of patients are treated without the need for further imaging. Diagnostic imaging, however, may play a role in selection of therapy. Firstly, there is an increasing tendency to treat patients with BPH medically, principally with α_1-blocking drugs that reduce the size of the hypertrophied prostate. The efficacy of treatment is largely assessed by resolution of symptoms, and, as stated earlier, the causes of prostatism are multifactorial and symptoms may be poorly related to prostate size. Nevertheless, it is common practice to record prostate size before and after treatment. In such studies, the basic method of determining prostate size from orthogonal transabdominal measurements may not be sufficiently accurate. The correlation between prostate weight estimated by transabdominal ultrasound and the weight of the surgically resected prostate is between 0.80 and 0.97.[59] Similar measurements using the transrectal approach are more accurate, with a correlation between 0.82 and 0.99 (Figure 11.19).[59–61] Measurement of volume from MRI scans is accurate and reproducible, provided that there are no movement artefacts (Figure 11.20).[62] Measurement of volume by transrectal ultrasound using multiple cross-sectional areas obtained while withdrawing the transducer by set increments using an external device is accurate but cumbersome (Figure 11.21). Using this method, accuracies of ±15% may be achieved.[63] Software is now available on some ultrasound machines that enable three-dimensional images of the prostate to be obtained. Visually acceptable images may be produced using a free-hand technique to move the transducer at a subjectively even rate. For volume measurement, however, manually

Although hypertrophy does occur in the outer gland, the cystic, necrotic, and calcified areas common in the inner gland do not often occur in the outer gland. The hypertrophied outer gland therefore has a similar appearance to normal outer glandular tissue. Thus, when cancer coincides with BPH, the two entities may be difficult to distinguish in the inner gland, but are not generally confused in the outer gland. The presence of heterogeneous BPH tissue in the inner gland largely explains the poorer sensitivity of both MRI and transrectal ultrasound in the detection of centrally placed cancers.[50,53–58]

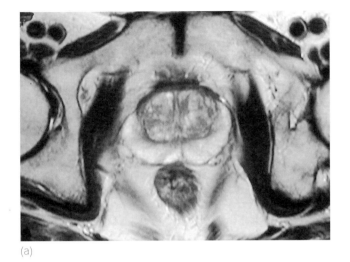

(a)

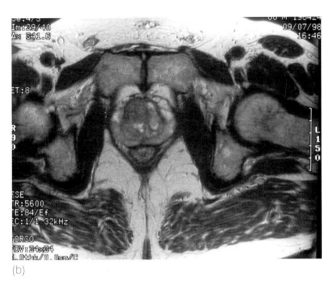

(b)

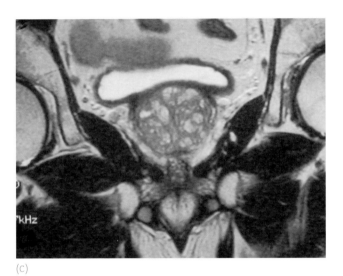

(c)

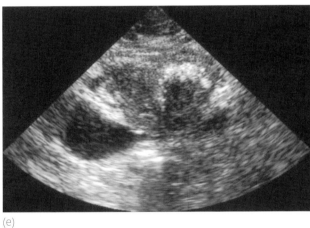

(e)

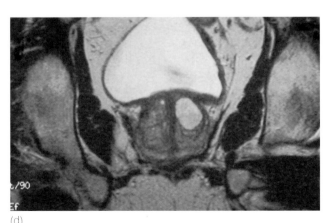

(d)

Figure 11.18

BPH: common signal patterns on magnetic resonance imaging (MRI) study. (a)–(d) show common patterns that are found.
(a) There is mixed signal in the inner gland. There is moderate thinning of the outer gland. (b) There is predominantly low signal. There is also loss of signal in the outer gland due to cancer. (c) There are high-signal nodules surrounded by medium-signal tissue. There is marked thinning of the outer gland. (d) shows a very high signal nodule on the left with a signal void at its periphery. In this case, a transrectal ultrasound scan of the same nodule (e) shows the peripheral nodule signal void is clearly due to the surrounding calcifications.

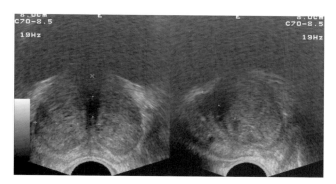

Figure 11.19
Prostate volume (weight) measurement on transrectal ultrasound. This shows the standard method of calculating the prostate volume from three orthogonal measurements.

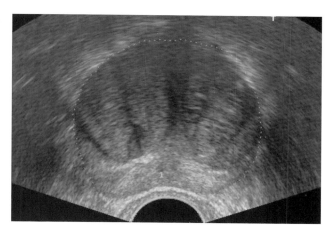

Figure 11.21
Prostate volume measurements by transrectal ultrasound. Multiple cross-sectional areas have been obtained at 5 mm intervals by withdrawing the transducer using a calibrated holder. The cross-sectional area of each section is measured and the volume is calculated from these. A single section is shown in which the cross-sectional area has been measured.

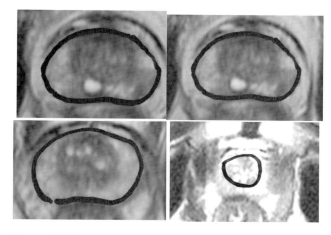

Figure 11.20
Prostate volume measurements on MRI study. Measurements of the cross-sectional areas of slices at 5 mm intervals are made and the volume is calculated from these.

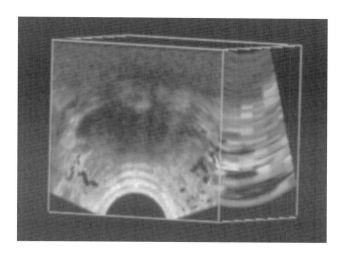

Figure 11.22
Prostate volume calculation from a three-dimensional (3D) ultrasound image. A 3D image of the prostate is shown. The volume is found using a computer programme that identifies the surface of the prostate and then calculates the volume.

controlled motion may be inaccurate because of variations in the speed of movement. This problem may be overcome by using an external device that senses the position of the transducer in space during the movement. Such a system may produce accurate estimations of prostate volume, provided that the patient does not move during the acquisition (Figure 11.22).

Urethral stents

Wire mesh stents inserted into the prostatic urethra have been used in the treatment of BPH, although they have not gained great popularity. This is largely due to difficulty in placing the stents accurately. Extension of permanent stents into the bladder predisposes to encrustation and calculus formation.

Projection of the stent below the verumontanum causes irritative symptoms and incontinence. Stents may be used as a temporary measure instead of catheterization or as a permanent treatment in patients who are unfit for surgery.[64] In such cases, transrectal ultrasound may be used to measure the length of the prostatic urethra and the size of the prostate when planning the procedure (Figure 11.23). The length of the stent, however, is usually determined cystoscopically using a calibrated urethral catheter. Stents are generally

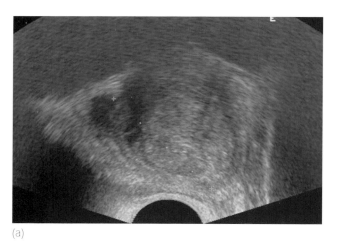

(a)

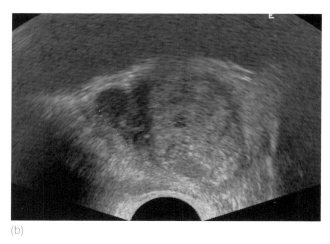

(b)

Figure 11.23
Urethral measurement for the placement of a urethral stent. The urethra has been measured from its orifice to a point just above the external sphincter. (a) A linear measurement has been taken. (b) The urethra is curved owing to BPH. A curved measurement has been taken.

positioned under urethroscopic control, although some centres use simultaneous transrectal ultrasound. This procedure enables visualization of stent placement in real time.

Finally, in patients with recurrence of symptoms, transrectal ultrasound may demonstrate displacement of the stent or growth of the prostate over the ends of the stent (Figure 11.24).

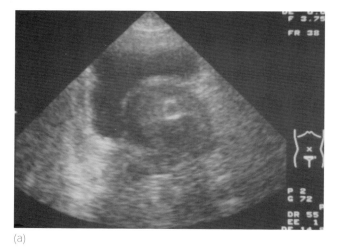

(a)

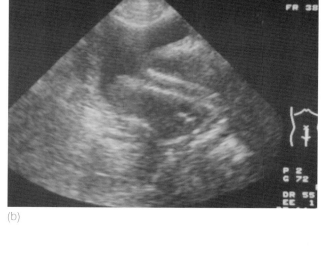

(b)

(c)

Figure 11.24
Permanent urethral stent: (a) axial plane; (b) sagittal plane. The stent is reasonably well placed, although the proximal (bladder) end is slightly short. The stent has been in place for 6 months, and epithelium is seen covering the mesh. (c) A poorly positioned permanent stent. Sagittal transrectal ultrasound shows that the wire is projecting into the bladder and has become encrusted with small stones (straight arrow). Shadowing from the stones (curved arrow) is noted. The image is orientated to correspond to a conventional voiding urethrogram. (c) is reproduced with permission from Rifkin MD. Ultrasound of the Prostate. Philadelphia: Lippincott-Raven, 1997.

A well-placed permanent stent has its proximal end lying against the bladder apex and its distal end just short of the sphincter. Temporary stents are designed to project into the bladder, and to minimize overgrowth of tissue so that they may be removed. Those designed for permanent use encourage epithelial growth over the wire mesh. In mature permanent stents, epithelium is seen as a cuff of medium-echodensity tissue about 3 mm thick surrounding the wire mesh. Nodular regrowth into the lumen may cause obstruction.[65–70]

Transurethral resection of the prostate

Transurethral resection of the prostate (TURP) is the traditional therapy for BPH, either as a primary treatment or in patients in whom medical treatment has failed. TURP is almost invariably carried out under direct cystoscopic vision. Simultaneous transrectal ultrasound has, however, been described, particularly in re-operations for regrowth.

Recurrence of symptoms following TURP is normally investigated in the same way as primary outflow tract obstruction. Transrectal ultrasound may, however, be used to evaluate the prostate. A TURP defect appears as an irregular channel of varying width along the proximal prostatic urethra, wider at the bladder base, and tapering in width toward the verumontanum (Figure 11.25). The defect may be seen on a passive study, but may only be visible if the bladder is sufficiently full. Compression of the bladder may be helpful. In some cases, the defect is only seen when the patient micturates. Regrowth of BPH tissue may present with narrowing of the channel (Figure 11.26) or by nodular regrowth into the lumen of the channel (Figure 11.27).[65] The recent trend has been to avoid extensive transurethral resections. Less extensive resections and even simple incision through the urethra into the prostatic tissue (transurethral incision of the prostate, TUIP) have been shown to be as effective, at least in smaller glands.[71] In the case of minimal resections and incisions, no change may be detected on subsequent ultrasound images. It is common following TURP for the ejaculatory duct to become obstructed. This may appear on the transrectal ultrasound image as enlargement of the ducts and seminal vesicles. It is usually of little significance, although some patients develop seminal vesiculitis with pain.

A number of newer methods designed to reduce the volume of periurethral prostatic tissue have become popular as alternatives to TURP. These utilize microwave heating, high-intensity focused ultrasound, transurethral needle ablation, and interstitial needle ablation.[72–74] Ultrasound imaging may be used in the planning, execution, and assessment of these treatments.

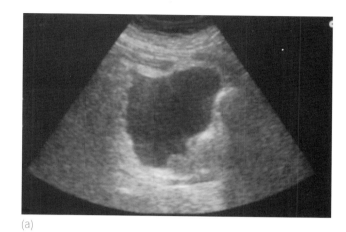

(a)

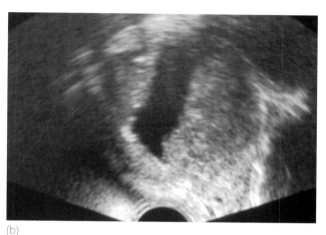

(b)

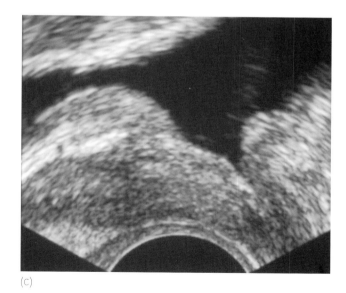

(c)

Figure 11.25
Transurethral resection (TURP) defect. (a) In this transabdominal view, the defect is poorly seen. In coronal (b) sagittal (c) transrectal ultrasound images, the TURP defect is clearly seen.

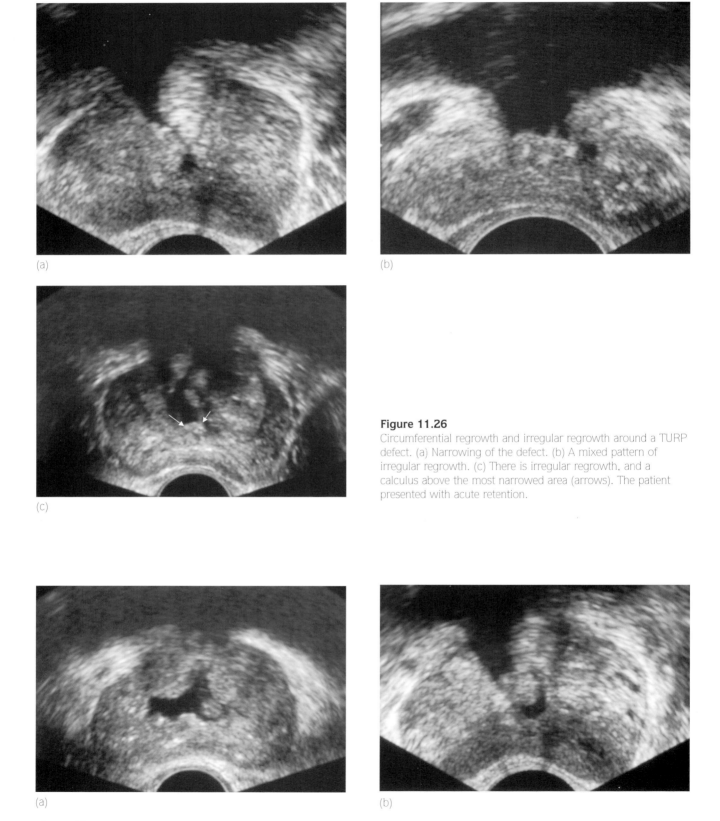

(a)

(b)

(c)

Figure 11.26
Circumferential regrowth and irregular regrowth around a TURP defect. (a) Narrowing of the defect. (b) A mixed pattern of irregular regrowth. (c) There is irregular regrowth, and a calculus above the most narrowed area (arrows). The patient presented with acute retention.

(a)

(b)

Figure 11.27
Nodular regrowth into a TURP defect. (a) A nodule is seen growing into the left side of the defect. (b) There is a central nodule.

Imaging in acute urinary retention

Patients with BPH frequently present with acute retention – an extremely painful condition relieved by bladder catheterization. Ultrasound may be requested to evaluate the upper tracts for hydronephrosis or to confirm an enlarged, nonemptying bladder. If symptoms are not relieved by catheterization, the position of the urinary catheter may be checked by ultrasound (Figure 11.28). If the catheter is misplaced, it may be repositioned under direct ultrasound control. In the unusual event of failure to catheterize the bladder via the urethra, suprapubic catheterization is performed. Although the latter is usually a straightforward procedure, previous abdominal surgery may result in adhesions. In such patients, it may be safer to perform suprapubic catheterization under direct ultrasound visualization.

BPH presenting with renal failure

Renal failure is diagnosed clinically and confirmed biochemically by measurement of serum creatinine, urea, and potassium. Ultrasound is then performed as a first investigation to determine the cause of the failure. In acute retention, the bladder will be full and often overdistended. The bladder does not empty on micturition or attempted micturition. There is often, although not invariably, hydronephrosis and hydroureter. The kidneys may be normal in size, or they may demonstrate age-related cortical loss, which will contribute to

the renal failure. When urinary retention is suspected as the cause of renal failure, repeat serum creatinine levels should be obtained following urinary catheterization. If the creatinine falls after catheterization, then outlet obstruction is proven to be at least a contributory cause.

In the setting of bladder outlet obstruction, hydronephrosis and hydroureter are usually bilateral, although not always to the same degree. Following relief of outlet obstruction by catheterization, there is a variability in reduction of the hydronephrosis. In some cases, notably those with more marked hydronephrosis, dilatation of the calyces may be permanent.

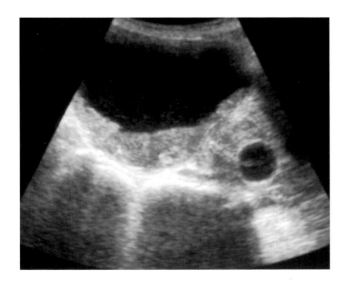

Figure 11.28
Misplaced urinary catheter. The catheter balloon is seen inflated in the prostated urethra.

References

1. McNeil JE. Origin and evolution of benign prostatic enlargement. Invest Urol 1978; 15: 340–5.
2. Garraway WM, Collins GN, Lee RJ. High prevalence of benign prostatic hypertrophy in the community. Lancet 1991; 388: 469–71.
3. Garraway WM, Russell EBAW, Lee RJ, Collins GM. Impact of previously unrecognised benign prostatic hyperplasia on the lives of middle-aged and elderly men. Br J Gen Pract 1992; 43: 318–21.
4. Diokno AC, Brown MB, Goldstein N, Herzog AR. Epidemiology of bladder emptying symptoms in elderly men. J Urol 1992; 148: 1418–21.
5. Schute CG, Ponser LA, Girman GC et al. The prevalence of prostatism: a population-based survey of urinary symptoms. J Urol 1993; 150: 85–9.
6. Gu FL. The incidence of benign prostatic hyperplasia and prostatic cancer in China. Chin J Surg 1993; 31: 323–6.
7. Sidney S, Quesenberry C, Sadler MC et al. Risk factors for surgically treated benign prostatic hyperplasia in a prepaid health care plan. Urology 1991; 38(Suppl): 13–19.
8. Morrison AS. Risk factors for surgery for prostatic hypertrophy. Am J Epidemiol 1992; 135: 974–80.
9. Glynn RJ, Campion EW, Bouchard GR, Silbert JE. The development of benign prostatic hyperplasia among volunteers of the Normative Aging Study. Am J Epidemiol 1985; 121: 78–90.
10. Daniel HW. More stage A prostatic cancers, less surgery for benign hypertrophy in smokers. J Urol 1993; 149: 68–72.
11. Denis L, Griffiths K, Khoury S et al. In: Proceedings of the 4th International Consultation on BPH. Paris: Health Publications, 1998.
12. Andersen JT. Prostatism: Clinical, radiological and urodynamic aspects. Neurourol Urodynam 1982; 1: 241–93.
13. Perys BJ, Machin DG, Woolfenden KA, Parsons KF. Chronic urinary retention – a sensory problem? Br J Urol 1988; 62: 546–9.
14. Lepor H, Machi G. Comparison of AUA symptom index in unselected males and females between fifty five and seventy years of age. Urology 1993; 42: 36–41.
15. Hald T, Elbadawi A, Horn T et al. The effects of obstruction and aging on the function of the lower urinary tract. In:

Proceedings of the 2nd International Consultation on Benign Prostatic Hyperplasia, Paris, 1993: 87–130.

16. Speakman MJ, Sethia KK, Fellows GJ et al. A study of the pathogenesis, urodynamic assessment and outcome of detrusor instability associated with bladder outflow obstruction. Br J Urol 1987; 59: 40–4.

17. Jones DA, George NJ, O'Reilly PH et al. Reversible hypertension associated with unrecognised high pressure chronic retention of urine. Lancet 1987; i: 1052–4.

18. Dowd JB, Ewert EE. Silent prostatism (unrecognised bladder neck obstruction.) JAMA 1961; 178: 296.

19. Cascione CJ, Bartone FF, Hussain MB. Transabdominal ultrasound versus excretory urography in preoperative evaluation of patients with prostatism. J Urol 1987; 137: 883–5.

20. Brandt TD, Neiman HL, Calenoff L et al. Ultrasound evaluation of the urinary system in spinal cord injured patients. Radiology 1981; 141: 473.

21. Griffiths CG, Murray A, Ramsden PD. Accuracy and repeatability of bladder volume measurement using ultrasound imaging. J Urol 1986; 136: 12.

22. Hakenberg OW, Ryall RL, Langois SL et al. A determination of bladder volume by sonocystography. J Urol 1983; 130: 249.

23. Kiely AE, Hartnell GG, Gibson RN et al. Measurement of bladder volume by realtime ultrasound. Br J Urol 1987; 60: 33.

24. McLean GK, Edell SL. Determination of bladder volumes by grey scale ultrasonography. Radiology 1978; 128: 181.

25. Abrams P, Blaivas J, Nodling J et al. The objective evaluation of bladder outflow obstruction. In: The 2nd International Consultation on Benign Prostatic Hyperplasia (BPH) Proceedings. Cockett AJK, Khoury S, Aso Y et al, eds. Scientific, 1993.

26. Schacterle R, Sullivan M, Yalla S. Combinations of maximum urinary flow rate and American Urological Association symptom index that are more specific for identifying obstructive and non-obstructive prostatism. Neurourol Urodyn 1996; 15: 459–70.

27. Speakman MJ, Sethia KK, Fellows GJ, Smith JC. A study of the pathogenesis, urodynamic assessment and outcome of detruser instability associated with bladder outflow obstruction. Br J Urol 1987; 59: 40–4.

28. Griffiths D, Hofner K, van Mastrigt R et al. Standardisation of terminology of lower urinary tract function: Pressure–flow studies of voiding, urethral resistance, and urethral obstruction. International Continence Society Sub-Committee on Standards of Terminology of Pressure–Flow Studies. Neurourol Urodyn 1997; 16: 1–18.

29. Drach GW, Layton TN, Binard WJ. Male peak urinary flow rate: relationship to volume voided and age. J Urol 1979; 122: 210.

30. Drach GW, Layton T, Bottaccini MR. A method of adjustment of male peak urinary flow rate for varying age and volume voided. J Urol 1982; 128: 960.

31. Ryall RL, Marshall VR. Normal peak urinary flow rates obtained from small voided volumes can provide a reliable assessment of bladder function. J Urol 1982; 127: 484.

32. Siroky MB, Olsson CA, Krane RJ. The flow rate nomogram: I. Development. J Urol 1979; 122: 65.

33. Siroky MB, Olsson CA, Krane RJ. The flow rate nomogram: II. Clinical correlation. J Urol 1980; 123: 200.

34. Susset JC, Picker P, Kretz M, Jorest R. Critical evaluation of uro-flow meters and analysis of normal curves. J Urol 1973; 109: 874.

35. Shaikin DC, Blaivos JG. Evaluation of the effects of neuromuscular disease of the urinary tract. In: Clinical Urography, 2nd edn. Pollack HM, Philadelphia: WB Saunders, 2000.

36. Gleason DM, Bottaccini MR, Lattimer JC. Some correlations between hydrodynamic and clinical findings in the urinary tract. J Urol 1968; 100: 783–6.

37. Gleason DM, Bottacini MR, Reilly RJ, Byrne JC. The residual stream energy as a diagnostic index of male urinary outflow obstruction. Invest Urol 1972; 10: 72–7.

38. Griffiths DJ. Urodynamic assessment of bladder function. Br J Urol 1977; 49: 29–36.

39. Schafer W. Urethral resistance? Urodynamic concepts of physiological and pathological bladder outlet function during voiding. Neurourol Urodyn 1985; 4: 161.

40. Bates CP, Corney LE. Synchronous cine/pressure/flow cystography: a method of routine urodynamic investigation. Br J Radiol 1971; 44: 44.

41. Blaivis JG, Fisher DM. Combined radiographic and urodynamic monitoring: advances in technique. J Urol 1981; 125: 541.

42. Blaivis JG. Multichannel urodynamic studies. Urology 1984; 23: 421.

43. McGuire EJ. Combined radiographic and manometric assessment of urethral sphincter function. J Urol 1977; 118: 632.

44. Abu-Yousef MM, Narayana AS. Transabdominal ultrasound in the evaluation of prostate size. J Clin Ultrasound 1982; 10: 275–8.

45. Henneberry M, Carter MF, Neiman HL. Estimation of prostatic size by suprapubic ultrasonography. J Urol 1979; 121: 615–16.

46. Roehrborn CG, Chinn HK, Fulgham PF et al. The role of transabdominal ultrasound in the preoperative evaluation of patients with benign prostatic hypertrophy. J Urol 1986; 135: 1190–3.

47. Roehrborn CG, Peters PC. Can transabdominal ultrasound estimation of postvoiding residue (PVR) replace catheterization? Urology 1988; 31: 445–9.

48. Abu Yousef MM. Benign prostatic hyperplasia: tissue characterisation using suprapubic ultrasound. Radiology 1985; 156: 169–73.

49. Gosling JA, Dickson JS. The structure and innervation of trabeculated detrusor smooth muscle. In: Proceedings of the 9th Annual Meeting of the International Continence Society, Rome, 1979; 9–13.

50. Sanders RC, Hamper UM, Dahnert WF. Update on prostatic ultrasound. Urol Radiol 1987; 9: 110–18.

51. Cascione CJ, Bartone FF, Hussain MB. Transabdominal ultrasound versus excretory urography in preoperative evaluation of patients with prostatism. J Urol 1987; 137: 883–5.

52. Minieri C, Carter SS, Romano G et al. The diagnosis of bladder outlet obstruction in men by ultrasound measurement of bladder wall thickness. J Urol 1998; 159: 761–5.

53. Roehrborn CG, Chinn HK, Fulgham PF et al. The role of transabdominal ultrasound in the preoperative evaluation of patients with benign prostatic hypertrophy. J Urol 1986; 135: 1190–3.

54. Greene DR, Egawa S, Hellerstein DK, Scardino PT. Sonographic measurements of transitional zone of prostate in men with and without benign prostatic hyperplasia. Urology 1990; 36: 293.

55. Hendrikx AJM, Doesburs WH, Reintjes AJM et al. Effectiveness of ultrasound in the preoperative evaluation of patients with prostatism. Prostate 1988; 13: 199.

56. Ngheim HT, Kellman GM, Sandberg SA, Kraig BM. Cystic lesions of the prostate. Radiographics 1990; 10: 635.

57. Scheibler ML, Tomaszewski JR, Bezzi M, et al. Prostatic carcinoma and benign prostatic hyperplasia: correlation of high resolution MR and histopathological findings. Radiology 1989; 172: 131–7.

58. Allen HS, Kressel HY, Arger PH et al. Age-related changes of the prostate evaluated by MR imaging. AJR 1989; 157: 77–81.

59. Roehrborn CG, Kurth KH, Leriche A et al. Diagnostic recommendations for clinical practice. In: Proceedings of the 2nd International Consultation on Benign Prostatic Hyperplasia, 1993; 289–90.

60. Littrup PJ, Williams CR, Egglin TK, Karne RA. Determination of prostatic volume with transrectal US for cancer screening. Part II. Accuracy of in vitro and in vivo techniques. Radiology 1991; 179: 49–53.

61. Watanabe H. Diagnosis of benign prostatic hypertrophy by ultrasound and outcome from surgery. Akt Urol 1993; 24: 127–30.

62. Gormley GJ, Stone RE, Bruskewitz RC et al. The effects of finasteride in men with benign prostatic hyperplasia. The Finasteride Study Group. N Engl J Med 1992; 327: 1185–1191.

63. Watanabe H, Igari D, Tanahasci Y et al. Measurements of size and weight of prostate by means of transrectal ultrasono-tomography. Tohoku J Exp Med 1974; 114: 277–285.

64. Smith PH, Marberger M, Conort P et al. Other non-medical therapies (excluding lasers) in the treatment of BPH. In: Proceedings of the 2nd International Consultation on Benign Prostatic Hyperplasia, Paris, 1993: 453–91.

65. Rifkin MD. Ultrasound of the Prostate, 2nd edn. Philadelphia: Lippincott-Raven, 1997.

66. Parikh AM, Milroy EJG. Precautions and complications in the use of the Urolume Wallstent. Eur Urol 1995; 563: 1–13.

67. Badlani G, Press SM, Oesterling JE, DeFalco K. Urolume endothelial prosthesis in the treatment of urethral stricture disease: longterm results of the North American Multi-Centre Urolume Trial. Urology 1995; 45: 846.

68. Milroy E, Allen A. Longterm results of Urolume urethral stent for recurrent urethral strictures. J Urol 1995; 155: 156–61.

69. Krogh J. Longterm complications of the Intraprostatic Spiral. Scand J Urol Nephrol 1992; 26: 191–92.

70. Chiu AW, Lin ATL, Lee Y-H et al. Stone encrustation: a relevant complication of the Intraprostatic Spiral. Eur Urol 1991; 19: 304–7.

71. Orandi A. Transurethral incision of prostate compared with transurethral resection of prostate in 132 matching cases. J Urol 1987; 138: 810–15.

72. Foster RS, Bihrle R, Sanghvi N et al. High intensity focussed ultrasound in the treatment of prostatic disease. Eur Urol 1993; 23(S1): 29–33.

73. Van Erps PM, Dourcy B, Denis LJ. Transrectal hyperthermia in benign prostatic hyperplasia. J Urol 1991; 145: 263A.

74. Schulman CC. Transurethral needle ablation (TUMA): safety, feasibility and tolerance of a new office procedure for treatment of benign prostatic hypertrophy (BPH). Eur Urol 1993; 24: 415–23 .

12

Prostatitis

Dennis Ll Cochlin

General considerations

The term prostatitis describes inflammation of the prostate that may be either bacterial or non-bacterial in nature. The condition may be acute or chronic. For the purpose of clinical diagnosis and management, Drach et al[1] have classified prostatitis into three categories:

- acute and chronic bacterial prostatitis;
- non-bacterial prostatitis;
- prostadynia.

For the purpose of management, the categories of non-bacterial prostatitis and prostadynia may be combined. For the discussion and interpretation of imaging in prostatitis, however, division into the categories of acute prostatitis, chronic prostatitis, and granulomatous prostatitis is more appropriate.

Only 5% of cases of prostatitis are proven to be due to a specific organism or secondary to urinary tract infections.[2] The vast majority of cases therefore are assumed to be non-bacterial prostatitis or prostadynia. Granulomatous prostatitis, a form of chronic prostatitis with focal masses, may be found more commonly with infections by specific organisms, but can occur secondarily to chronic infection with any organism. Imaging appearances of granulomatous prostatitis differ from those of non-granulomatous prostatitis, and therefore warrant special attention. Prostadynia is a term that describes chronic pain arising from the prostate, in which no abnormality is demonstrated and no organisms are identified.

Acute prostatitis

Acute prostatitis may present with sudden onset of fever, dysuria, frequency, urgency, nocturia, or pain in the lower back, perineum, and rectum. There may also be general malaise, arthralgias, myalgias, and bladder outlet obstruction. Symptoms range from mild to extremely severe. Acute prostatitis often occurs concomitantly with acute cystitis with symptoms of severe dysuria. A large number of organisms have been identified as causing acute prostatitis, but most are the Gram-negative organisms normally associated with urinary tract infections, 80% being *Escherichia coli*. Acute prostatitis often follows urinary tract infections (Table 12.1).[3]

Chronic bacterial prostatitis

Chronic bacterial prostatitis presents with frequency, dysuria, urgency, low back pain, pelvic pain, genital pain and occasionally post-ejaculatory pain, and haematospermia. The severity of symptoms is variable, and in some men symptoms are few or absent, presentation being that of recurrent or (more accurately) relapsing urinary tract infections. With the increasing frequency of prostatic biopsy for suspected prostatic cancer, evidence of chronic prostatitis is often found in the biopsy specimens of men with no symptoms or history of prostatitis. Chronic prostatitis is often caused by the same organisms that cause acute prostatitis, most often *E. coli*. Chronic prostatitis may be the most common cause of relapsing urinary tract infections in men. Because antibiotics do not penetrate well into the alkaline environment of the prostate, prostatitis may be incompletely treated, resulting in chronic infection. Calcifications or calculi within the prostate, particularly when found in young men, are often caused by chronic prostatitis. It is thought that these calcifications may act as a nidus for infection, making chronic prostatitis difficult to eradicate.[4,5]

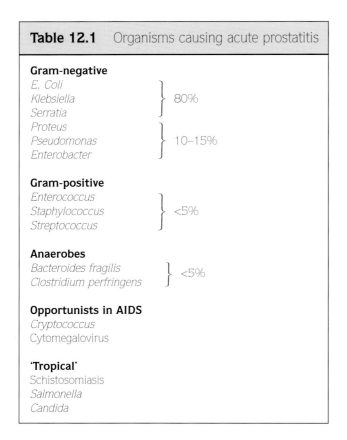

Table 12.1   Organisms causing acute prostatitis

Gram-negative
E. Coli
Klebsiella   } 80%
Serratia

Proteus
Pseudomonas   } 10–15%
Enterobacter

Gram-positive
Enterococcus
Staphylococcus } <5%
Streptococcus

Anaerobes
Bacteroides fragilis   } <5%
Clostridium perfringens

Opportunists in AIDS
Cryptococcus
Cytomegalovirus

'Tropical'
Schistosomiasis
Salmonella
Candida

Table 12.2   Causes of chronic prostatitis

- Chronic form of acute prostatitis
- Non-bacterial – probably due to chemical prostatitis caused by reflux of urine into the prostate
- Possibly due to:
    Chlamydia trachomatis
    Trichomonas vaginalis
    Ureoplasma ureolyticum

Imaging has little place in the diagnosis of chronic prostatitis. The echotexture of the gland may appear heterogeneous, but these changes are non-specific. Transrectal ultrasound, however, may be requested in order to exclude an abscess.

Granulomatous prostatitis

Granulomatous prostatitis is a specific form of chronic prostatitis characterized by granulomatous masses within the prostate. It is a particularly important condition for those imaging the prostate, since it causes hard, hypoechoic, low-signal T2-weighted MRI lesions that resemble prostatic cancer on digital rectal examination, transrectal ultrasound, and MRI. The true diagnosis may only be possible with biopsy. There are a number of possible causes of granulomatous prostatitis (Table 12.3).

Granulomatous prostatitis may be caused by *Mycobacterium tuberculosis*, and may be associated with miliary tuberculosis. Infection of the prostate secondary to renal tuberculosis does not seem to occur.[13] Tuberculous infection of the prostate is, however, uncommon – or at least uncommonly proven – in the Western world, presumably due to the relatively low prevalence or tuberculosis there. Whether tuberculous granulomatous prostatitis is more common in countries where tuberculosis is more common is not documented. The most common cause of granulomatous prostatitis in developed countries is infection from bacille Calmette-Guérin (BCG) instilled into the bladder for the treatment of bladder cancer.[14] Other infec-

However, this hypothesis may not be true, since prostatic calcifications are common in older men[6] and the majority clearly cause no harm. Those calcifications found in patients with chronic prostatitis, however, may have a different aetiology, and certainly infection within the calculi has been documented.[5,6]

Chronic non-bacterial prostatitis

Although chronic prostatitis is often non-bacterial, as judged by failure to grow organisms from expressed prostatic secretions, it may follow acute infection with the common organisms. The symptoms of non-bacterial prostatitis, are the same as those of chronic bacterial prostatitis and are equally variable. Painful ejaculation appears to be a symptom more common in chronic non-bacterial prostatitis. The cause of non-bacterial prostatitis is not known with certainty. It has been suggested that *Chlamydia trachomatis*, *Trichomonas vaginalis*, and *Ureaplasma urealyticum* may be causative (Table 12.2).[7,8] Most workers, however, believe that these organisms are not truly causative agents.[7,9–11] It is more likely that the disease in most or all patients is a chemical prostatitis caused by intraprostatic reflux of urine.[12]

Table 12.3   Causes of granulomatous prostatitis

- Idiopathic
- Tuberculosis
- BCG therapy
- Blastomycosis
- Coccidioidomycosis
- *Cryptococcus*

tions, notably blastomycosis and coccidioidomycosis have been implicated in granulomatous prostatitis.[15] Eosinophilic prostatitis[16] and malakoplakia[17] are also causes.

In the majority of cases of granulomatous prostatitis, however, no organism is identified. In these cases, granulomatous prostatitis may represent a reaction to chronic bacterial prostatitis after the causative organism has been eradicated. Another possible cause that has been postulated is ductal obstruction, with extravasation of ductal contents into the prostatic parenchyma causing a granulomatous reaction.[18] Whatever the cause, the majority of cases of granulomatous prostatitis are, in effect, idiopathic.

Iatrogenic prostatitis

Biopsy of the prostate may lead to prostatitis due to secondary infection, often with anaerobic bacteria.[19] With appropriate antibiotic coverage, however, few patients are affected. Those who do develop such infections tend to get symptoms of septicaemia rather than prostatitis.

Urethral catheterization is a common cause of prostatitis, particularly with repeated catheterization, self-intermittent catheterization, long-term catheterization, or condom drainage.[20] 'Granulomatous' prostatitis from the use of BCG in the treatment of bladder cancer has already been discussed.

Prostadynia

Prostadynia is, by definition, idiopathic. The diagnosis of prostadynia is made when there is prostatic pain but a normal digital rectal examination, and no organisms are identified in expressed prostatic secretions. Some would add to this a normal transrectal ultrasound examination.[21] The failure to detect organisms, however, does not exclude infection as the cause, and some clinicians will treat the condition with a trial of antibiotics.

Diagnosis

The diagnosis of prostatitis is traditionally based upon the clinical symptoms described earlier, with or without urethral discharge and with or without a history of preceding or concomitant urinary tract infection. Digital rectal examination reveals a hard or sometimes boggy, oedematous tender prostate. Expressed prostatic secretions are obtained during the examination, and are examined microscopically for white cells and by bacteriological culture.

Increasingly, prostatitis is discovered with few or no symptoms. When serum prostatic-specific antigen (PSA) is measured as a screening test for prostate cancer, evidence of prostatitis is often found on the transrectal ultrasound image or on histological examination of biopsy specimens. Evidence of prostatitis does not preclude the need for biopsy, since both prostatitis and cancer may be present in the same gland. Nonetheless, it is important to document the presence of prostatitis, since, if no cancer is found, this may explain the elevated PSA.[22] When cancer is found with coexisting prostatitis, the PSA level is not a reliable indicator of the extent of disease. Active prostatitis may be associated with high PSA levels, which should return to normal after effective treatment. Evidence of previous prostatitis is often found on histology of specimens obtained by transurethral resection of the prostate (TURP) performed for outlet obstruction due to benign prostatic hypertrophy. Asymptomatic prostatic infection is relatively common in older men.[23]

Imaging appearances of prostatitis

Acute prostatitis

In acute prostatitis, the prostate is often palpably enlarged and oedematous, usually feeling firm on digital rectal examination, although sometimes feeling boggy. Transrectal ultrasound demonstrates an image of the prostate that appears either normal or non-specifically enlarged.[22] Periurethral and periglandular hypoechoic regions have been described, and are probably due to oedema,[23] but are uncommon (Figure 12.1). In some cases, subtle areas of focal, usually slightly hypoechoic, abnormality may be seen (Figure 12.2). MRI studies show enlargement of the gland, with decreased signal on T1-weighted images and increased signal on T2-weighted images in the inflamed areas. These findings are usually in the outer gland and the periurethral areas[24–26] (Figures 12.3 and 12.4). There is also increased enhancement of the inflamed tissue with gadolinium (Figure 12.5). Focal findings on imaging studies may represent areas of focal change in generalized prostatitis, although in most cases the prostatitis is probably truly focal (Figure 12.6).[27–29] It is only in severe cases that definite well-circumscribed focal areas and abscesses are seen (Figures 12.7–12.9). Acute prostatitis causes a variable degree of prostatic hyperaemia. The inflamed areas are hyperaemic (Figure 12.10). Sometimes a large proportion of the gland or the whole gland may be hyperaemic (Figure 12.11), and sometimes the periprostatic plexus may be hyperaemic (Figures 12.10 and 12.11).[30,31]

Prostatic abscesses are now uncommon, although they were very common in the pre-antibiotic era. They now tend to occur in elderly, diabetic, or immunosuppressed patients.

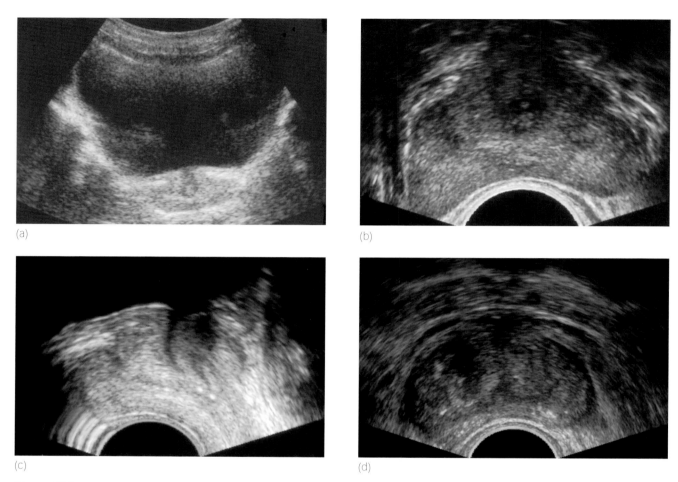

(a)

(b)

(c)

(d)

Figure 12.1
Acute prostatitis. (a) Periurethral low echodensity is seen on this transabdominal scan. (b) There is periurethral low echodensity
in this case, seen on an axial-view transrectal scan. (c) Sagittal view demonstrates periurethral oedema along the proximal urethra.
(d) Periglandular low echodensity is seen in this case along the lateral margins of the gland.

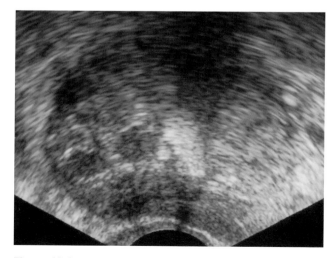

Figure 12.2
Acute prostatitis. Hypoechoic areas are seen throughout the
right side of the prostate. The whole gland is swollen.

Figure 12.4
Acute prostatitis secondary to placement of a Foley catheter:
(a) proton density and (b) T2-weighted sagittal images. The
prostate (P) is enlarged owing to benign prostatic hyperplasia. A
Foley catheter balloon (F) is wrongly inflated within the prostatic
urethra. Inflammatory change is shown as diffuse high signal
intensity on the T2-weighted image (arrow). B is the urinary
bladder and the curved arrow indicates air in the bladder.
Reproduced with permission from Hricak H, Carrington BM.
MRI of the Pelvis. London: Martin Dunitz, 1991.

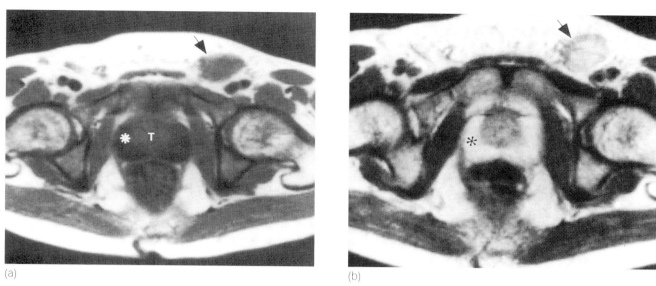

(a)

(b)

Figure 12.3

Acute prostatitis: (a) T1-weighted and (b) T2-weighted axial images. The prostate is enlarged, and the peripheral zone (asterisk) is of lower signal intensity than the adjacent transitional zone (T). The peripheral zone shows marked increase in signal intensity on T2-weighted images. The prostatitis was a sequel to acute epididymitis. Enlargement of the spermatic cord is seen (arrow). Reproduced with permission from Hricak H, Carrington BM. MRI of the Pelvis. London: Martin Dunitz, 1991.

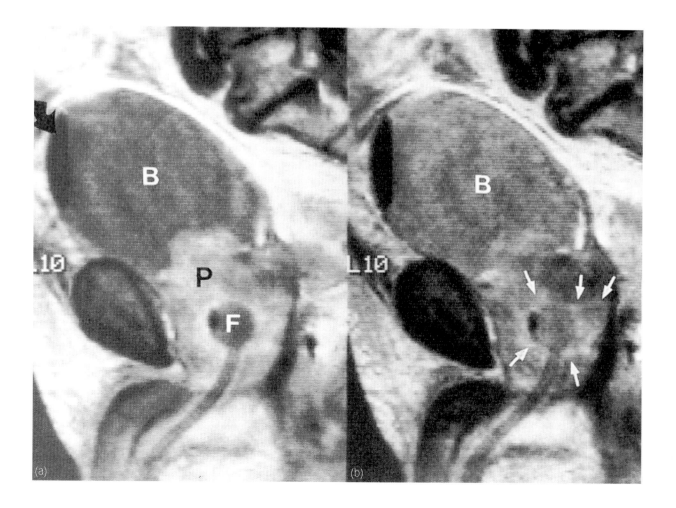

(a)

(b)

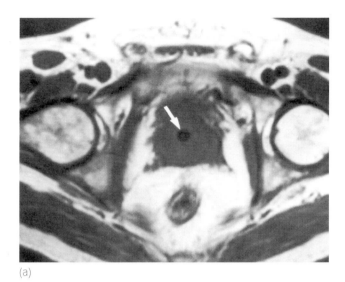

(a)

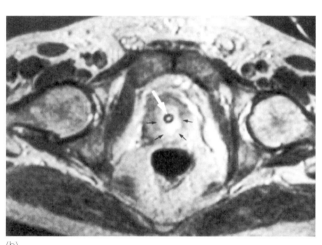

(b)

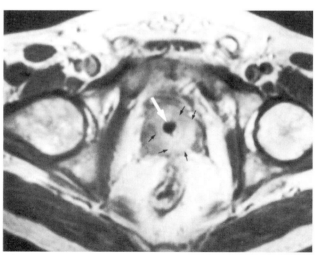

(c)

Figure 12.5
Acute prostatitis secondary to a long-term indwelling catheter: (a) T1-weighted, (b) T2-weighted, and (c) Gd-DTPA-enhanced T1-weighted images. On the T2-weighted and Gd-enhanced T1-weighted images the periurethral region shows an increase in signal intensity (small black arrows), but the enhancing tissue on the Gd-enhanced image is of greater volume than seen in the T2-weighted image, and extends into the peripheral zone. The white arrow indicates the urethral catheter. Reproduced with permission from Hricak H, Carrington BM. MRI of the Pelvis. London: Martin Dunitz, 1991.

Figure 12.6
Prostatis: MRI study. (a) Sagittal section, SE 2000/20. There is enlargement of the prostate (P) and thickening of the adjacent bladder and mucosa (arrows) due to cystitis. B is the bladder, S the symphysis pubis, and R the rectum. (b) Sagittal section, SE 3000/80. There are numerous high-intensity foci (arrowheads) throughout the prostate. The inflamed bladder mucosa is less obvious because of the intensity of urine on this pulse sequence. Reproduced by permission from McCarthy S, Fritzsche PJ. Male pelvis. In: Magnetic Resonance Imaging (Stark DD, Bradley WG Jr, eds). St Louis, MO: Mosby, 1988.

Figure 12.7
Prostatic abscess. (a) An abscess is beginning to form (arrows) Note also the calcification due to underlying chronic prostatitis. (b) A more advanced abscess. (c,d) An abscess beginning to extend through the pseudocapsule.

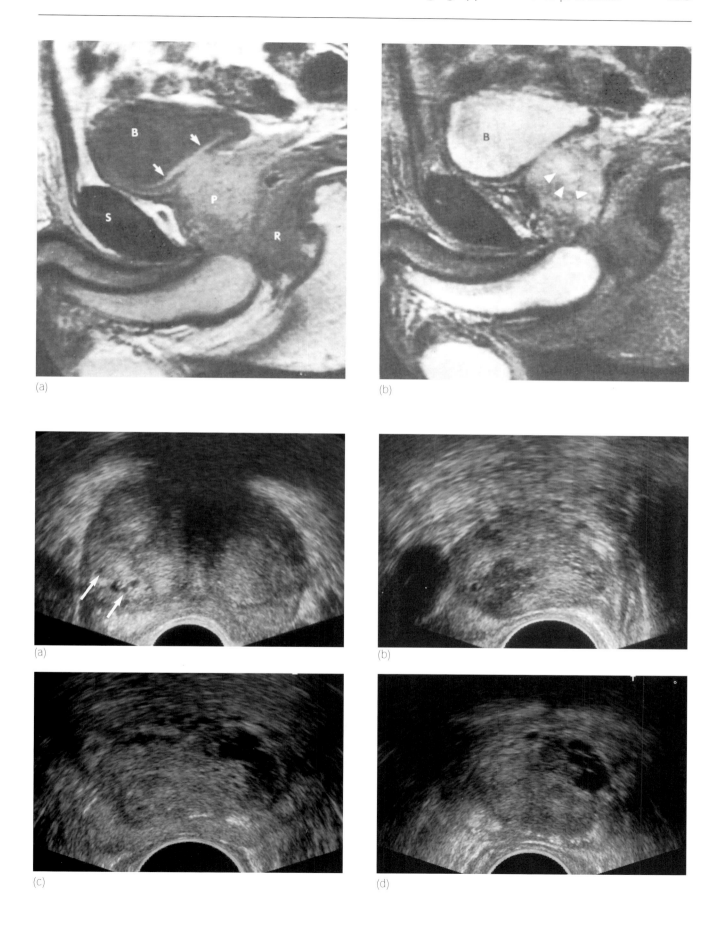

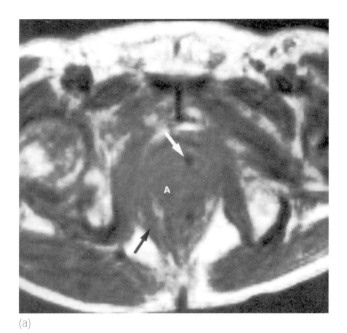

(a)

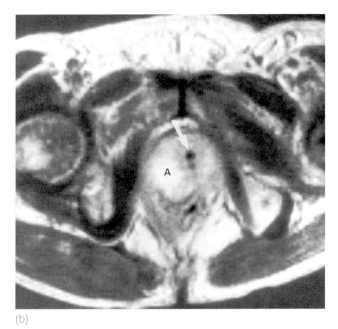

(b)

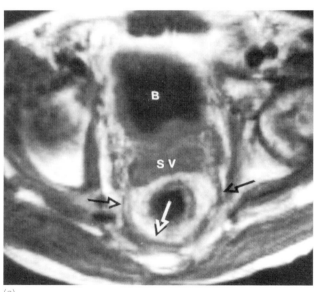

(c)

Figure 12.8

Prostatic abscess: MRI studies: (a) T1-weighted and (b) T2-weighted axial images, with (c) a T1-weighted image at the level of the seminal vesicles. On the T1-weighted image, the prostate shows asymmetrical enlargement and infiltration of the periprostatic fat (black arrow). The urethra and Foley catheter (arrow) are displaced. The abscess (A) is of medium signal intensity on the T1-weighted images, but markedly increases in signal intensity on the T2-weighted image, where it displays an indistinct margin. Inflammation has spread to the seminal vesicles (SV), which are enlarged and demonstrate an ill-defined margin. The perirectal fascia is indicated by black open arrows and the presacral space by the white open arrow. Reproduced with permission from Hricak H, Carrington BM. MRI of the Pelvis. London: Martin Dunitz, 1991.

Figure 12.9

Prostatic abscess: CT scan. An ill-defined low density region (arrow) is seen within the prostate gland. Reproduced with permission from Hricak H, Carrington BM. MRI of the Pelvis. London: Martin Dunitz, 1991.

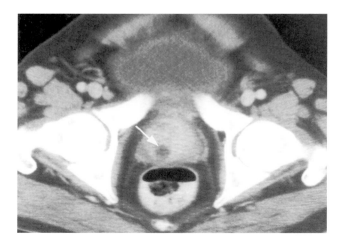

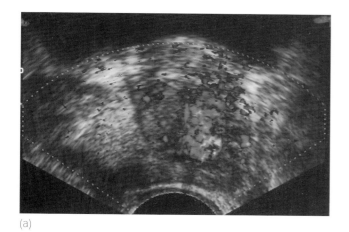

(a)

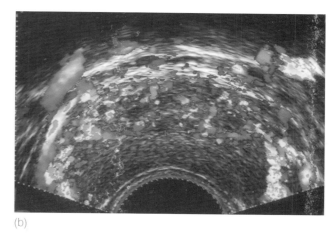

(b)

Figure 12.10
(a) Dense hyperaemia is seen in this developing abscess on a power-domain Doppler study. (b) There is marked hyperaemia around an extensive abscess within the gland, and also hyperaemia of the periprostatic plexus.

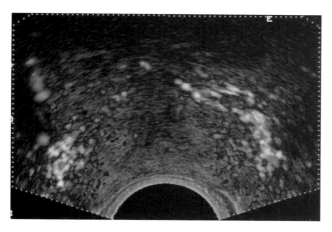

Figure 12.11
Chronic prostatitis. There is marked hyperaemia of the whole outer gland and the periprostatic plexus.

Descriptions of the appearance of prostatic abscesses are few. The imaging characteristics of a prostate abscess are similar to those of abscesses in other organs, ranging from areas of subtle altered echodensity to obvious fluid collections and, sometimes, fluid–fluid levels.[32–35] Gas has been described in prostatic abscesses seen on X-ray and computed tomography.[36] There are no descriptions of gas-containing prostatic abscesses on ultrasound, but these would presumably show areas of shadowing and comet-tail artefact. CT may be useful in the diagnosis and follow-up of prostatic abscesses, being less painful and invasive than transrectal ultrasound. The CT appearance of an abscess in the prostate is similar to that of any other abscess, except for the site. Abscesses may be confined to the prostate or may spread through the prostate capsule to involve the periprostatic tissues and seminal vesi-

cles. Abscess cavities contain pus and may be unilocular or multilocular.[37]

Chronic non-granulomatous prostatitis

Chronic non-granulomatous prostatitis, both bacterial and non-bacterial, often presents with a normal appearance on transrectal ultrasound and MRI. In other cases non-specific areas of decreased echodensity may be seen within the prostate (Figure 12.12).[28] There is a tendency in this condition to produce areas of dystrophic calcification. The

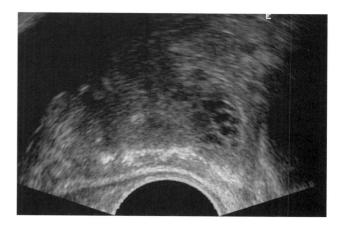

Figure 12.12
Chronic prostatitis. There are hypoechoic areas throughout the gland. Appearances are non-specific. Biopsy proved the clinical diagnosis of chronic prostatitis.

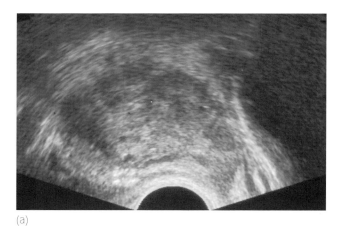

(a)

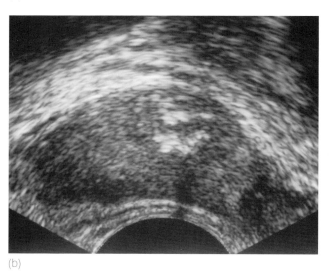

(b)

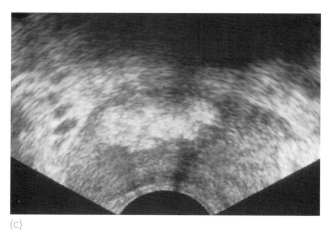

(c)

Figure 12.13
Calcification of chronic prostatitis. (a) A group of calcifications are seen in the outer gland. Biopsy revealed chronic prostatitis. (b) There are calcifications in the inner gland. This was also biopsy-proven chronic prostatitis. (c) A large group of calcifications are present in this patient with intractable chronic prostatitis. Prostatectomy was performed and the calcified area proved to be infected.

calcifications occur in the parenchyma of the prostate, and tend to form in circumscribed groups (Figure 12.13) as opposed to calcified corpora amylacea (Figure 12.14), which tend to be periurethral, in the surgical capsule, or scattered (see Chapter 13). The individual calcifications associated with prostatitis may show a subtle difference from those of calcified corpora, being rather more angular.[5, 6] As with acute prostatitis, hyperaemia is common, particularly hyperaemia of the periprostatic plexus (Figure 12.15).[30]

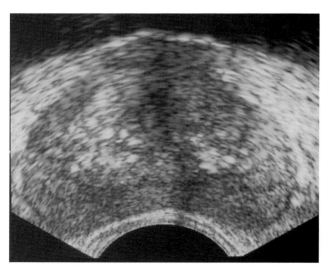

Figure 12.14
Calcified corpora amylacea.

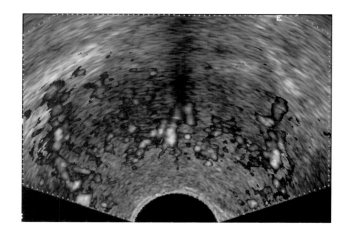

Figure 12.15
Chronic prostatitis. There is hyperaemia of the periprostatic plexus, although it is less marked than may be seen in acute prostatitis.

Granulomatous prostatitis

Granulomatous prostatitis causes well-circumscribed significantly hypoechoic lesions, usually in the outer gland, but occasionally in the inner gland (Figure 12.16). MRI demonstrates well-circumscribed areas of low signal on T2-weighted images (Figure 12.17). These focal lesions may deform the capsule and cause asymmetry of the gland (Figure 12.18). The appearances closely mimic that of prostatic cancer, and biopsy is usually necessary for diagnosis.[18,38]

Tuberculous infection of the prostate may produce granulomatous prostatitis, with multiple well-circumscribed, hypoechoic areas. Tuberculous prostatitis may also demonstrate multiple prostatic or periurethral abscess cavities that communicate with the urethra and fill with contrast during urethrography (Figure 12.19). Although a solitary abscess may be found with any type of infection, multiple abscesses strongly suggest tuberculosis.[13] Calcification within the prostate may occur in any form of chronic prostatitis, but tuberculosis can result in extensive calcification that involves the whole gland, often causing widespread destruction of the glandular tissue. The classic appearance of calcifications with tuberculosis is of extensive calcification, often with a linear pattern (Figure 12.20).

Periglandular fluid may be seen with tuberculous prostatitis. This fluid tends to be moderately echogenic. The seminal vesicles are frequently involved, and may contain echogenic material as well as calcification in the walls (see Chapter 14).[39–42]

Malakoplakia is a condition of unknown aetiology, although it appears to be a granulomatous reaction to infection in the

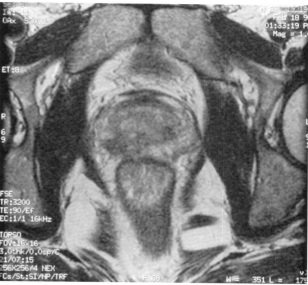

(a)

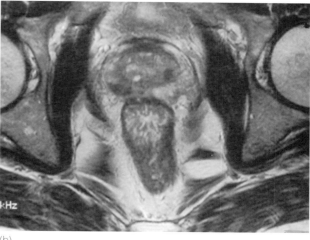

(b)

Figure 12.17
Granulomatous prostatitis. MRI scans, with (a) TR = 5620, TE = 90 and (b) TR = 3200, TE = 90, show an area of low signal in the outer gland. Biopsy revealed granolomatous prostatitis.

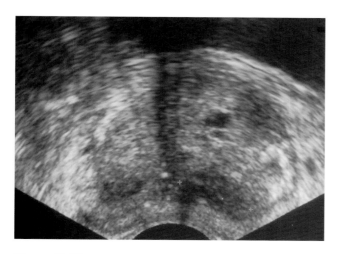

Figure 12.16
Granulomatous prostatitis. A hypoechoic area is seen in the outer gland, suggesting cancer. Biopsy revealed granulomatous prostatitis. There is calcification in the rest of the gland, possibly due to chronic prostatitis.

urinary tract, notably *E. coli* infection. As such, it is logical to classify it as a form of granulomatous prostatitis. Its appearance is similar to that of other forms of granulomatous prostatitis, although it tends to be multifocal and to cause marked irregularity of the prostatic pseudocapsule, resembling stage T3 prostatic cancer (Figure 12.21). Malakoplakia may be reported in biopsy of the prostate, although it is quite uncommon in developed countries, where recurrent urinary infections are treated more effectively than in developing countries.[43–48]

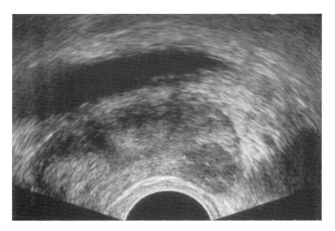

Figure 12.18
Granulomatous prostatitis. A hypoechoic area is seen bulging the capsule. Biopsy revealed granulomatous prostatitis.

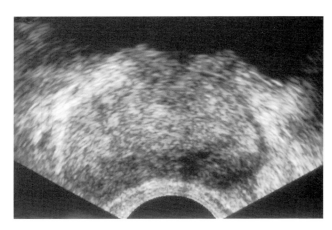

Figure 12.21
Malakoplakia. There are ill-defined hypoechoic areas throughout the gland, simulating cancer. Biopsy showed extensive malakoplakia.

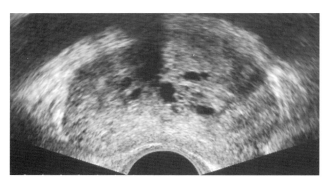

Figure 12.19
Periurethral abscess. Multiple small abscesses due to tuberculosis are seen around the urethra.

Imaging in the treatment of prostatitis

The majority of patients with prostatitis are treated with antibiotic therapy alone. Prostatic abscesses, however, may need to be drained. This may be achieved periurethrally via a urethroscope, transperineally, or transrectally. Ureteroscopic drainage is most often used. However, drainage through the urethra entails a risk of cystitis. Transrectal ultrasound-guided drainage or drainage via the transperineal approach reduce the risk of cystitis. It is possible to insert a drain into the abscess by a catheter-over-wire technique, but simple aspiration is usually effective.[49,51]

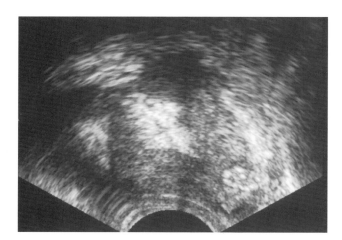

Figure 12.20
Tuberculous calcification. There was dense calcification throughout a large part of the gland in this case of tuberculous prostatitis. See also Figure 13.13 in Chapter 13.

References

1. Drach GW, Fair WR, Mears EM Jr, Stamey TA. Classification of benign diseases associated with prostatic pain: prostatitis or prostatodynia? J Urol 1978; 120: 266.
2. Brunner H, Weidner W, Schiefer H-G. Studies of the role of *Ureaplasma urealyticum* and *Mycoplasma hominis* in prostatitis. J Infect Dis 1983; 147: 807.
3. Mears EMJ. Acute and chronic prostatitis: diagnosis and treatment. Infect Dis Clin North Am 1987; 1: 855.
4. Eykyn S, Bultitude MI, Mayo ME et al. Prostatic calculi as a source of recurrent bacteriuria in the male. Br J Urol 1976; 7: 169.
5. Meares EM Jr. Chronic bacterial prostatitis: role of transurethral prostatectomy (TURP) in therapy. In: Therapy of Prostatitis (Weidner W, Brunner H, Krause W, Rothauge CF, eds). Munich: W Zuckschwerdt Verlag, 1986; 193–7.
6. Peeling WB, Griffiths GJ. Imaging of the prostate by ultrasound. J Urol 1984; 132: 217.

7. Shortliffe LMD, Elliott KM, Sellers RG et al. Measurement of chlamydial and ureaplasmal antibodies in serum and prostatic fluid of men with nonbacterial prostatitis. J Urol 1985; 133: 276A.

8. Berger RE, Alexander ER, Harnisch JP et al. Etiology, manifestations and therapy of acute epididymitis: prospective study of 50 cases. J Urol 1979; 121: 750.

9. Meares EM Jr. Bacterial prostatitis versus 'prostatitis': a clinical and bacteriological study. JAMA 1973; 224: 1372.

10. Mardh P-A, Colleen S. Search for uro-genital tract infections in patients with symptoms of prostatitis. Studies on aerobic and strictly anaerobic bacteria, mycoplasmas, fungi, trichomonads and viruses. Scand J Urol Nephrol 1975; 9: 8.

11. Berger RE, Krieger JN, Kessler D et al. Case–control study of men with suspected chronic idiopathic prostatitis. J Urol 1989; 141: 328.

12. Kirby RS, Lowe D, Bultitude MI, Shuttleworth KED. Intra-prostatic urinary reflux: an aetiological factor in bacterial prostatitis. Br J Urol 1982; 54: 729.

13. Gow JG. Genitourinary tuberculosis. In: Campbell's Urology (Walsh PC, Retic AB, Vaughan ED, Wein AJ, eds). Philadelphia: WB Saunders, 1998: 817.

14. Rifkin MD, Tessler FN, Tublin ME, Ross JS. US case of the day. Granulomatous prostatitis resulting from BCG therapy. Radiographics 1998; 18: 1605–7.

15. Chen KTK, Schiff JJ. Coccidioidiomycysis of prostate. Urology 1985; 25: 82.

16. Towfighi J, Sadeghee S, Wheeler JE et al. Granulomatous prostatitis with emphasis on eosinophilic variety. Am J Clin Pathol 1972; 58: 630.

17. Stanton MJ, Maxted W. Malakoplakia: a study of the literature and current concepts of pathogenesis, diagnosis and treatment. J Urol 1981; 125: 139.

18. Clements R, Gower TK, Griffiths GJ, Peeling WB. Transrectal ultrasound appearances of granulomatous prostatitis. Clin Radiol 1993; 47: 174–6.

19. Sohlberg OE, Chetner M, Platch N, Brawer MM. Prostatic abscess after transrectal guided prostatic biopsy. J Urol 1991; 146: 420–2.

20. Fincke B, Friedland G. Prevention and management of infection in the catheterised patient. Urol Clin North Am 1976; 3: 313.

21. Mears EMJ. Prostadynia: clinical findings and rationale for treatment. In: Therapy of Prostatitis (Weider W, Brenner H, Krause W, Rathauge CF, eds). Munich: W Zuckschwerdt Verlag, 1986; 207–11.

22. Dalton D. Elevated serum prostate specific antigen due to acute bacterial prostatitis. Urology 1989; 33: 645.

23. Griffiths G, Crooks A, Roberts E et al. Ultrasonic appearance associated with prostatic inflammation: a preliminary study. Clin Radiol 1984; 35: 343–5.

24. Secaf E, Nuruddin RN, Hricak H et al. MR imaging of the seminal vescicles. AJR Am J Roentgenol 1991; 156: 989–94.

25. Bryan DJ, Butler HE, Nelson AO et al. Magnetic resonance imaging of the prostate. AJR 1986; 146: 543–8.

26. Lee JKT, Rholl KS. MRI of the bladder and prostate. AJR 1986; 147: 732–6.

27. McNeal J. Regional morphology and pathology of the prostate. Am J Pathol 1986; 49: 347–57.

28. Di Trapani D, Pavone C, Serretta V et al. Chronic prostatitis and prostatodynia: ultrasonic alterations of the prostate, bladder neck, seminal vesicle and periprostatic venous plexas. Eur Urol 1988; 15: 230.

29. Doble A, Carter S. Ultrasonographic findings in prostatitis. Urol Clin North Am 1989; 16: 763–73.

30. Cho IR, Keener TS, Nghiem HV et al. Prostatic blood flow characteristics in the chronic prostatitis/pelvic pain syndrome. J Urol 2000; 163: 1130–3.

31. Rifkin M, Sudakoff G, Alexander A. Color Doppler imaging of the prostate. Technique, results and potential applications. Radiology 1993; 186: 509–13.

32. Rabii R, Rais H, Joual A et al. Prostatic abscesses. A review. Ann Urol 1999; 33: 271–73.

33. Papanicolaou N, Pfister RC, Stafford SA, Parkhurst EC. Prostate abscess: Imaging with transrectal sonography and MR. AJR 1987; 149: 981.

34. Thornhill BA, Morehouse HT, Coleman P, Hoffman-Tretin JC. Prostatic abscess: CT and sonographic findings. AJR 1987; 148: 899.

35. Rorvik J, Daehlin L. Prostatic abscess: imaging with transrectal ultrasound. Scand J Urol Nephrol 1989; 23: 307.

36. Rifkin M. Ultrasound of the Prostate, 2nd edn. Philadelphia: Lippincott-Raven, 1997.

37. Rifkin MD. Inflammation of the lower genitourinary tract: the prostate, seminal vesicles and scrotum. In: Clinical Urography, 2nd edn (Pollack HM, McClellan BL, eds). Philadelphia: WB Saunders, 2000.

38. Bude R, Bree RL, Adler RS, Jafri SZ. Transrectal ultrasound appearance of granulomatous prostatitis. J Ultrasound Med 1990; 9: 677.

39. Christensen WI. Genitourinary tuberculosis: review of 102 cases. Medicine 1974; 53: 377.

40. Wolf LE. Tuberculous abscess of the prostate in AIDS. Ann Intern Med 1996; 125: 156.

41. Wang J, Chang T. Tuberculosis of the prostate: CT appearance. J Comput Assist Tomogr 1991; 15: 269.

42. Hamrick-Turner J, Abbitt PL, Ros PR. Tuberculosis of the lower genitourinary tract: findings on sonography and MR. AJR 1992; 158: 919.

43. Stanton MJ, Maxted W. Malakoplakia: a study of the literature and current concepts of pathogenesis, diagnosis and treatment. J Urol 1981; 125: 139.

44. Anderson T, Kristiansen W, Ruge S, Hansen JPH. Malakoplakia of the prostate causing fatal fistula to rectum. Scand J Urol Nephrol 1986; 20: 153.

45. Chantelois AE, Parker SH, Sims JE, Horne DW. Malakoplakia of the prostate sonographically mimicking carcinoma. Radiology 1990; 177: 193.

46. McClure J. Malakoplakia of the prostate: a report of two cases and a review of the literature. J Clin Pathol 1979; 32: 629.

47. Koga S, Arakaki Y, Matsouka M, Ohyama C. Malakoplakia of the prostate. Eur Urol 1985; 11: 137.

48. Lou TY, Teplitz C. Malakoplakia: pathogenesis and ultra-structural morphogenesis: a problem of altered macrophase (phagolysosomal) response. Hum Pathol 1974; 5: 191.

49. Gan E. Transrectal ultrasound-guided needle aspiration for prostatic abscesses: an alternative to transurethral drainage? Techn Urol 2000; 6: 178–84.

50. Lim JW, Ko YT, Lee DH et al. Treatment of prostatic abscess: the value of transrectal ultrasonographically guided needle aspiration. J Ultrasound Med 2000; 19: 609–17.

51. Collado A, Palou J, Garcia-Penit J et al. Ultrasound-guided needle aspiration in prostatic abscess. Urology 1999; 53: 548–52.

13

Prostatic calculi and calcifications

Dennis Ll Cochlin

General considerations

The terms calculus and calcification are often used loosely for the same entity. Strictly speaking, however, calculi form in hollow organs or cavities whereas calcifications form in solid tissues. Both may occur in the prostate. Prostatic calculi and calcifications may be classified as primary, which occur in an otherwise-normal gland, or secondary, which accompany a pathological process (usually benign prostatic hypertrophy (BPH), prostatitis, or cancer). In practice, however, there is overlap between these two groups.

Prostatic calculi and calcifications are very common in older men, and are found incidentally in 50% of transrectal ultrasound examinations for suspected prostatic cancer. Larger calcifications are often seen on plain abdominal X-rays. Such calcifications are more common in patients with upper urinary tract calculi, probably due to hypercalcaemia.[1] Postmortem autopsy studies, however, show that microscopic calculi are far more common than those seen on diagnostic imaging, occurring in 30% of all adult prostates.[2] It is only in a small minority of older men that prostatic calculi or calcifications are clinically significant. In younger men, however, calculi and calcifications are less common, and more often indicate significant pathology.

Aetiology

The periurethral glands in young men are situated adjacent to the urethra and the ejaculatory ducts. In older men, hyperplasia of the inner gland may displace some periurethral glands outwards so that they lie in the junction between the enlarged inner gland and the outer gland, commonly known as the surgical capsule. This distribution of the periurethral glands that changes with hyperplasia and age determines the distribution of prostatic calculi.[2]

Periurethral glands secrete a proteinaceous material, which forms bodies called corpora amylacea. Calculi form within these bodies inside periurethral glands. Following the normal distribution of periurethral glandular tissue, these calculi typically form linear strings along the urethra above the verumontanum (Figure 13.1), and particularly in the region of the verumontanum (Figure 13.2). Similar strings of calculi may also form along the line of the ejaculatory ducts (Figure 13.3). In older men with BPH, linear calcification is commonly seen along the surgical capsule (Figure 13.4). Obstruction of periurethral glandular elements within the prostate by BPH may lead to further calculus formation.[2] Calcifications in the periurethral area, along the ejaculatory ducts, and along the surgical capsule are rarely of clinical significance, although they may be associated with prostatitis in young men. Calculi within the lumen of the urethra or ejaculatory duct, however, are significant and are often very difficult to distinguish from periurethral or periductal calculi[4] (Figures 13.5 and 13.6). Calculi may also occur in Müllerian duct cysts and ejaculatory duct cysts. These are discussed in Chapter 10.

Calcifications in other parts of the prostate have a different aetiology. They occur when calcium salts impregnate secretions that collect around groups of desquamated epithelial cells in the follicles of the prostatic glandular tissue. They may therefore occur anywhere in the prostate, although they are more common in the inner gland than the outer gland. When they occur in a scattered pattern in older men, they are of no clinical significance[5] (Figure 13.7). When grouped together, however, and particularly when unilateral and occurring in younger men, they suggest prostatitis, which may be active or resolved (Figure 13.8). Although calcifications may occur in any type of prostatitis, they are more common in granulomatous prostatitis.[6] Calculi associated with bacterial prostatitis

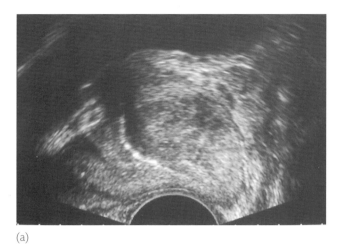

(a)

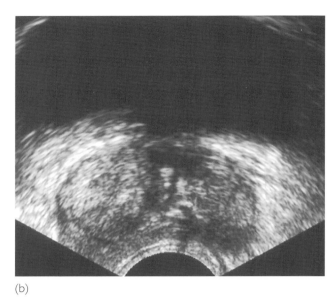

(b)

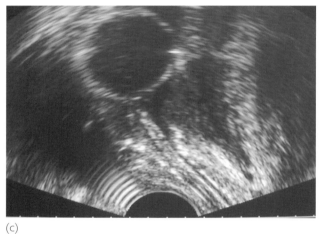

(c)

Figure 13.1
Periurethral calculi. (a) Sagittal and (b) axial views showing a typical pattern of a row of calculi lying along the urethra above the level of the verumontanum. (c) Sagittal view with a urethral catheter in situ, showing the periurethral situation of the calculi.

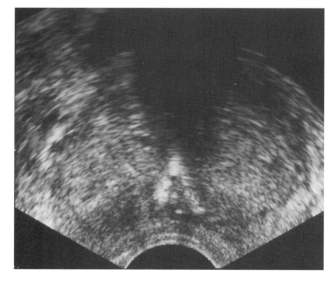

Figure 13.2
Calculi at the verumontanum. Calculi are shown around the verumontanum with a characteristic 'inverted-V' pattern. They should not be misinterpreted as ejaculatory duct cysts.

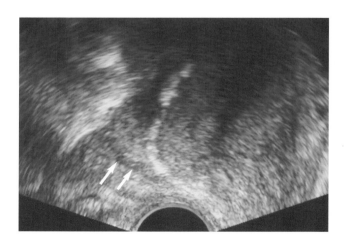

Figure 13.3
Peri-ejaculatory duct calculi. This sagittal view shows peri-ejaculatory duct calculi (arrows) posterior to the periurethral calculi.

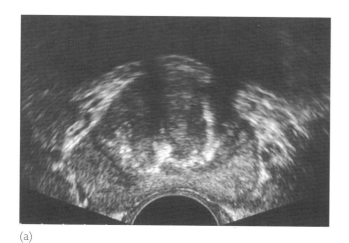

(a)

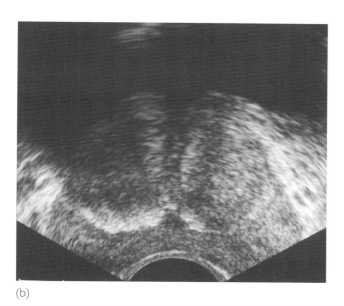

(b)

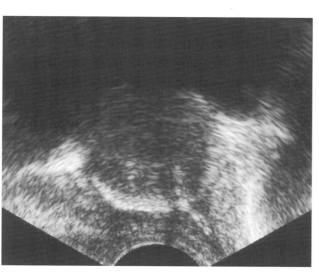

(c)

Figure 13.4
Calculi in the surgical capsule. (a) Axial scan showing calculi in the surgical capsule of a patient with moderate benign prostatic hypertrophy (BPH). (b) Coronal and (c) sagittal scans showing calculi in the surgical capsule of a patient with marked BPH.

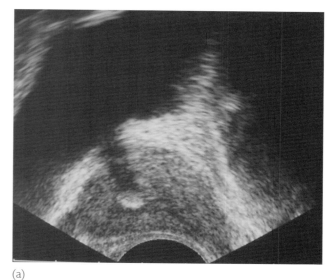

(a)

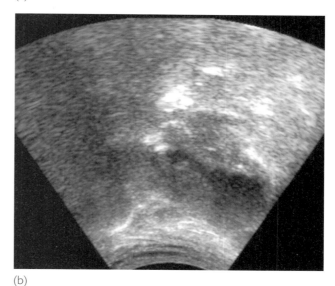

(b)

Figure 13.5
Urethral calculus. (a) This sagittal scan in a patient with suspected prostatitis shows a urethral calculus. This was later proven by urethrography. (b) This transabdominal scan of a man in acute retention shows a calculus in the urethra. There is also a transurethral resection (TURP) defect.

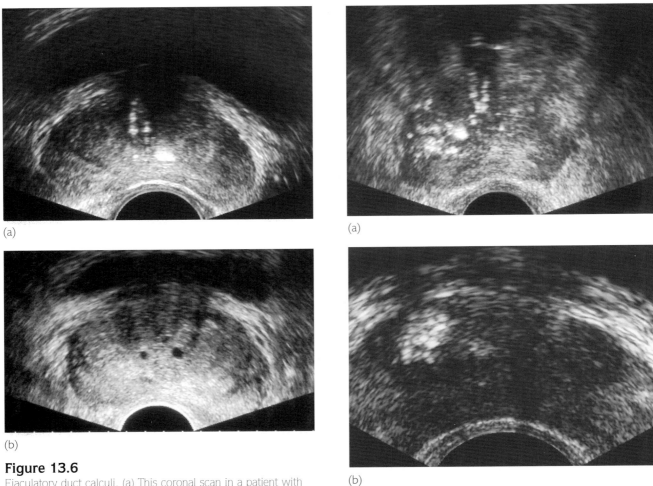

(a)

(b)

Figure 13.6
Ejaculatory duct calculi. (a) This coronal scan in a patient with haematospermia shows a small ejaculatory duct calculus on the right and a larger one on the left. (b) A coronal scan at a more cranial level shows dilated ejaculatory ducts.

(a)

(b)

Figure 13.8
Calculi due to prostatitis. (a) A closely packed group of calcifications are seen in the right inner gland, with a surrounding hypoechoic area. These are typical of the calculi of prostatitis. (b) Closely packed calculi within a hypoechoic area due to prostatitis in a young man.

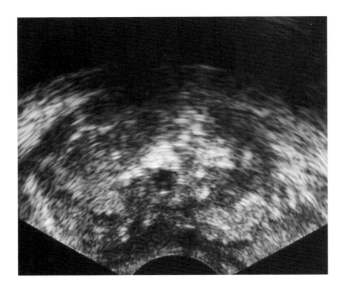

Figure 13.7
Scattered parenchymal calcifications. Scattered calcifications are seen throughout the inner and outer gland.

may act as a nidus of infection, complicating the eradication of infection. In refractory cases of infection, it may be useful to remove such a nidus from the prostate.[7,8] This relationship between calculi and continuing infection is not clearly established, and remains controversial.

Calculi within the prostate are sometimes packed very closely. High-resolution ultrasound units may resolve individual calculi that may appear as a single calculus on transabdominal ultrasound or plain X-rays (Figure 13.9). Low-resolution imaging is probably responsible for reports in the literature of prostatic calculi up to several centimetres in size. Such large calculi may actually represent closely packed groups of smaller calculi.

Calcifications rarely occur in prostate cancers. More commonly, cancers may develop in areas of previous benign

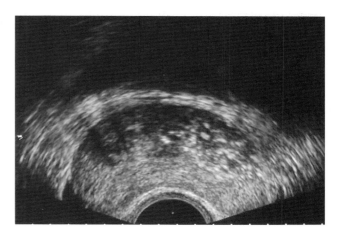

Figure 13.10

Cancer surrounding calculi. A hypoechoic cancer is seen with calcifications within it. There are also other calcifications in the gland, and it is likely that the cancer has formed around pre-existing benign calculi.

calcification. Cancer may grow to surround areas of benign calcification, particularly in the inner gland (Figure 13.10). Less commonly, dystrophic calcification may arise in areas of tumour necrosis. Calcifications that form within a cancer demonstrate a far finer pattern than benign calculi[7] (Figures 13.11 and 13.12). Thus, in patients undergoing transrectal ultrasound-guided biopsy of the prostate for suspected prostatic cancer, directed biopsy should be performed into areas of fine calcification.

Even in patients with suspected prostate cancer, areas of coarse calcification in the inner gland almost always represent benign disease. However, biopsy of these areas may demonstrate active prostatitis. In the absence of cancer, such biopsy results may be useful to explain a high serum prostate-specific antigen (PSA) level. In such patients with coexisting cancer and prostatitis, the PSA level may not be correlated with the volume of the tumour.

Several other rare causes of prostatic calculi deserve mention. Tuberculous prostatitis often presents with focal masses, but only rarely causes calcification. The calcification of tuberculous prostatitis when it does occur is quite dense, and may involve the entire gland[9] (Figure 13.13). Schistosomiasis may rarely cause prostatic calcifications, which are scattered throughout the gland and are due to calcified ova in the prostatic acini and ducts[10] (Figure 13.14).

Dense calcification may occur following radiotherapy when this procedure is performed shortly after transurethral resection[11] (Figure 13.15). This complication is now rarely seen, since awareness of it has led to radiotherapy being delayed for a sufficient period following surgery.

Ochronosis with alkaptonuria is a rare cause of prostatic calculi. The calculi are due to precipitation of homogentisic acid.[12]

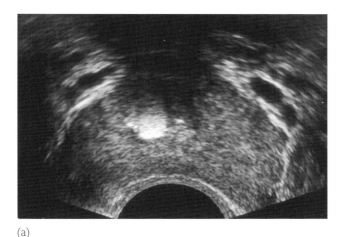

(a)

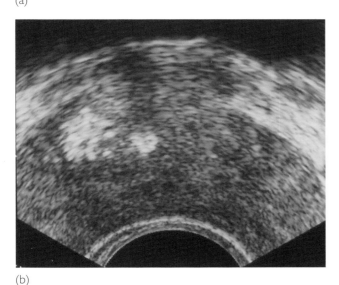

(b)

Figure 13.9

'Large' calculi. (a) An apparently large calculus that is in reality a group of closely packed small calculi. (b) Two 'large' calculi: in this case, a high-resolution scan clearly defines these as numerous closely packed separate small calculi.

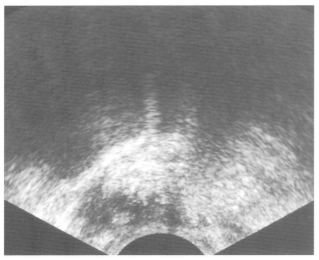

(a)

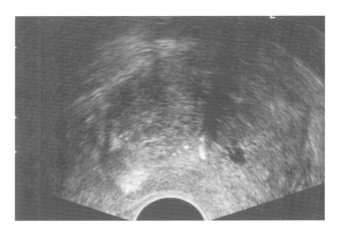

Figure 13.12
Calcification in a cancer. Calcifications are seen within this peripheral cancer. The calcifications are typically finer than those seen in benign calcification.

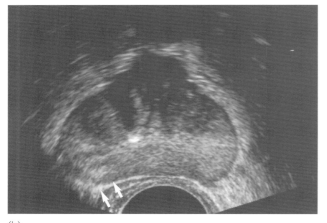

(b)

Figure 13.11
Calcification in a cancer. (a) The outer gland cancer contains a group of calcifications. (b) This cancer contains calculi with a linear pattern (arrows).

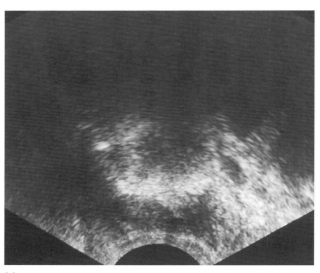

(a)

Figure 13.13
Tuberculosis. (a) In this relatively early case, there is dense calcification occupying much of the gland along with areas of necrosis. (b) X-ray film of an advanced case showing dense linear calcification of the prostatic fossa. At cystoscopy, no prostatic tissue was seen. Presumably, the glandular portions of the gland had sloughed and passed. The calcification lined the surface of the remaining prostatic fossa. Reproduced by kind permission from Kim SH. Genitourinary tuberculosis. In: Clinical Urography, 2nd edn (Pollack HM, McClellan BL, eds). Philadelphia: WB Saunders, 2000.

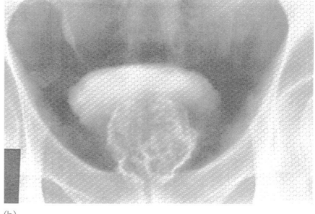

(b)

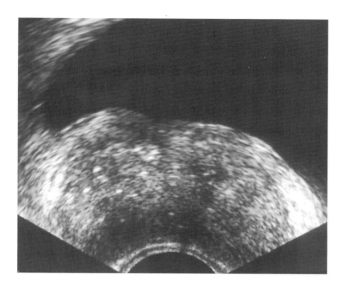

Figure 13.14

Schistosomiasis. Rounded calcifications are seen throughout the gland, representing calcified ova in the prostatic ducts.

The significance of prostatic calculi

Idiopathic calculi may occur at any age. However, in a young man, prostatic calculi occurring in any pattern suggest prostatitis. Closely grouped calculi are more suggestive of prostatitis, particularly if unilateral. In a small minority of men, the calculi may possibly act as a nidus of infection. Removal of these calculi may be necessary for eradication of the prostatitis.

Fine calcifications may be rarely found in cancers. When fine calcifications are seen, they should be biopsied. Areas of calcification near the posterior border of the gland may produce hard palpable areas on digital rectal examination (Figure 13.16). Such calcifications should be reported on transrectal ultrasound of the prostate, as they may explain the findings on digital rectal examination, and may negate the significance of the digital rectal examination findings for staging prostate cancer.

Calcifications may hide parts of the anterior gland on transrectal ultrasound study owing to shadowing (Figure 13.17). This is rarely a significant problem, since most cancers occur in the outer gland, which is rarely obscured.

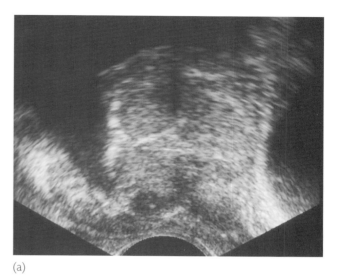

(a)

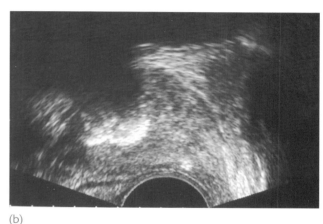

(b)

Figure 13.15

Post-radiotherapy calcification. (a) Sagittal and (b) coronal views showing farly dense calcification around a TURP defect. The patient had received a course of radiotherapy commencing two weeks after the transurethral resection.

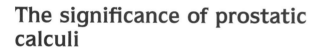

Figure 13.16

Peripheral calcification clinically simulating cancer. The peripheral calcification on the right of the prostate presented as a hard nodule on digital rectal examination. It was clinically thought to be cancer. Transrectal ultrasound-guided biopsy of this area and the rest of the gland showed no evidence of cancer.

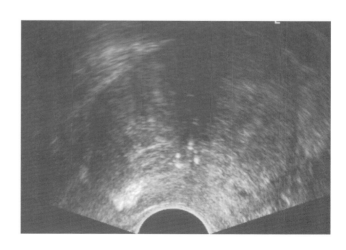

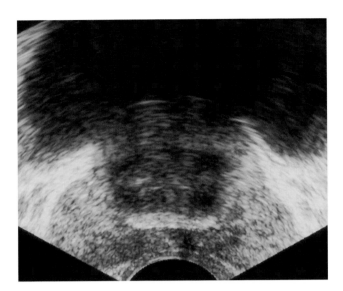

Figure 13.17
Calcification obscuring part of the gland. The dense surgical capsule calcification obscures a large part of the gland.

Calculi within the urethra and ejaculatory ducts are difficult to distinguish from periurethral and periductal calculi unless there is significant dilatation of the urethra or duct (Figure 13.5 and 13.6). When this distinction is important, the diagnosis of urethral calculi may be made by urethrography – either conventional contrast urethrography or sonourethrography. Ejaculatory duct calculi are confirmed in some centres by contrast studies of the ducts. Calculi in Müllerian duct cysts and ejaculatory duct cysts are rare. They are discussed in Chapter 10.

References

1. Sutor DJ, Wooley SE. The crystalline composition of prostate calculi. Br J Urol 1974; 46: 533.
2. Fox M. The natural history and significance of stone formation in the prostate gland. J Urol 1963; 89: 716.
3. Littrup PJ, Lee F, McLeary RD et al. Transrectal US of the seminal vesicles and ejaculatory ducts: clinical correlation. Radiology 1988; 168: 625.
4. Peeling WB, Griffiths GJ. Imaging of the prostate by ultrasound. J Urol 1984; 132: 217.
5. Clements R, Thomas KG, Griffiths GJ, Peeling WB. Transrectal ultrasound appearances of granulomatous prostatitis. Clin Radiol 1993; 47: 174.
6. Eykyn S, Bultitude MI, Mayo ME, Lloyd-Davies RW. Prostatic calculi as a source of recurrent bactiurea in the male. Br J Urol 1974; 46: 527.
7. Mears EMJ. Infected stones of the prostate gland. Laboratory diagnosis and clinical management. Urology 1974; 4: 560.
8. Egawa S, Wheeler TM, Greene DR, Scardino PT. Unusual hypoechoic appearance of prostate cancer on transrectal ultrasonography. Br J Urol 1992; 69: 169.
9. Roylance J, Penry JB, Rhys Davies E, Roberts M. The radiology of tuberculosis of the urinary tract. Clin Radiol 1970; 21: 163.
10. Al-Ghorab MM. Radiological manifestations of genito-urinary bilharziasis. Clin Radiol 1968; 19: 100.
11. Jones WA, Miller EV, Sullivan LD, Chapman WH. Severe prostatic calcification after radiation therapy for cancer. J Urol 1979; 121: 828.
12. Douenias R, Rich M, Badlani G et al. Predisposing factors in bladder calculi: review of 100 cases. Urology 1991; 37: 240–3.

14

The seminal vesicles, ejaculatory ducts and vasa deferentia

Dennis Ll Cochlin

General considerations

The seminal vesicles develop as lateral outpouchings of the Wolffian ducts during the 13th to 19th weeks of gestation.[1,2] These symmetrical structures lie at the superior aspect of the prostate, behind the bladder. They are separated from the rectum and bladder by fibrofatty tissue and neurovascular structures of the hypogastric sheath. The shape of the seminal vesicles is variable. They may be long and narrow, or short and wide, but should appear symmetrical (Figures 14.1 and 14.2). They may lie horizontally or they may be orientated in a 'V' pattern, sometimes extending quite steeply in a cephalad direction from the bladder base. Three anatomic patterns of tubular structures are recognized in the seminal vesicles. In the majority of men, each seminal vesicle consists of a single tightly folded tube, 10–18 cm in (unfolded) length, with short side branches, 3–4 mm in diameter. Variations of this branching pattern have little importance when interpreting diagnostic images. The typical seminal vesicle measures 0.4–1.4 cm in width and 1.9–4.1 cm in length.[3,4]

Imaging of the seminal vesicles

The seminal vesicles may be visualized on transabdominal ultrasound studies through the full bladder. However, transrectal sonography provides superior anatomic detail. The best images are produced in the axial/coronal plane with a transrectal transducer (Figure 14.2). In patients with prostatic hyperplasia, the seminal vesicles are displaced superiorly, and an end-firing transducer may be required (Figure 14.1). High-frequency transrectal ultrasound may visualize the seminal vesicle as a tightly folded tube, with luminal contents of variable echodensity. The junction of the seminal vesicle with the ampullary portion of the vas deferens forms the ejaculatory duct (Figure 14.3). A wedge-shaped area of fat is found between the prostate and the seminal vesicles, but may be obliterated in cases of seminal vesicle invasion by prostate cancer (Figure 14.9).

As the seminal vesicles lie at a variable angle to the true coronal plane, it is sometimes advantageous to angle the transducer in order to image each vesicle separately along its length. Large seminal vesicles may extend outside the field of view of a transrectal transducer positioned in the midline. In these cases, the lateral tips of the seminal vesicles need to be

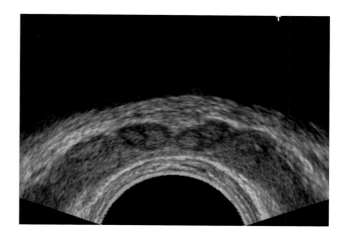

Figure 14.1
Normal seminal vesicles. These were imaged in an angled coronal plane with an end-firing transducer. Some of the walls are seen as hypoechoic rings, and some are merged with the medium-echodensity luminal contents. The tips lie out of the field of view.

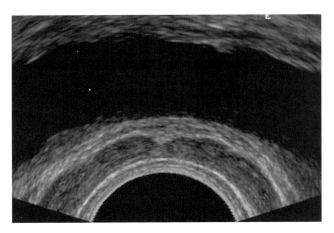

Figure 14.2
Normal seminal vesicles. These were imaged in the axial plane with a side-firing transducer. The plane is similar to that shown in Figure 14.1, but is a true axial plane and gives somewhat more detail.

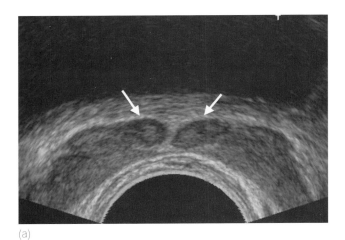

(a)

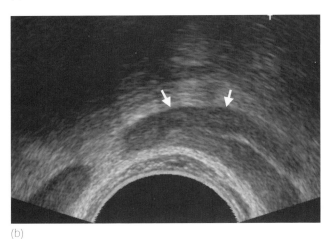

(b)

Figure 14.3
Junction of seminal vesicles and vasa deferentia. (a) The ampullae of the vasa deferentia are seen (arrows), with the seminal vesicles extending laterally. (b) An oblique view shows the left vas deferens in greater length (arrows).

imaged separately (Figure 14.4). The normal tapered appearance of the seminal vesicle is well visualized in the oblique sagittal plane as it approaches the base of the prostate (Figures 14.1–14.5). The fat triangle between the prostate and the seminal vesicle should also be visible in this plane

Magnetic resonance imaging (MRI) produces excellent images of the seminal vesicles, but it is doubtful whether MRI has any advantage over ultrasound for imaging of the seminal vesicles. Very detailed images are produced with a transrectal coil, although a good phased-array pelvic coil may produce images that are as good, without the invasiveness and costs of a transrectal coil (such coils are for single-use only). Seminal vesicles are seen on T2-weighted MRI as multiple ovoid areas of high signal, representing the lumen cut at various angles, surrounded by low-signal rings representing the walls of the tube. The signal intensity of luminal contents varies with age, and probably reflects androgen status. In men below the age of about 70 years, the signal intensity of the luminal contents is equal to or greater than that of fat. In prepubertal boys and older men, the signal intensity is equal to or less than that of fat. The walls and narrower lumen of the vas deferens are also demonstrated by MRI (Figure 14.6). T1-weighted MRI demonstrates lower signal in the lumen, often similar to the signal intensity of muscle. Computer tomography (CT) scans of the pelvis also demonstrate the seminal vesicles and vasa deferentia, but with less detail than sonography and MRI (Figure 14.7).

Vasography and seminal vesiculography can be used to test the patency of the vasa deferentia and ejaculatory ducts by injection of saline, methylene blue, or radiographic contrast into the vas deferens. Much of the information that was previously obtained by this invasive technique may now be obtained by transrectal ultrasound or MRI. The technique of vasography involves exposing the vas deferens in the scrotal sac via a small incision and cannulating it. Saline is usually

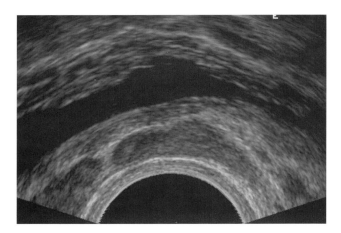

Figure 14.4
Normal seminal vesicles. An axial view at an angle producd by rotating the transducer shows the tip of the left seminal vesicle.

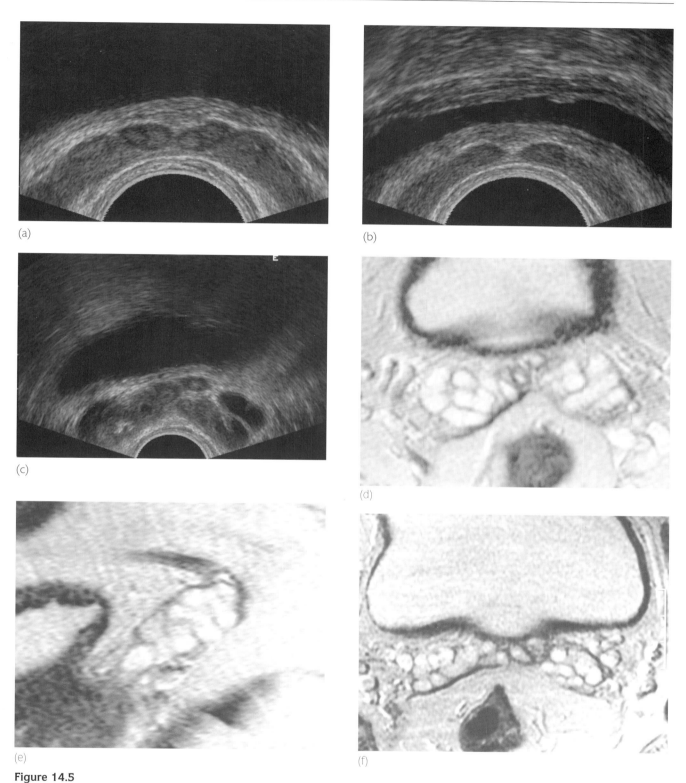

Figure 14.5

Variations in the pattern of the normal seminal vesicles with age. (a) Transrectal ultrasound study in a 30-year-old man: the seminal vesicles are of normal size, with medium-echodensity luminal contents. (b) A 65-year-old man: the luminal contents are of higher echodensity and the walls are ill defined. (c) A 71-year-old man: the vesicles are dilated and there is layering of the luminal contents. (d–f) T2-weighted axial and sagittal MRI of the seminal vesicles of a 40-year-old man: the luminal contents are homogeneously high-signal; the walls are low-signal. (g) A 9-year-old boy shows small, low-signal seminal vesicles. (h) A 60-year-old man shows rather large lumina, which are common at this age: this is probably due to an element of obstruction from benign prostatic hypertrophy.

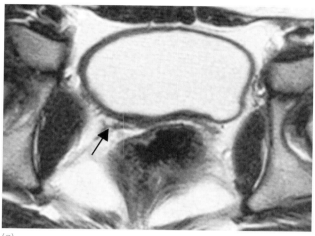

(g)

Figure 14.5
Continued

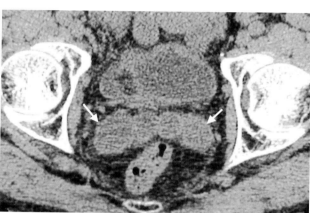

(h)

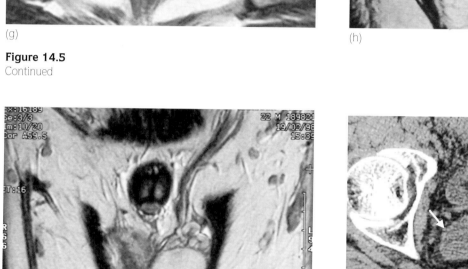

Figure 14.6
Normal vasa deferentia : MRI study. In this T2-weighted coronal study, a long length of the vas deferens is demonstrated.

Figure 14.7
Normal seminal vesicles: CT scan. The seminal vesicles are clearly seen (arrows). The images lack the detail of transrectal ultrasound or MRI studies.

injected first in both directions, towards the epididymis and towards the ejaculatory duct. Flow without resistance suggests patency. In a patent system, methylene blue injected towards the ejaculatory duct is observed to flow into the urethra. Observation is achieved by direct visualization via a ureteroscope or by seeing flow through a Foley catheter inserted into the bladder. In cases of obstruction when the level of obstruction remains in doubt, injection of radiographic contrast under fluoroscopic control will outline the ejaculatory structures and define the point of obstruction, as well as any cysts that communicate with the system. The seminal vesicle is demonstrated by vasography as a fine tightly folded tube.[5]

An alternative method of studying the seminal vesicles and ejaculatory ducts is by transrectal ultrasound-guided injection of contrast into the seminal vesicles. This approach is less invasive than conventional vasography and does not run the risk of damaging the vas. This technique outlines the lumina of the seminal vesicles and the normal ejaculatory ducts, but not the proximal vasa deferentia[6] (Figure 14.8).

Seminal vesicle involvement in prostate cancer

Seminal vesicle involvement in prostate cancer has an impact on staging, treatment options, and prognosis. The seminal

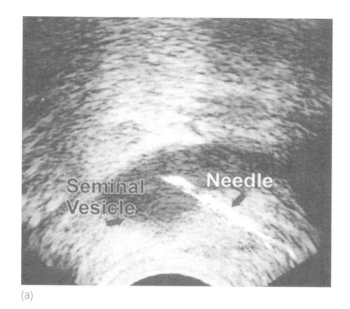

(a)

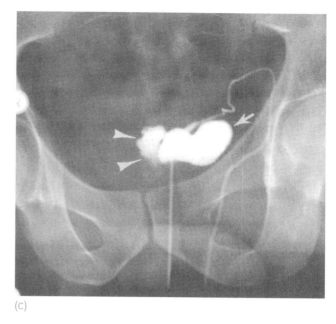

(c)

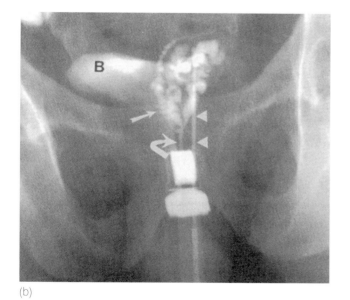

(b)

Figure 14.8

Seminal vesiculography. (a) Transrectal ultrasound image shows the seminal vesicle puncture. (b) Normal study. Contrast has been injected through the needle (arrowheads) to opacify the left seminal vesicle, the ampulla of the vas deferens (straight arrow), and the ejaculatory duct (curved arrow). Contrast is seen in the bladder (B), indicating patency of the ejaculatory duct. (c) In this study, the left seminal vesicle (arrow) and the ampulla of the vas deferens (arrowheads) are dilated. Retrograde filling of the vas deferens, a common finding with this technique, is also shown. The ejaculatory duct and bladder have not filled, indicating obstruction. Reproduced with permission from Jones TR, Zagara RJ, Jarrow JP. Transrectal US-guided seminal vesiculography. Radiology 1997; 205: 276–8.

vesicles are always examined as part of the transrectal ultrasound-guided biopsy procedure, although sonographic diagnosis of seminal vesicle invasion is difficult. One well-known sign is obliteration of the triangles of fat that lie between the base of the prostate and the seminal vesicles due to spread of tumour through the fat (Figure 14.9). Invasion of the seminal vesicle itself may be manifest as a loss of the normal tapered appearance as the vesicle approaches the prostate. Increased echogenicity of part of the seminal vesicle, particularly the proximal part, is highly suspicious (Figure 14.10). Altered echodensity of the lumina of the seminal vesicles is common in older men, and is not a reliable sign of cancer involvement.[7,8] Asymmetry of the seminal vesicles is also suspicious. The confirmation of seminal vesicle

involvement is obtained by direct biopsy of the seminal vesicles via the transrectal approach. Biopsy of the seminal vesicles does not add significantly to the complication rate of prostate biopsy, although haematospermia is more common than when the prostate alone is biopsied.

MRI is more sensitive than transrectal ultrasound in detecting seminal vesicle involvement in prostate cancer, although its specificity is low. MRI may demonstrate low signal-areas in the seminal vesicles that are suspicious for cancer[9] (Figure 14.11). When such areas are in direct continuity with a low-signal tumour within the prostate, it is highly probable that they represent invasion of the seminal vesicles (Figure 14.12). Suspicion of tumour invasion may be confirmed by biopsy (Figure 14.13). In the author's centre,

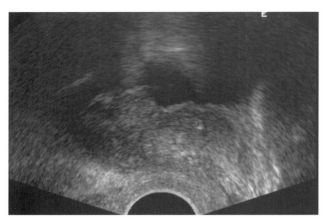

Figure 14.9
Prostate cancer involving the seminal vesicles: transrectal ultrasound study, sagittal view. The seminal vesicle is invaded by prostatic tumour. The position of the normal fat angle is obliterated.

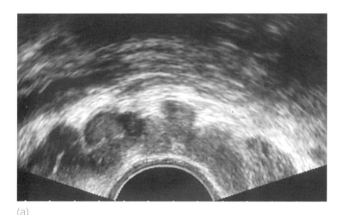

(a)

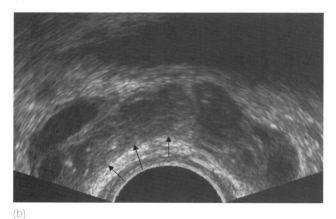

(b)

Figure 14.10
Prostate cancer involving the seminal vesicles. (a) The medial parts of the seminal vesicles show increased echodensity and loss of definition of the walls and lumina due to prostatic tumour invasion. The lateral part of the right seminal vesicle is obstructed by the tumour. (b) A different case. Some of the architecture of the seminal vesicles is preserved, but there is tumour in the posterior part (arrows).

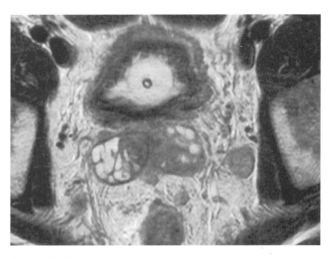

Figure 14.11
Prostate cancer involving the seminal vesicle: T2-weighted MRI study, with TR = 5601, TE = 84. The tumour is seen in the medial parts of both seminal vesicles.

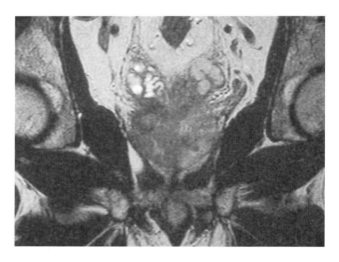

Figure 14.12
Prostate cancer involving the seminal vesicles: T2-weighted MRI study, with TR = 2600, TE = 98. There is medium to low signal in the medial part of the left seminal vesicle. In this case, it is in continuity with the prostate tumour. The loss of signal in the lumen of the seminal vesicle above the tumour is a feature that is often seen. The cause is not known – it may be related to obstruction by the tumour.

we perform three biopsies of each seminal vesicle (distal, mid, and proximal), including the part of the seminal vesicle seen on the MRI to be abnormal. Many such cases show no specific histologic abnormality on the biopsy core. Abnormal MRI signal may be related to alterations in the contents of the vesicle lumen related to age, or perhaps to reduced sexual activity.

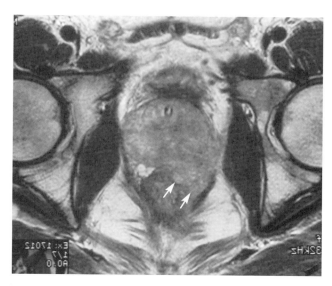

Figure 14.13

Prostate cancer involving the seminal vesicles: T2-weighted MRI study, with TR = 600, TE = 84. There is low signal throughout the left seminal vesicle (arrows). Biopsy showed this to be tumour, but this pattern is of low specificity and may be seen in older men owing to age-related changes.

Amyloid

Amyloidosis frequently affects the seminal vesicles of older men, and is found on autopsy studies in 20% of men over 76 years of age.[10] Usually, amyloid involvement is of very small areas that are not detected on imaging. Occasionally amyloidosis causes solid areas large enough to be visible on ultrasound or MRI studies (Figure 14.14). Such cases may mimic involvement of the seminal vesicles with prostate cancer. The true diagnosis may only be revealed by biopsy of the seminal vesicles.[11]

Seminal vesicle cysts

True cysts of the seminal vesicle are rare, and most are congenital.[16] Some may be acquired after episodes of infection or obstruction.[17,18] Hydatid cysts of the seminal vesicles have also been described.[19,20] Congenital cysts are often associated with other mesonephric duct abnormalities, including ectopic insertion of the ureter into the seminal vesicle and ipsilateral renal abnormalities such as agenesis of the kidney (Zinner syndrome) or ureter.[15,19,21–23] Some are associated with adult (autosomal dominant) polycystic kidney disease.[24]

Most seminal vesicle cysts are small and asymptomatic, although cysts of any size may present with chronic haematospermia or painful ejaculation. Some cysts, however, reach a considerable size, some even filling the whole pelvis.[24] These present with symptoms due to their pressure effects. Pressure on the bladder may produce frequency or outlet obstruction, while pressure effects on the rectum can result in tenesmus.[25]

Most seminal vesicle cysts are unilateral, but bilateral cysts have been described. Cysts may be unilocular, septate, or multilocular. Larger cysts involve the whole seminal vesicle, with no normal vesicular structures remaining (Figure 14.15). Malignant change has been described in seminal vesicle cysts, but is exceedingly rare[21]. The usual treatment for a symptomatic simple seminal vesicle cyst is aspiration.

Large cysts of the seminal vesicle may be seen on an ultrasound study, CT, or MRI of the pelvis. Smaller cysts are best demonstrated by transrectal ultrasound (Figure 14.15) or seminal vesicle MRI using a phased-array coil (Figure 14.16). The imaging features of uncomplicated cysts of the seminal vesicles are the same as those of any other simple cyst.

Seminal vesicle cysts may become infected, and present with the symptoms of prostatitis, or with pressure symptoms on the bladder or rectum. Aspiration and antibiotic therapy are the recommended treatments for infected cysts.

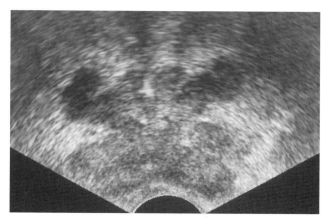

Figure 14.14

Seminal vesicle amyloidosis. Seminal vesicles show solid contents within their lumena. This was thought to be involvement with prostatic cancer, but biopsy revealed amyloidosis.

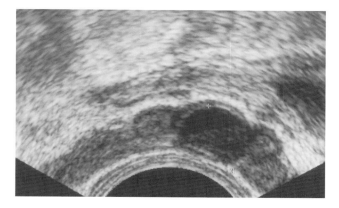

Figure 14.15

Seminal vesicle cyst. Transrectal ultrasound study. This is a typical seminal vesicle cyst. There is some layering, which suggested the possibility of infection, but aspiration revealed a sterile cyst.

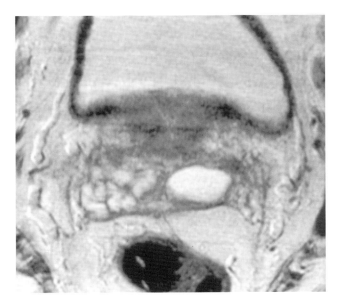

Figure 14.16
Seminal vesicle cyst: T2-weighted MRI study. Axial view showing a typical seminal vesicle cyst.

Sonography of infected cysts may demonstrate complex patterns of echogenicity, sometimes with layering (Figure 14.17). MRI may also demonstrate a pattern of change in the signal of the cyst contents. Imaging appearances of infected cysts, however, may be identical to those of uninfected cysts. In patients with symptoms suggestive of infection, cyst aspiration should be performed regardless of the appearance.

Seminal vesicle and vas deferens calcifications and calculi

Calcifications of the vasa deferentia and seminal vesicles are often related to diabetes, but may develop owing to degenerative changes in older men.[26] Calcifications also occur in the chronic diseases of tuberculosis or schistosomiasis. Typically, tuberculous calcification is coarse and asymmetrical, while schistosomiasis calcifications are also coarse but symmetrical.[27] Calcifications may be seen on plain X-ray films or CT, where they follow the anatomic paths of the vasa and seminal vesicles (Figure 14.18). These calcifications are of little clinical significance.

Calculi may be seen within the lumina of the seminal vesicles. Their cause is not known for certain. Some may be secondary to reflux of urine into the seminal vesicles, following surgery or secondary to obstruction.[28] Calculi are found in a minority of patients with haematospermia and infertility, although they are not necessarily causative.[29] Most are found incidentally and do not cause symptoms. Transrectal ultrasound demonstrates the typical appearance of calculi (Figure 14.19)

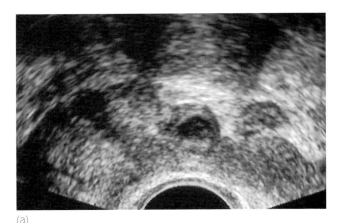

(a)

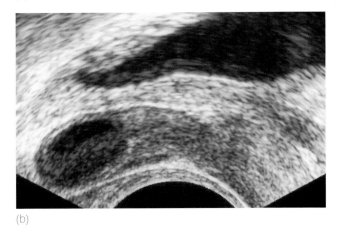

(b)

Figure 14.17
Infected seminal vesicle cyst. (a) This patient had symptoms of prostatitis, a high temperature, and a high white cell count. There is a thick-walled seminal vesicle cyst with echogenic contents. Aspiration showed infection. (b) A different case, but with similar symptoms. Here there is layering within the cyst. This sign is, however, of low specificity – compare Figure 14.15

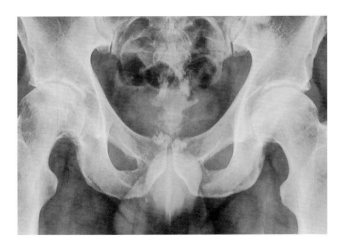

Figure 14.18
Calcification of the seminal vesicles. An X-ray shows calcification in both the seminal vesicles in a young diabetic.

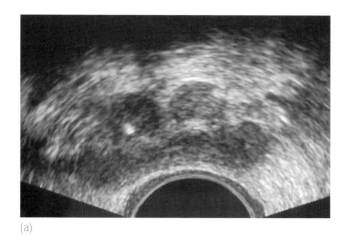
(a)

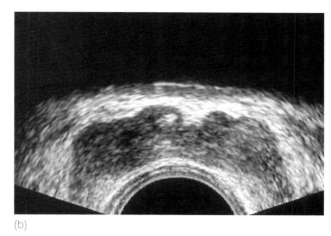
(b)

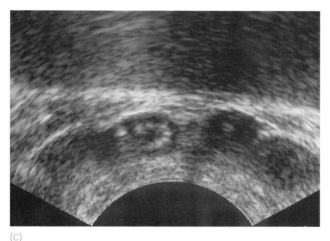
(c)

Figure 14.19
Seminal vesicle calculi. (a)–(c) show different patterns of seminal vesicle calculi: patient (a) was asymptomatic, and a transrectal ultrasound study was performed because of an elevated prostate-specific antigen level; patient (b) had painful ejaculations; patient (c) had persistent haematospermia.

Infection of the seminal vesicles

Acute infection of the seminal vesicles (seminal vesiculitis) is uncommon in developed countries, although in some parts of the world, tuberculosis and schistosomiasis of the seminal vesicles are relatively common. Bacterial seminal vesiculitis occurs almost invariably in the presence of prostatitis.[29,31] Diagnostic imaging has little role to play in uncomplicated acute seminal vesiculitis, since the seminal vesicles show no specific imaging abnormality. Rarely, seminal vesiculitis may progress to seminal vesicle abscess. Abscesses usually occur in diabetics or immunocompromised patients, in patients with indwelling catheters, and in patients who have had instrumentation of the genitourinary tract. An early abscess may present as asymmetric enlargement of the seminal vesicles on transrectal ultrasound, MRI, or CT (Figure 14.20). A developed abscess may demonstrate cavities with echogenic contents, layering and thick walls. Larger abscesses may spread outside the seminal vesicles into surrounding tissues[31–34] (Figure 14.20).

Chronic infection, notably tuberculosis, initially causes debris within the lumina of the vesicles with vesicular wall thickening, and later intraluminal calcifications[27,36,37] (Figure 14.21).

Schistosomiasis of the urinary tract may affect the seminal vesicles before affecting the kidneys, ureters, and bladder. In these cases, the presenting symptom is haematospermia. Examination of the ejaculate reveals blood and *Schistosoma* ova (oospermia).[27,38] The appearance of the seminal vesicles in the early stages of such infection has not been documented. In the later stages of the disease, there is calcification of the seminal vesicles along with small round calcifications in the prostatic ducts due to calcified ova (Figure 14.22).

Obstruction of the seminal vesicles and ejaculatory ducts

A seminal vesicle may be obstructed at the level of the vesicle itself or along the ejaculatory duct. The seminal vesicles themselves may be obstructed by post-infective fibrosis or by cysts. The ejaculatory ducts may be obstructed owing to congenital aplasia, infection (prostatitis), Müllerian or ejaculatory duct cysts, or calculi. The ejaculatory ducts of older men often become obstructed as a result of compression by the enlarged inner gland of benign prostatic hypertrophy.

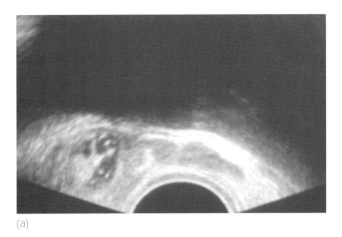

(a)

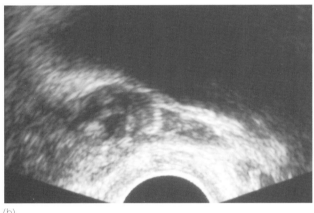

(b)

Figure 14.20
Seminal vesicle abscess. (a,b). Two separate cases. In each there is a mixed-echodensity lesion with anechoic areas within the seminal vesicle, representing an abscess.

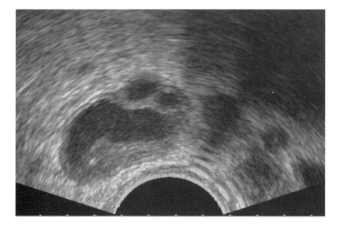

Figure 14.21
Seminal vesicle tuberculosis. The vesicles are very dilated and contain debris in this patient with tuberculous vesiculitis.

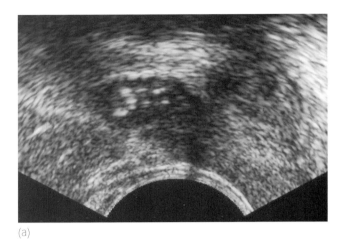

(a)

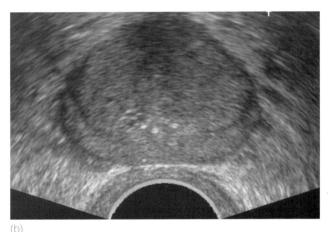

(b)

Figure 14.22
Seminal vesicle schistosomiasis. A group of rounded calcifications are seen (a) in the right seminal vesicle and (b) in the prostate of this patient who had haematospermia, oospermia, and proven urogenital schistosomiasis.

As a consequence of obstruction, the lumina of the ducts dilate and the seminal vesicle enlarges. The ampullary portion of the vas deferens may also dilate. Enlargement of the ductal lumen to more than 4 mm or an increase in the width of the seminal vesicle to more than 20 mm are indicative of obstruction. The luminal contents may be of homogeneous low echodensity and homogeneous high signal on T2-weighted MRI, or they may be of mixed echodensity and mixed MRI signal. Obstruction of the seminal vesicles or ejaculatory ducts may be unilateral or bilateral, depending on the cause (Figure 14.23). The cause is often demonstrated by transrectal ultrasound or MRI. If further workup is needed, classical vasography or seminal vesiculography will demonstrate the level of obstruction.

Obstruction of the seminal vesicles is often associated with infertility. In older men, in whom fertility is not usually an issue, obstruction is often demonstrated incidentally on transrectal ultrasound or MRI, and is of no clinical significance.

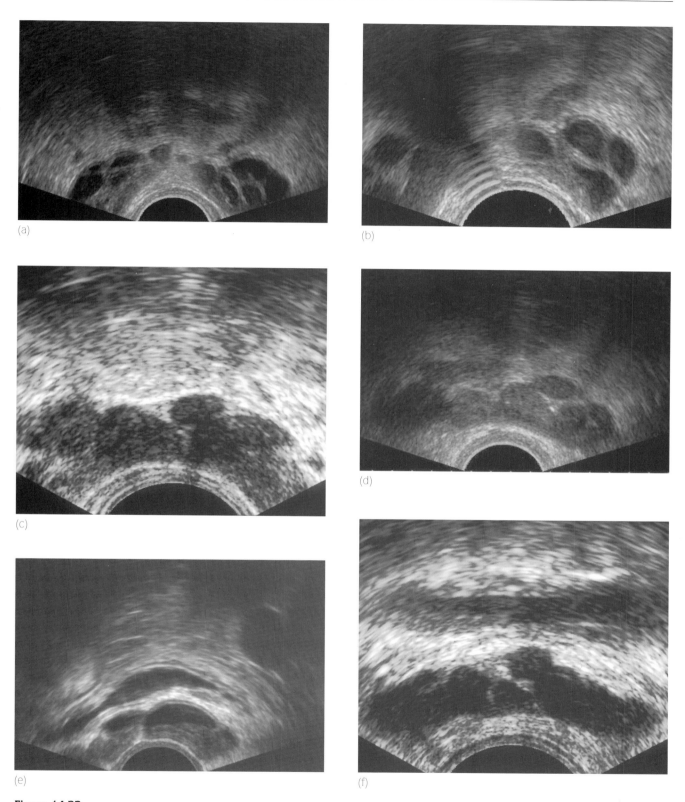

Figure 14.23

Obstruction of the seminal vesicles. (a)–(f) show different patterns of obstruction in the seminal vesicles, all of which were uncomplicated cases of obstruction: (a) dilated seminal vesicles with anechoic contents; (b) slightly more echoic contents; (c) echoic contents within the lumen; (d) areas of relatively high echodensity simulating tumour; (e) layering simulating infection; (f) loss of definition of the walls. (g) T2-weighted MRI study of obstructed seminal vesicles.

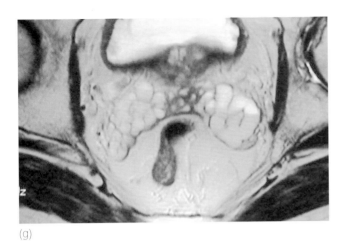

(g)

Figure 14.23
Contionued.

The normal ejaculatory ducts are visible as subtle structures in young men evaluated with transrectal sonography. The lumen is often not visible, and the ducts appear as fine linear structures just posterior and lateral to the urethra (Figure 14.24). A luminal diameter of more than 1 mm indicates dilatation of the ducts. Dilated ducts are more easily seen on the ultrasound image (Figure 14.25), and may also be seen on axial MRI scans.

Strictures may be fibrous or calcified, and may occur anywhere along the length of the duct. They may be unilateral or bilateral, and may be congenital or secondary to infection.[38–41] The stricture itself is often not visible sonographically. Calcified strictures may be seen (Figure 14.26), but may be indistinguishable from the more common periductal calcifications.

Müllerian duct cysts may cause obstruction of the ejaculatory ducts because the ducts enter the cyst or because the cyst compresses the ends of normally positioned ducts.[39,42–46]

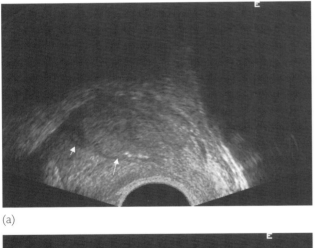

(a)

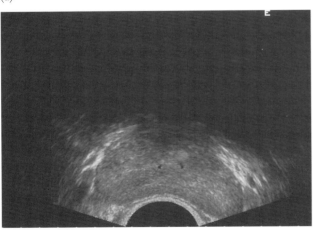

(b)

Figure 14.24
Normal ejaculatory ducts: (a) sagittal view; (b) coronal view. The normal ejaculatory duct is seen, with a narrow lumen of less than 1 mm.

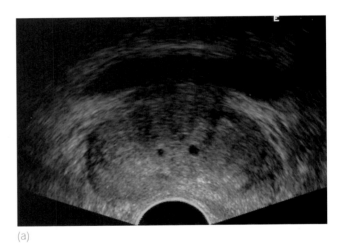

(a)

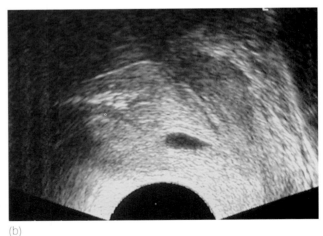

(b)

Figure 14.25
Obstructed ejaculatory ducts. (a) Axial view showing bilateral ejaculatory duct dilatation. (b) Sagittal view of the right ejaculatory duct. The cause of the obstruction has not been shown.

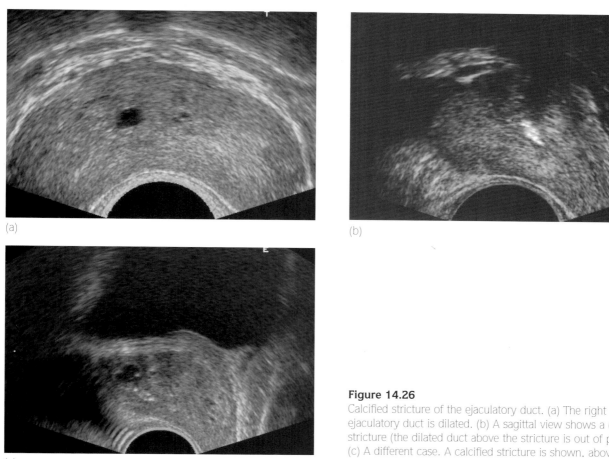

(a)

(b)

(c)

Figure 14.26
Calcified stricture of the ejaculatory duct. (a) The right ejaculatory duct is dilated. (b) A sagittal view shows a calcified stricture (the dilated duct above the stricture is out of plane). (c) A different case. A calcified stricture is shown. above which there is a dilated duct with a pseudocystic appearance.

Usually, both ducts are dilated (Figure 14.27). Cysts of the ejaculatory ducts themselves may be associated with obstruction of the ducts (Figure 14.28). The obstruction, however, is probably due to an associated aplasia rather than to the cyst itself.

Hypoplasia of the ejaculatory ducts is difficult to diagnose on transrectal ultrasound by the appearance of the ducts themselves. Such hypoplasia, however, is always associated with hypoplasia of the ipsilateral seminal vesicle. Recognition

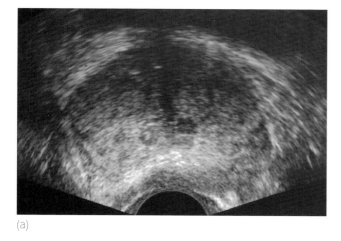

(a)

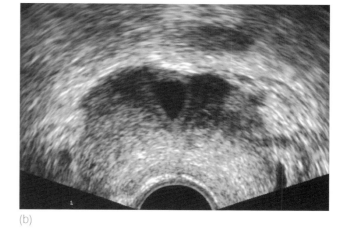

(b)

Figure 14.27
Ejaculatory duct obstruction due to a Müllerian duct cyst. (a) Both ejaculatory ducts are dilated with echogenic material. seen in the lumen of the right duct. (b) A view in the lower axial plane shows the Müllerian duct cyst that is causing the obstruction.

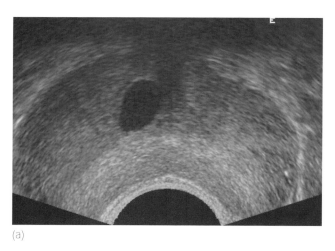

(a)

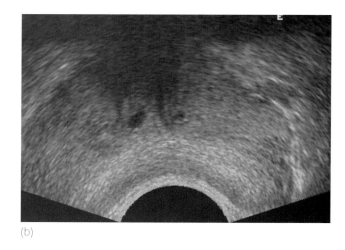

(b)

Figure 14.28
Ejaculatory duct cyst causing obstruction. (a) An ejaculatory duct cyst is shown. In this case, it is clearly situated slightly to the right of the midline. Often, however, ejaculatory duct cysts appear to be midline. (b) A higher section shows the obstructed right ejaculatory duct.

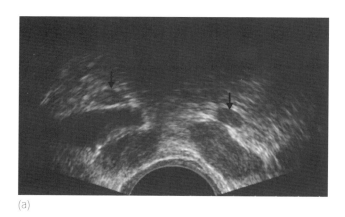

(a)

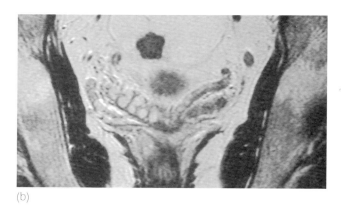

(b)

Figure 14.29
Atrophy of the seminal vesicles. (a) An axial-view transrectal ultrasound study shows an absent left seminal vesicle. The right seminal vesicle is obstructed. The vasa deferentia are both present (arrows). (b) T2-weighted MRI study showing an atrophic left seminal vesicle.

of the hypoplastic seminal vesicle establishes the diagnosis[45–47] (Figure 14.29).

Calculi within the ejaculatory ducts appear as echodense foci, and may demonstrate posterior acoustic shadowing. Calculi may be present without obstruction. Obstruction is suggested when a calculus is seen with a more proximal dilated duct. In many patients, the relationship of a calculus to the ejaculatory duct is not clearly defined, and it may be difficult to distinguish ejaculatory duct calculi from calculi in the adjacent prostatic ducts or parenchyma[48] (Figure 14.30).

Benign prostatic hyperptrophy is often associated with ejaculatory duct obstruction. Ductal ectasia involving the ejaculatory ducts and seminal vesicles is generally found as an incidental observation in older men undergoing transrectal ultrasound for suspected cancer.[49]

Absence or hypoplasia of the seminal vesicles and vasa deferentia

The seminal vesicles and vasa deferentia develop from the same embryonic anlage. Congenital absence or hypoplasia often affect both structures simultaneously, and are frequently associated with absence of the distal two-thirds of the ipsilateral epididymis. These conditions may be unilateral or bilateral, and are often associated with infertility.[15,16,45] Renal tract anomalies are also often associated with absence of the seminal vesicle, mainly renal aplasia, and ectopic insertion of the ureter into the vas deferens.[16] There is also a strong association with the cystic fibrosis gene, often in the

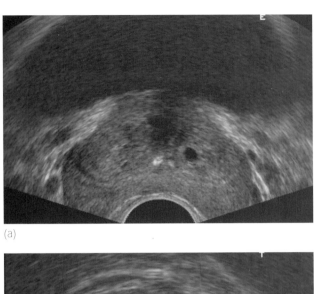

(a)

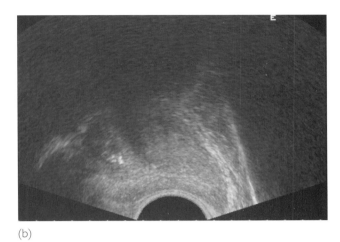

(b)

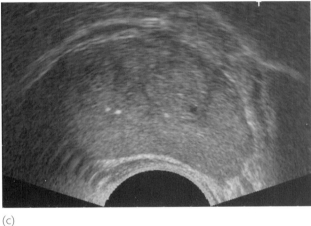

(c)

Figure 14.30
Ejaculatory duct calculi. (a) Calculi are seen near the lower ends of both ejaculatory ducts. There is also a cyst in a nodule of benign prostatic hypertrophy on the left. (b) Axial and (c) sagittal views of two calculi in the left ejaculatory duct. The patient presented with painful ejaculation. Removal of the calculi alleviated the symptoms.

absence of clinical disease. Absence or hypoplasia of the seminal vesicles causes infertility based upon reduction of ejaculatory volume, even when unilateral and not associated with a hypotrophic vas deferens.

Bilateral atrophy of the vasa deferentia is usually associated with the cystic fibrosis gene.[50] Unilateral atrophy is usually congenital and associated with ipsilateral renal agenesis. Unilateral aplasia is not associated with the cystic fibrosis gene.[51] Acquired atrophy of the vas deferens is not associated with anomalies of the epididymis or the seminal vesicles, although the vesicles are often dilated secondarily to the atrophy. In some cases there is also ectasia of the rete testis and multiple epididymal cysts (Figure 14.31).

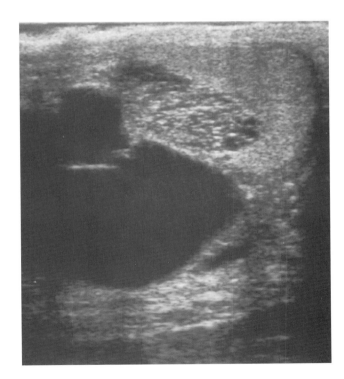

Figure 14.31
Ectasia of the rete testis and epididymal cysts. The rete testis is very ecstatic and there are large epididymal cysts in this patient with obstructed ejaculatory ducts.

Imaging appearances

Unilateral absence or hypoplasia of the seminal vesicles is easy to appreciate because of the loss of normal symmetry. Bilateral change is more difficult to interpret. The normal seminal vesicles vary in their orientation. When the seminal vesicle extends in a steeply cephalad direction from the base of the prostate, it may be erroneously interpreted as hypoplastic on transverse sonography. MRI may be easier to interpret in such cases. Associated absence of the vas deferens is diagnosed when there is absence of the ampulla of the vas on imaging or by absence of the scrotal portion of the vas deferens on physical examination.

Absence of the vasa deferentia often presents as a more subtle finding than absence of the seminal vesicle, although absence of the ampulla of the vas should be noted (Figure 14.32). Absence of the distal two-thirds of the epididymis, if present, is often detected by physical examination. Interpretation of the ultrasound image is more difficult because of the variability of the normal epididymis.

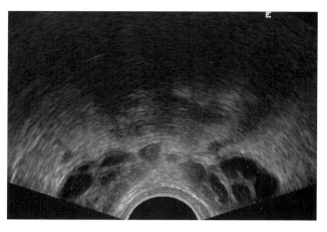

Figure 14.33
Dilated seminal vesicles due to diabetes. The dilatation found in diabetics is shown. The dilatation in these cases is not related to obstruction.

Dilatation of the seminal vesicles

Dilatation of the seminal vesicles may occur in diabetics without obstruction. The imaging features, however, are indistinguishable from those of obstruction (Figure 14.33).

Reduplication and ectopia of the seminal vesicles and ectopia of the vas deferens

Reduplication of the seminal vesicles is a rare congenital anomaly in which two apparently normal seminal vesicles are seen on the same side (Figure 14.34). Crossed ectopia may also occur, accompanied by crossed ectopia of the vas deferens. Alternatively, crossed ectopia of the vas deferens may occur as an isolated anomaly with the seminal vesicle remaining in its normal position. Ectopia of the seminal vesicle may also occur with one or both of the seminal vesicles lying on the correct side but in an abnormal position relative to the prostate. This form of ectopia is less common. All forms of

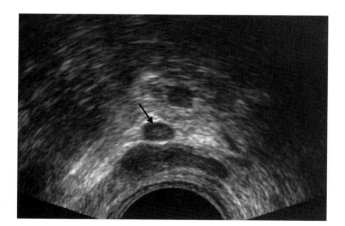

Figure 14.32
Absence of the vas deferens. The right vas deferens is seen (arrow); the left is absent.

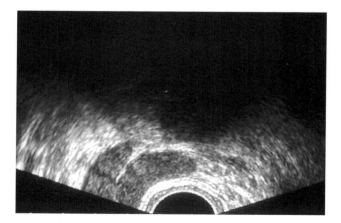

Figure 14.34
Reduplication of the seminal vesicles. The right seminal vesicle is duplicated.

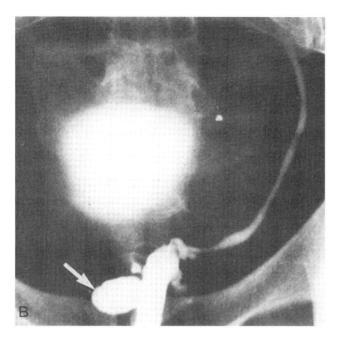

Figure 14.35
Ectopic ureter entering the vas deferens. An ectopic ureter is seen to enter the vas deferens (common duct). Reproduced with permission from: Nilop Murcia M, Friedland GW, de la Vries P. Congenital anomalies of the male genitalia. In: Clinical Urography 2nd edn (Pollack HM, McClellan BL eds). Philadelphia: WB Saunders, 2000: 868–91.

seminal vesicle ectopia may be associated with ipsilateral renal agenesis or abnormal insertion of the ureter into the vas deferens, often referred to as the common duct (Figure 14.35). As part of the same complex, a duplicated urethra may drain the seminal vesicle and there may be diverticulae of the seminal vesicle.[52,53]

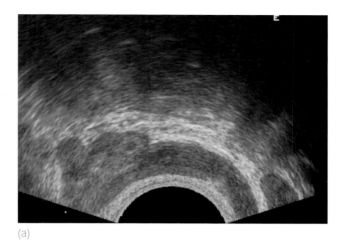

(a)

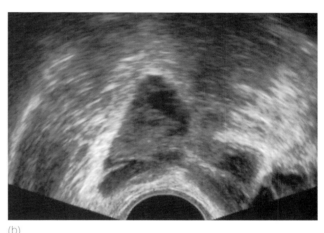

(b)

Figure 14.36
Adenocarcinoma of the seminal vesicle. (a) This patient presented with persistent haematospermia. A tumour is seen at the tip of the right seminal vesicle. Biopsy revealed adenocarcinoma. (b) This patient presented with pelvic pain. There is an adenocarcinoma in the right seminal vesicle, proven by biopsy.

Tumours of the seminal vesicles

Tumours of the seminal vesicles are exceedingly rare. The most common malignant tumour is adenocarcinoma, followed by sarcomas.[16,21,50–61] Carcinoid, primary seminoma fibromas, myxomas, and cystic adenomas have all been described. Any of these tumours may cause pain and haematospermia, as well as obstruction of the seminal vesicles (Figure 14.36). It is not possible to distinguish between these tumours on the basis of imaging characteristics (Figure 14.37). For illustrative purposes, however, a selection of tumours is included (Figures 14.38–14.40).

Adenocarcinoma and sarcoma may be locally invasive and present with symptoms of a pelvic tumour.

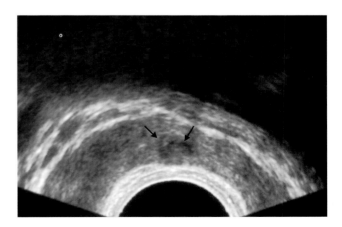

Figure 14.37
Adenoma of the seminal vesicle. The tumour (arrowed) was found on biopsy to be an adenoma.

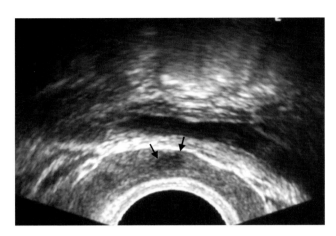

Figure 14.38
Fibroma of the seminal vesicle. The tumour (arrowed) was found on biopsy to be a benign fibroma.

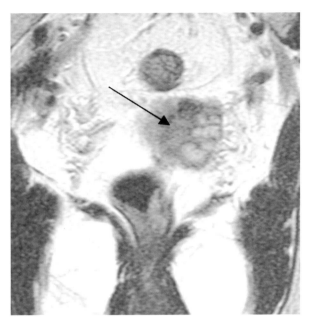

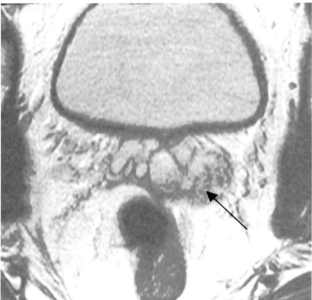

Figure 14.39
Ectopic prostatic tissue within the seminal vesicles. This 37-year-old man presented with persistent haematospermia. The tumour is shown within the seminal vesicle (arrows) in this T2-weighted MRI scan. Surgical excision revealed ectopic prostatic tissue. Ectopic prostatic tissue may occur anywhere in the male genitourinary tract, and commonly presents with haematospermia.

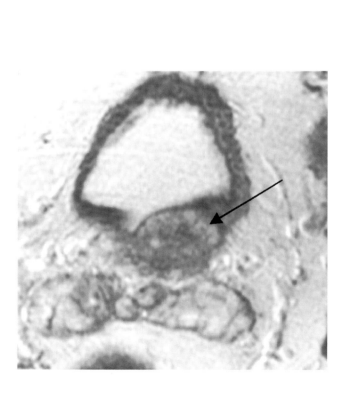

Figure 14.40
Mass due to atrophic tissue in the seminal vesicle. A T2-weighted MRI study in a patient with prostate cancer. A solid tumour was thought to be seminal vesicle involvement with prostatic cancer. Biopsy revealed non-malignant atrophic tissue.

REFERENCES

1. Arey LB. The urinary system. In: Developmental Anatomy. Philadelphia: WB Saunders, 1965: 313.
2. Brewster SF. The development and differentiation of human seminal vesicles. J Anat 1985; 143: 45.
3. Aboul-Azm TE. Anatomy of the human seminal vesicles and ejaculatory ducts. Arch Androl 1979; 3: 287.
4. Jarow JP. Transrectal ultrasonography in infertile men. Fertil Steril 1993; 60: 1035–9.
5. Al-Omari H, Girgis SM, Hanna AZ. Diagnostic value of vaso-seminal vesiculography. Arch Androl 1985; 15: 187.
6. Meyer JJ, Hartig PR, Koos GW, McKinley CR. Transrectal seminal vesoculography. J Urol 1979; 121: 129.
7. Hardeman SW, Causey JQ, Hickey DP, Soloway MS. Transrectal ultrasound for staging prior to radical prostatectomy. Urology 1989; 34: 175–80.
8. Langlotz C, Schnall M, Pollack H. Staging of prostatic cancer. Accuracy of MR imaging. Radiology 1995; 194: 645–6.
9. Rifkin MD, Zerhouni EA, Gatsonis CA et al. Comparison of magnetic resonance imaging and ultrasonography in staging early prostatic cancer – results of a multi-institutional cooperative trial. N Engl J Med 1990; 323: 621–6.
10. Pitkanen P, Westermark P, Cornwell GG III, Murdoch W. Amyloid of the seminal vesicles: a distinctive and common localised form of senile amyloidosis. Am J Pathol 1983; 110: 64.
11. Ramchantani P, Schnall MD, LiVolsi VA et al. Senile amyloidosis of the seminal vesicles mimicking metastatic spread of prostatic carcinoma on MR images. AJR 1993; 161: 99.
12. King BF, Hattery RR, Lieber MN et al. Congenital cystic disease of the seminal vesicles. Radiology 1991; 178: 207.
13. Parsons RB, Fisher AM, Bar-Chama N, Mitty HA. MR imaging in male infertility. Radiographics 1997; 17: 627–37.
14. Kuligowska E, Fenlon HM. Transrectal US in male infertility: spectrum of findings and role in patient care. Radiology 1998; 207: 173–81.
15. Kenny PJ, Spirt BA, Leeson MD. Genitourinary anomalies: radiologic–anatomic correlations. Radiographics 1984; 4: 233–66.
16. Kenny PJ, Leeson MA. Congenital anomalies of the seminal vesicles: spectrum of computed tomographic findings. Radiology 1983; 149: 247–51.
17. Conn IG, Peeling WB, Clements R. Complete resolution of a large seminal vesicle cyst – evidence for an obstructive aetiology. Br J Urol 1992; 69: 636–9.
18. Lynch MJ, Flannigan GM. Seminal vesicle cyst, renal agenesis and epididymitis in a 50 year old patient. Br J Urol 1992; 69: 98.
19. Friedrichs R, Ebert T, Yol TJ et al. Use of endorectal surface coil magnetic resonance imaging for diagnosis of a multicystic seminal vesicle with ipsilateral renal agenesis. Urol Int 1996; 57: 115–18.
20. Kuyumcuoglu U, Erol D, Germiyanoglu C, Balcaci L. Hydatid cyst of the seminal vesicle. Int Urol Nephrol 1991; 23: 479.
21. Okada Y, Tanaka H, Takeychi H et al. Papillary adenocarcinoma in a seminal vesicle associated with ipsilateral renal agenesis: a case report. J Urol 1992; 148: 1543—5.
22. Shieh CP, Liao YJ, Li YW et al. Seminal vesicle cyst associated with ipsilateral renal malformation and hemivertebra: report of two cases. J Urol 1993; 150: 1214–15.
23. Rappe BJ, Mueleman EJ, Bebryune FM. Seminal vesicle cyst with ipsilateral renal agenesis. Urol Int 1993; 50: 54–6.
24. Keenan JF, Rifkin MD. Ultrasonographic diagnosis of seminal vesicle cysts in polycystic kidney disease. J Ultrasound Med 1996; 15: 343.
25. Cakewart P, De Costa M, Buylsteke P et al. Anal tenesmus caused by seminal vesicle cyst. Urology 1997; 49: 139–41.
26. Kellett MA. The radiological features of diabetes mellitus. Radiol Clin North Am 1967; 5: 239.
27. Jorulf H, Lindsdorf E. Urogenital schistosomiasis: CT evaluation. Radiology 1985; 157: 745.
28. Wilkinson AG. Case report: calculus in the seminal vesicle. Pediatr Radiol 1983; 23: 327.
29. Worischeck JH, Parra RO. Chronic hematospermia: assessment by transrectal ultrasound. Urology 1994; 46: 515–20.
30. Christiansen E, Purvis K. Diagnosis of chronic bacterial prostovesiculitis by rectal ultrasonography in relation to symptoms and findings. Br J Urol 1991; 67: 173.
31. Fender D, Hamdy FC, Neil DE. Transrectal ultrasound appearance of schistosomal prostato-semin-vesiculitis. Br J Urol 1996; 77: 166.
32. Chandra I, Doringer E, Sarica K et al. Bilateral seminal vesicle abscesses. Eur Urol 1991; 20: 164.
33. Doringer E, Chandra I, Sarica K et al. MRI of bilateral seminal vesicle abscesses. Eur J Radiol 1991; 12: 60.
34. Kang YS, Fishman EK, Kuhlman JE et al. Seminal vesicle abscesses: spectrum of computed tomographic findings. Urol Radiol 1989; 11: 182.
35. Sue DE, Chikola C, Brant-Zawadzki MN et al. MR imaging in seminal vesiculitis. J Comput Assist Tomogr 1989; 13: 662.
36. Birnbaum BA, Friedman JP, Lubat E et al. Extrarenal genitourinary tuberculosis: CT appearance of calcified pipe-stem ureter and seminal vesicle abscess. J Comput Assist Tomogr 1990; 14: 653.
37. Premkumar A, Newhause JH. Seminal vesicle tuberculosis: CT appearance. J Comput Assist Tomogr 1988; 12: 676.
38. Honig SC. Use of ultrasonography in the evaluation of the infertile man. World J Urol 1993; 11: 102–10.
39. Honig SC. New diagnostic techniques in the evaluation of anatomic abnormalities of the infertile male. Urol Clin North Am 1994; 21: 417–32.
40. Carter SS, Shinohara K, Lipshultz LI. Transrectal ultrasonography in disorders of the seminal vesicles and ejaculatory ducts. Urol Clin North Am 1989; 16: 772–90.
41. Kim ED, Lipshultz LI. Role of ultrasound in the assessment of male infertility. J Clin Ultrasound 1996; 24: 437–53.
42. Jarow JP. Transrectal ultrasonography of infertile men. Fertil Steril 1993; 60: 1035–9.
43. Hendry WF, Pryor JP. Müllerian duct (prostatic utricle) cyst: diagnosis and treatment in subfertile males. Br J Urol 1992; 69: 79–82.
44. Stricker HJ, Kunan JR, Foerber GJ. Congenital prostatic cyst causing ejaculatory duct obstruction: management by transrectal cyst aspiration. J Urol 1993; 149: 1141–3.
45. Parsons RB, Fisher AM, Bar-Chama N, Mitty HA. MR imaging in male infertility. Radiographics 1997; 17: 627–37.
46. Kuligowska E, Fenlon HM. Transrectal ultrasound in male infertility: spectrum of findings and role in patient care. Radiology 1998; 207: 173–81.

47. Choi IR, Lee MS, Rah KH et al. Magnetic resonance imaging in hemospermia. J Urol 1997; 157: 258–62.

48. Littrup PJ, Lee F, McCleary RD et al. Transrectal ultrasound of the seminal vesicles and ejaculatory ducts: clinical correlation. Radiology 1988; 168: 625.

49. Vertby GW. Vaso-seminal vesiculography in hypertrophy and carcinoma of the prostate with special reference to the ejaculatory ducts. Acta Radiol 1960; 199: 1–194.

50. Kaplan E, Chwachman H, Perlmutter AD et al. Reproductive failure in males with cystic fibrosis. N Engl J Med 1968; 279: 65–9.

51. Trigaux VP, Van Beers B, Delchambre F. Male genital tract malformations associated with ipsilateral renal agenesis: sonographic findings. J Clin Ultrasound 1981; 19: 3–10.

52. Wakatsuki A, Oda T, Ocki K. Case profile: crossed ectopia of seminal vesicles and blind-ending ureter. Urology 1984; 24: 291–2.

53. Watanabe M, Hirani J, Numasawa K et al. Crossed ectopia of the left vas deferens leaving ipsilateral seminal vesicle in normal position. J Urol 1992; 148: 886–8.

54. Tanaka T, Takeuchi T, Oguchi K et al. Primary adenocarcinoma of the seminal vesicle. Hum Pathol 1987; 18: 200.

55. Davis NS, Merguerian PA, DiMarco PL et al. Primary adenocarcinoma of the seminal vesicles presenting as bladder tumour. Urology 1988; 32: 466.

56. Amirkhan RH, Molberg KH, Wiley EL et al. Primary leimyosarcoma of the seminal vesicle. Urology 1994; 44: 132.

57. Lamont JS, Hesketh PJ, de las Morenas A, Babayan RK. Primary angiosarcoma of the seminal vesicle. J Urol 1991; 146: 165.

58. Laurila P, Leivo I, Makisalo H et al. Müllerian adenosarcoma-like tumor of the seminal vesicle. Arch Pathol Lab Med 1992; 116: 1072.

59. Chiou RK, Limas C, Lange PH. Hemangiosarcoma of the seminal vesicle: case report and literature review. J Urol 1985; 134: 37.

60. Kawahara M, Matsuhashi M, Tajima M et al. Primary carcinoma of the seminal vesicle. Urology 1988; 32: 269.

61. Benson RC Jr, Clark WR, Farrow GM. Carcinoma of the seminal vesicle. J Urol 1984; 132: 483.

15

Imaging of male infertility

Dennis Ll Cochlin

Introduction

The investigation of male infertility requires a detailed clinical history and physical examination followed by semen analysis. In the appropriate clinical circumstances, imaging tests may assist in determining the cause of infertility and directing treatment. A detailed description of the investigation of male infertility by history, physical examination, semen analysis, hormone profile, and testicular biopsy is beyond the scope of this book. For more detail, the reader is referred to 'Campbell's Urology'.[1] This chapter will examine the place of imaging of the prostate, ejaculatory ducts, seminal vesicles, and vasa deferentia in the investigation of infertility. All the anomalies associated with infertility are described in detail in the other chapters of this book. This chapter brings them together in the context of male infertility. Some references are made to scrotal imaging where appropriate, but a complete discussion of the role of scrotal imaging in infertility is not included. For this, the reader is referred to 'Imaging of the Scrotum and Penis'.[2]

General considerations

The commonly accepted definition of infertility is the inability to conceive after one year of unprotected intercourse. By this definition, the condition affects 10–15% of couples in the USA, and a similar percentage in the UK, Ireland, and mainland Europe.[3–6] It is estimated that a male factor is entirely responsible for the infertility in 20% of cases and partly responsible for another 30%.[7] Historically, infertility investigations concentrated largely on the female partner, with only cursory regard for male infertility. In the 1980s, there was increasing awareness of the importance of investigating both male and female partners. However, increased reliance on in vitro fertilization (IVF) and assisted reproduction techniques during the 1980s, diminished the incentive to find the cause of infertility. More recently, however, there has been increasing awareness that assisted reproduction techniques have drawbacks, in terms of both their high cost and medical complications. Some cases of male infertility are easily cured and therefore the investigation of possible male infertility is well worthwhile.

Investigation of male infertility

The first step is to obtain a thorough history and physical examination. Both of these should be general, but with particular emphasis on aspects relating to infertility. Jarow[8] makes the point that lack of a thorough history and examination may lead to missing serious pathology presenting as infertility. The history and examination will identify causes of infertility such as Klinefelter syndrome, hormonal abnormalities, and testicular pathology such as maldescent or injury. Physical examination may reveal small testes, although ultrasound study is more accurate at assessing testicular size and texture. A soft testis is likely to be poor at producing sperm. Large varicoceles may be palpated, although small ones may not be palpable and may only be detected on ultrasound study. Physical examination is used to assess the presence or absence of the scrotal portion of the vas deferens. Some authorities advocate a digital rectal examination of the prostate and seminal vesicles in order to detect a tender prostate that would suggest prostatitis, cystic dilatation of the seminal vesicles, or a large midline cyst. Digital rectal examination is not, however, routinely performed in all fertility clinics.

The next step is semen analysis. At this stage, testicular biopsy is often performed in order to assess spermatogenesis, and for sperm retrieval. These procedures may reveal a great deal about the cause of infertility. For more detailed information on this subject, the reader is referred to 'Campbell's Urology'.[1] In many cases, history, physical examination, and semen analysis will establish a definitive diagnosis. In other cases, further investigation by imaging of the sperm transport system is required.

Based upon analysis of this data, the causes of male infertility may be divided broadly into one of two groups. The first group includes impaired spermatogenesis. The second group includes infertility due to obstruction or other abnormalities of the sperm transport system. The 'plumbing' problems in the second group are potentially curable by surgery. Diagnostic imaging may have a role to play in the investigation of both groups. Impaired spermatogenesis may be further investigated by scrotal imaging. Suspected abnormalities of the sperm transport system require imaging of the vasa deferentia, seminal vesicles, and ejaculatory ducts. It is this group that is the subject of this chapter.

Abnormalities of the vas deferens

The combination of azoospermia and low-volume ejaculate suggests an abnormality of the vasa deferentia and an associated abnormality of the seminal vesicles. The vas deferens may be congenitally absent or there may be partial agenesis, which may be unilateral or bilateral. Agenesis of the vas deferens is always associated with ipsilateral agenesis or hypotrophy of the seminal vesicle.[7,9] There is frequently (but not invariably) absence of the distal two-thirds of the ipsilateral epididymis. Congenital absence or agenesis of the vasa deferentia accounts for 1–2.5% of cases of male infertility and 4.4–17% of cases of azoospermia.[6,9,10] Atrophy of the vas deferens may also occur secondary to infection or obstruction, although this cause is rare. In these post-infective cases the distal part of the vas is atrophied while the proximal part remains normal. The seminal vesicles are not atrophic in these cases, and are often secondarily dilated. The epididymes are not atrophic. There is sometimes tubular ectasia of the rete testes associated with multiple epididymal cysts.

The vas deferens may become obstructed due to a fibrotic or calcified stricture, or due to calculi or obstructive cysts. 'Cysts' of the vas deferens may actually represent dilatation of the vas secondary to obstruction rather than true cysts. Their pathogenesis is not known. They are often bilateral and associated with cysts in the seminal vesicles. The multifocal nature of this anomaly suggests a congenital cause, although low-grade infection has also been suggested as a cause.

The portion of the vas deferens that lies in the scrotum is best assessed by palpation. This examination is straightforward in most patients, but may be difficult if the testes lie high, if there is a small taut scrotal sac or if the cord is thickened. In these cases imaging is often requested. The scrotal portion of the vas deferens may be surprisingly difficult to visualize by sonography in such cases, since the same factors that make physical palpation difficult tend to make the ultrasound study difficult. When it is not possible to assess the distal portion of the vas deferens by transrectal ultrasound, a magnetic resonance imaging (MRI) study will demonstrate the whole length of the vas deferens.

When the vasa deferentia are absent from the scrotum on physical examination, the cause of the infertility is established, and in many centres no further confirmation is required. Some centres, however, will request a transrectal ultrasound study in order to confirm absence of the distal portions of the vasa deferentia, and to confirm associated absence or hypotrophy of the seminal vesicles. When the vasa deferentia are palpated within the scrotum, a transrectal ultrasound study is necessary to detect the rare cases of secondary atrophy of the distal vas, or to detect obstruction by calculi and cysts.

Anomalies of the seminal vesicles are often associated with anomalies of the ipsilateral renal tract. Between 16% and 43% of these patients will have renal agenesis, crossed renal ectopia, or a pelvic kidney. Such renal anomalies are more common on the left.[11–19] In some cases, a history of renal anomalies may suggest the cause of infertility. In other cases, investigation of the infertility may be the first indicator of renal abnormalities. It is therefore customary to perform a renal tract ultrasound study on these patients.

There is a strong association between anomalies of the vasa deferentia and cystic fibrosis. All men with cystic fibrosis have bilateral agenesis of the vasa deferentia. About 80% of men with bilateral agenesis of the vasa deferentia will carry at least one allele for the cystic fibrosis gene. Patients with unilateral agenesis and obstruction of the contralateral vas may also carry a cystic fibrosis gene anomaly.[20] This fact is important, since these patients should be offered genetic counselling and informed that their offspring may carry the gene for cystic fibrosis.

Anomalies of the seminal vesicles

The seminal vesicles contribute 80–90% of the volume of the ejaculate. They alkalinize the ejaculate and add fructose. A low-volume ejaculate with a low pH and low fructose levels suggests seminal vesicle anomalies. Agenesis and hypoplasia of the seminal vesicles have already been mentioned in association with agenesis and hypoplasia of the vas deferens.[19] The seminal vesicles may be occluded by areas of fibrosis or calcification, usually regarded as congenital but occasionally due to infection. These occlusions are often associated with similar occlusions of the vas deferens. Calculi may be seen in the seminal vesicles, but are probably secondary to obstruction rather than its cause. Seminal vesicle cysts are rare, but are associated with obstruction due to discontinuity of the vas and seminal vesicle. A large cyst in one seminal vesicle may also obstruct the opposite seminal vesicle and vas. Seminal vesicle cysts are often associated with ipsilateral renal, ureteric, and bladder anomalies. Bilateral seminal vesicle cysts are strongly associated with polycystic kidneys, with important implications for genetic counselling. True cysts of the seminal vesicles are different from dilatation secondary to ejaculatory duct obstruction, although these entities may be difficult to distinguish on diagnostic imaging.

Anomalies of the ejaculatory ducts

Azoospermia with normal testes suggests bilateral obstruction of the sperm transport system. This may occur at the level of the vasa deferentia or the ejaculatory ducts.

The most common cause of obstruction of the ejaculatory ducts is compression by the enlarged inner prostate gland of benign prostatic hypertrophy (BPH). This condition tends to affect older men in whom fertility in not usually an issue. Less commonly, BPH may present in younger men as well. Evidence of BPH is visible on the transrectal ultrasound study, and when the seminal vesicles are dilated, obstructed ejaculatory ducts are assumed.

Ejaculatory duct obstruction may be associated with midline prostatic cysts, although not all cysts cause obstruction. Müllerian duct cysts may cause bilateral obstruction, either when the ducts enter the cyst or when the cyst compresses the distal ends of the ducts. Cysts of the ejaculatory ducts themselves tend to occur distally along the course of the ducts. Although not strictly midline, they often appear to lie in the midline and may be indistinguishable from Müllerian duct cysts. They are usually associated with obstruction, although it is usually unclear whether they are the cause or the result of obstruction.

Some ejaculatory ducts contain calculi, which may cause obstruction. Other ejaculatory ducts may be obstructed by a fibrous stricture, which may calcify. In these cases of acquired obstruction, the proximal duct and seminal vesicle are usually dilated. Finally, the ejaculatory ducts may be hypoplastic or absent. In these cases, there is coexisting hypoplasia or agenesis of the seminal vesicles. The small seminal vesicles associated with a hypoplastic ejaculatory duct stand in contrast to the dilated seminal vesicles found with acquired obstruction of the ejaculatory ducts.[7,8,11–14,21]

Treatment

Although obstruction of the sperm transport system only accounts for a minority of cases of male infertility, this type of obstruction may be surgically correctable at a far lower cost than assisted fertilization. Furthermore, correction of the obstruction should provide a permanent cure. Surgically correctable cases are those with obstruction at the level of the distal two-thirds of the ejaculatory ducts. Cysts compressing the ducts may be aspirated under ultrasound guidance with relief of the obstruction. As a backup measure, any sperm aspirated from the cysts may be stored for possible use. Other causes of ductal obstruction are treated by transurethral cutdown to expose the patent part of the duct.[21–31]

References

1. Sigman M. Howards SS. Male infertility. In: Campbell's Urology (Walsh PC, Retik AB, Vaughan ED Jr, Wein AJ, eds). Philadelphia: WB Saunders, 1998.
2. Rifkin MD, Cochlin DL (eds). Imaging of the Scrotum and Penis. London: Martin Dunitz, 2002
3. Spira A. Epidemiology of human reproduction. Hum Reprod 1986; 1: 111–15.
4. de Kreser DM. Male infertility. Lancet 1997; 349: 787–90.
5. Templeton A. Infertility: epidemiology, aetiology and effective management. Health Bull (Edin) 1995; 53: 294–8.
6. Abyholm T. Azoospermia and oligozoospermia: etiology and clinical findings. Arch Androl 1983; 10: 57–61.
7. Kuligowska E. Transrectal ultrasonography in diagnosis and management of male infertility. In: Imaging in Infertility and Reproductive Endocrinology (Jaffe R, Pierson RA, Abramowiz JS, eds). Philadelphia: JB Lippincott, 1994: 217–29.
8. Jarow JP. Role of ultrasonography in the evaluation of the infertile male. Semin Urol 1994; 12: 274–82.
9. Kuligowska E, Baker CE, Oates RD. Male infertility: role of transrectal US in diagnosis and management. Radiology 1992; 185: 353–60.
10. Moore KL. The Developing Human: Clinically Oriented Embryology, 3rd edn. Philadelphia: WB Saunders, 1991: 365–82.
11. Carter SStC, Shinohara K, Lipshultz LI. Transrectal ultrasonography in disorders of the seminal vesicles and ejaculatory ducts. Urol Clin North Am 1989; 16: 773–88.
12. Abbitt PL, Watson L, Howards S. Abnormalities of the seminal tract causing infertility: diagnosis with endorectal sonography. AJR 1991; 157: 337–9.
13. Jarow JP. Transrectal ultrasonography of infertile men. Fertil Steril 1993; 60: 1035–9.

14. Honig SC. Use of ultrasonography in the evaluation of the infertile man. World J Urol 1993; 11: 102–10.

15. Parsons RB, Fisher AM, Bar-Chama N, Mitty HA. MR imaging in male infertility. Radiographics 1997; 17: 627–37.

16. Tanagho EA. Embryologic basis for lower ureteral anomalies: a hypothesis. Urology 1976; 7: 451–64.

17. Jequier AM, Ansell ID, Bullimore NJ. Congenital absence of the vasa deferentia presenting with infertility. J Androl 1985; 6: 15–18.

18. Pereira JK, Chait PG, Daneman A. Bilateral persisting mesonephric ducts. AJR 1993; 160: 367–9.

19. Trigaux JP, Van Beers B, Delchambre F. Male genital tract malformations associated with ipsilateral renal agenesis: sonographic findings. J Clin Ultrasound 1991; 19: 3–10.

20. Mulhall JP, Oates RD. Vasal aplasia and cystic fibrosis. Curr Opin Urol 1995; 5: 316–19.

21. Meacham RB, Hellerstein DK, Lipshultz LI. Evaluation and treatment of ejaculatory duct obstruction in the infertile male. Fertil Steril 1990; 59: 393–7.

22. Malatinsky E, Labady F, Lepies P et al. Congenital anomalies of the seminal ducts. Int Urol Nephrol 1987; 19: 189–94.

23. Lucon AM, Nahas WC, Wroclawski ER et al. Congenital cyst of the seminal vesicle. Eur Urol 1983; 9: 362–3.

24. Jevenois PA, Van Sinoy ML, Sintzoff SA et al. Cysts of the prostate and seminal vesicles: MR imaging findings in 11 patients. AJR 1990; 155: 1021–4.

25. Poore RE, Jarow JP. Distribution of intraprostatic hyperechoic lesions in infertile men. Urology 1995; 45: 467–9.

26. Hamilton S, Fitzpatrick JM. Ultrasound diagnosis of a prostatic cyst causing acute urinary retention. J Ultrasound Med 1987; 6: 385–7.

27. Namiki M. Recent concepts in the management of male infertility. Int J Urol 1996; 3: 249–55.

28. Costabile RA. Infertility – Is there anything we can do about it? J Urol 1997; 157: 158–9.

29. Sokol RZ. The diagnosis and treatment of male infertility. Curr Opin Obstet Gynaecol 1995; 7: 177–81.

30. Madgar I, Seidman DS, Levran D et al. Micromanipulation improves in-vitro fertilization results after epididymal or testicular sperm aspiration in patients with congenital absence of the vas deferens. Hum Reprod 1996; 11: 2151–4.

31. Schlegel PN, Girardi SK. Clinical review 87: In vitro fertilization for male factor infertility. J Clin Endocrinol Metab 1997; 82: 709–16.

16

Haematospermia

Dennis Ll Cochlin

General considerations

Haematospermia (haemospermia) is a condition in which altered or fresh blood appears in the ejaculate. The condition may occur as an isolated incident, as a small number of recurrent incidents, or at every ejaculation. Traditional teaching states that haematospermia is seldom of clinical significance, and that the patient should be reassured.[1–4] Recurrent or continuous haematopsermia, however, may be associated with important pathology. It is increasingly common practice to investigate these cases.

The first step in investigating haematospermia is to obtain a detailed history. Associated symptoms may indicate the cause of the condition. Pelvic and perineal pain suggests seminal vesiculitis, usually associated with prostatitis. Tuberculosis and gonorrhoea are particularly likely to cause haematospermia.[5] In countries where schistosomiasis is endemic, haematospermia is often the first symptom of urogenital infection. The diagnosis is confirmed by examination of the ejaculate, which contains blood and *Schistosoma* ova (oospermia).[6] Vasculitis and hypertension may cause haematospermia,[7] and a relevant history may suggest these conditions. Many cases of haematospermia, however, have no associated symptoms. Their causes are investigated by transrectal ultrasound study, sometimes supplemented by or replaced by magnetic resonance imaging (MRI).

Aetiology of haematospermia

Most of the causes of haematospermia have been described and illustrated elsewhere in this book. Bleeding may occur in any part of the ejaculatory system, from the testes to the urethra. It has been stated that urethral bleeding causes fresh blood while bleeding from more proximal parts of the system causes brown discolouration. This distinction, however, is not always clear-cut. Urethral bleeding often causes post-ejaculatory haematuria as well as haematospermia. Therefore, the combination of post-ejaculatory haematuria with haematospermia strongly suggests a urethral cause.

Furuya et al[8] advocate needle aspiration of the seminal vesicles and any midline cysts to determine the source of the bleeding. Because bleeding from the vas deferens or testes may accumulate in the seminal vesicles, a positive seminal vesicle tap may result from bleeding in the seminal vesicle itself, as well as from the vas deferens or the testis. A negative tap indicates bleeding from a more distal source. Altered blood or fresh blood from a midline cyst indicates that this is the source.

A number of papers have reported finding a cause for chronic or recurrent haematospermia in a large proportion of cases[2,9,10] (Table 16.1). In many of these series the most common 'cause' reported is dilatation of the seminal vesicles. Haematospermia is more common in infertile men. In this group, ejaculatory duct anomalies and obstruction are often the cause. Obviously, the bleeding must originate distal to the obstruction, or the obstruction must be incomplete in order for blood to enter the ejaculate.

Seminal vesicle pathology

As noted above, isolated dilatation of the seminal vesicles is often found in men with haematospermia. However, it is debatable whether dilatation itself can cause haematospermia. Other pathological processes in the seminal vesicles are less common, but include cysts, adenocarcinoma, ectopic prostatic tissue, and amyloidosis. It is likely that any of these

Table 16.1   Causes of haematospermia: pathology found in patients with haematospermia and its associated significance.

Scrotum	
Carcinoma of the rete testis	Presenting symptom is haematospermia; very rare
Testicular cancer	Only found in advanced locally invasive tumours
Trauma	Bleed into seminal vesicles
Seminal vesicles	
Dilatation	Probably not a cause per se, but may indicate vesiculitis or other related pathology
Seminal vesiculitis	
Calcification	May indicate vesiculitis
Seminal vesicle cyst	
Adenocarcinoma	Very rare
Ectatic prostatic tissue	Probably rare
Amyloidosis	Common in older men, and probably an incidental finding
Prostate	
Prostate cancer	Should be suspected in men over 40 years of age
Prostatatis	Usually there are other symptoms of prostatitis
Prostatic calcification	In young men suggests prostatitis
Ejaculatory duct calculi	There may be associated infertility
Midline cysts	Uncommon cause
Prostatic hyperplasia and calcification	Probably an incidental finding in men over 40 years of age
Urethra	
Polyp	Causes haematospermia and haematuria
Ectopic prostatic tissue	Causes haematospermia and haematuria
Engorged urethral vein	Rare
Bladder	
Bladder cancer	Unusual cause

pathologies may cause haematospermia, with the possible exception of amyloidosis. Although cases of seminal vesicle amyloidosis have been found in patients with haematospermia, amyloidosis of the seminal vesicles is very common in older men, is normally asymptomatic and may be an incidental finding in older men with haematospermia. Seminal vesiculitis is thought to be one of the more common causes of haematospermia.[11] Calcifications within the seminal vesicles have been reported in cases investigated for haematospermia. These calcifications may result from chronic seminal vesiculitis, which also causes the haematospermia. Littrup et al[12] have suggested that these patients often have self-limiting haematospermia that may be caused by passing of calcareous material.[12]

Prostate pathology

Prostate cancer may cause haematospermia. Haematospermia usually appears only in advanced cancer of the prostate, but it may occasionally be a presenting symptom. The diagnosis of prostate cancer should be considered in men over the age of 40 years.[13]

Acute or chronic prostatitis may also cause haematospermia, although it is likely in some cases that the haematospermia is due to an associated seminal vesiculitis.[2,11]

Midline cysts, most commonly Müllerian duct cysts but also ejaculatory duct cysts, are found in a proportion of patients with haematospermia. Altered blood found in the aspirate from a Müllerian duct cyst is undoubtedly a cause of haematospermia.[14,15] Benign prostatic hypertrophy and prostatic calcifications have been reported in patients with haematospermia in some series.[10,13] These are so common in older men, however, that in most or all cases they are probably incidental findings. Prostatic calcifications in younger men often indicate chronic prostatitis, which may be the cause of the haematospermia. Calculi in the ejaculatory ducts are a more definite cause of haematospermia.[10,14,15] They are more frequently found in patients with haematospermia and infertility.

Testicular pathology

Although haematospermia may occur with any testicular tumour, it is normally a late symptom, occurring with locally invasive disease. The exception is carcinoma of the rete testis in which haematospermia may be the presenting symptom.[16—18] Carcinoma of the rete testis is rare. Nonetheless, physical examination of the testes should be performed in patients with haematospermia, and an ultrasound study of the scrotum may be advised.

Scrotal trauma occasionally causes bleeding into the epididymis that results in haematospermia for a variable period following the injury. Haemorrhage into the epididymis may cause non-specific enlargement or may be seen on ultrasound study or MRI as marked enlargement of the epididymal tubules.

Urethral pathology

Many pathologies of the urethra, including trauma, may cause haematospermia. Urethral pathology most often causes haematuria, but occasionally is associated with haematospermia. Occasionally, urethral pathology may cause haematospermia without haematuria, or post-ejaculatory haematuria.[13,19] The urethral condition that most often causes recurrent haematospermia is urethral polyps.[20,21] Post-ejaculatory haematurea has been reported to be caused by polyps containing ectopic prostatic tissue within the urethra,[8,22] haemangioma of the prostatic urethra,[23] and engorged urethral veins.[24] A somewhat bizarre condition has been described in which the ejaculate is coloured black owing to the presence of a melanoma.[25] Diagnosis of suspected urethral pathology is usually obtained by urethrography or urethroscopy.

Bladder pathology

Bladder cancer is a rare cause of haematospermia.[10]

Iatrogenic causes

Transrectal biopsy of the prostate causes haematospermia in a large proportion of patients. This symptom can be quite prolonged, especially if sexual activity is infrequent. Haematospermia is more likely to occur if the seminal vesicles are biopsied. Patients should be warned of the possibility of haematospermia and reassured that the symptom is harmless. Haematospermia also occurs for a variable period following surgery to the prostate.

Conclusions

The cause of haematospermia may be determined in many cases from the history and accompanying symptoms. In other cases, the cause is not evident. Solitary episodes of haematospermia are rarely significant and probably do not require investigation. Recurrent or persistent episodes or haematospermia associated with infertility strongly suggest pathology in the sperm transport system that may require investigation. Cases not associated with infertility and without a relevant history of accompanying symptoms have traditionally been labelled idiopathic and seldom investigated. A number of recent studies have shown that abnormalities of the sperm transport system are found in a large majority of such cases. It must be stated, however, that the majority of the pathologies found, even if causative, have no practical treatment available for them.

Malignancy of the prostate should be considered in men over the age of 40 years. These men should have their serum prostatic-specific antigen (PSA) measured. If elevated, transrectal ultrasound and prostate biopsy is indicated. If the PSA is normal, the need for transrectal ultrasound is debatable. Apart from the rare cancer of the rete testis, cancers of the testis only cause haematospermia in advanced cases, when the diagnosis is usually obvious at the time of examination. Physical examination of the testes is indicated in cases of haematospermia, but the need for further imaging of the testes is arguable. While adenocarcinomas of the seminal vesicles and rete testes undoubtedly cause haematospermia as an early symptom, both are extremely rare. Nevertheless, patient expectations often dictate that all symptoms should be investigated and that all pathologies, however rare, should be excluded. Thus, a greater number of patients with haematospermia are now investigated by transrectal ultrasound of the prostate and seminal vesicles, or with MRI, urethroscopy and cystoscopy.

References

1. Marshall VF, Fuller NL. Hemospermia. J Urol 1983; 129: 377–98.
2. Fletcher MS, Herzberg Z, Pryor JP. The aetiology and investigation of haemospermia. Br J Urol 1981; 53: 669–71.
3. Yu HH, Wong KK, Lim TK, Leong CH. Clinical study of hemospermia. Urology 1977; 10: 562–3.
4. Leary FJ, Aguilo JJ. Clinical significance of hematospermia. Mayo Clin Proc 1974; 49: 815–17.
5. Gow JG. Genitourinary tuberculosis. In: Urology (Blandy JP, ed). Oxford: Blackwell Science, 1976.
6. Corachan M, Valls ME, Gascon J et al. Hematospermia: a new etiology of clinical interest. Am J Trop Med Hyg 1994; 50: 580.
7. Brendler CV. In: Campbell's Urology (Walsh PC, Retik AB, Vaughan ED Jr, Wein AJ, eds). Philadelphia: WB Saunders, 1998.

8. Furuya S, Ogura H, Saitoh N et al. Hematospermia: an investigation of the bleeding site and underlying lesions. Int J Urol 1999; 6: 539–47.

9. Worischeck JH, Parra RO. Chronic hematospermia: assessment by transrectal ultrasound. Urology 1994; 43: 515–20.

10. Amano T, Kunimi K, Ohkawa M. Transrectal ultrasonography of the prostate and seminal vesicles with hemospermia. Urol Int 1994; 53: 139–42.

11. Weidner W, Jantos Ch, Schumacher F et al. Recurrent haematospermia – underlying urogenital anomalies and efficacy of imaging procedures. Br J Urol 1991; 67: 317–23.

12. Littrup PJ, Lee F, McLeary RD et al. US of the seminal vesicles and ejaculatory ducts: clinical correlation. Radiology 1988; 168: 625–8.

13. Ganabathi K, Chadwick D, Feneley RSL, Gingell JC. Haemospermia. Br J Urol 1992; 69: 225–30.

14. Neustein P, Hein PS, Goergen TG. Chronic hematospermia due to müllerian duct cyst: diagnosis by magnetic resonance imaging. J Urol 1989; 142: 828.

15. Van Poppel H, Vereecken R, Greeter PDE, Verduyn H. Hematospermia owing to utricular cyst: embryological summary and surgical review. J Urol 1982; 129: 608–9.

16. Smith SJ, Vogelzang RL, Smith WM, Moran MJ. Papillary adenocarcinoma of the rete testis: sonographic findings. AJR 1987; 148: 1147–8.

17. Mostofi FK, Sabin LH, International Histological Classification of Tumors of Testis, No. 16. Geneva: World Health Organization, 1977.

18. Jacobellis U, Ricco R, Ruotolo G. Adenocarcinoma of the rete testis 21 years after orchiopexy: case report and review of the literature. J Urol 1981; 125: 429–30.

19. Yu HHY, Wong KK, Lim TK, Leong CH. Clinical study of hematospermia. Urology 1977; 10: 562–3.

20. Ross JC. Haemospermia. Practitioner 1969; 203: 59–62.

21. Stein AJ, Prioleau PG, Catalona WJ. Adenomatous polyps of the prostatic urethra: a cause of hemospermia. J Urol 1980; 124: 298–9.

22. Hiraishi K, Fujisawa A, Kumagai H. A case of benign polyp with prostatic-like epithelium of the urethra. Jpn J Clin Urol 1988; 42: 431–3.

23. Furuya S, Ogura H, Tanaka Y et al. Hemangioma of the prostatic urethra: hematospermia and massive post-ejaculation hematuria with clot retention. Int J Urol 1997; 4: 524–6.

24. Cattolica EV. Massive hemospermia: a new etiology and signified treatment. J Urol 1982; 128: 151–2.

25. Smith GW, Griffith DP, Pranke DW. Melanospermia: an unusual presentation of malignant melanoma. J Urol 1973; 110: 314–16.

Section IV

Therapy

17

Image-guided therapy of prostate disease

Ehab A el-Gabry and Leonard G Gomella

Introduction

Traditional management of benign prostatic hyperplasia (BPH) and prostate cancer has included invasive procedures such as transurethral resection of the prostate for BPH and radical prostatectomy for localized prostate cancer. Advances in less-invasive alternative therapies for these diseases have resulted primarily from the development and adaptation of ultrasound imaging for the prostate. These newer therapies can be broadly classified as ultrasound-guided or ultrasound-ablative, and are summarized in Table 17.1. This chapter will focus on the mechanisms of action, applications, and outcomes of cryosurgery and high-intensity focused ultrasound for PC and transurethral microwave thermotherapy for BPH. Radiation therapy is discussed in Chapter 18.

Cryosurgery for prostate cancer

Therapeutic options for localized prostate cancer include observation, hormonal therapy, cryotherapy, radiation therapy, and radical prostatectomy. Of these options, cryotherapy is perhaps the most controversial. Nonetheless, it is applied to patients with primary and radio-recurrent prostate cancer at many centers in the USA and abroad.

Mechanisms of action

Contemporary principles of cryosurgery (also called cryotherapy and cryoablation) include rapid cooling, slow thawing,

and repetition of the process to create an ice ball exceeding the limits of the tumor. The basic mechanisms of cryogenic tissue ablation are summarized in Table 17.2. A double

Table 17.1 Minimally invasive therapies for the treatment of prostate diseases. Treatments where the ultrasound monitoring is essential for the therapy are noted in bold.

- **Cryosurgery**
- **Brachytherapy**
- **Transurethral microwave therapy (TUMT)**
- Interstitial laser therapy/interstitial laser coagulation (ILC)
- Water induced thermotherapy (WIT)
- **High-intensity focused ultrasound (HIFU)**
- Transurethral needle ablation

Table 17.2 Basic mechanisms of cryogenic ablation of tissues.

Cellular level
- Destabilization of lipid cell membrane
- Cellular dehydration secondary to an osmotic gradient created by extracellular ice crystal formation
- Denaturation of cellular proteins secondary to pH changes
- Cellular distension and subsequent membrane rupture due to fluid shift during thawing

Parenchymal level
- Vascular thrombosis
- Subsequent coagulative and ischemic necrosis

Table 17.3 Commonly used cryotherapy devices.

Device	Freezing source	Cooling temperature
Candela (Wayland, MA)	Liquid nitrogen	−186° C
CMS (Rockville, MD)	Liquid nitrogen	−195° C
Endocare (Irvine, CA)	Liquid argon	−130°C

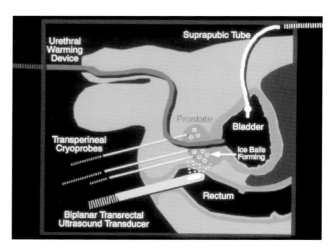

Figure 17.1.

Positioning of the cryotherapy probes using a biplanar ultrasound transducer. Courtesy of Dr. Jack Long.

freeze/thaw cycle is recommended for maximum tissue ablation. Currently, liquid nitrogen and argon gas are the most frequently used cryogens. Argon gas provides improved delivery of the cryogen to the probe tip, and allows the use of smaller-diameter probe tips. Although argon-based cryosurgical systems do not achieve temperatures as low as nitrogen-based systems, they offer a more rapid freeze/thaw cycle and similar ice-ball sizes. Currently available cryosurgical devices are listed in Table 17.3.

Technique

Adequate cryoablation is difficult to achieve with a gland mass above 50 g. Neoadjuvant hormonal therapy is recommended for such patients to reduce the size of the gland prior to cryosurgery. Hormonal regimens typically include an injectable luteinizing hormone-releasing hormone (LHRH) analogue (leuprolide or goserelin) along with an oral anti-androgen such as flutamide or bicalutamide for 3–4 months.

Cryosurgery is performed in the operating room under proper sterile conditions using either general or spinal anesthesia. The patient is prepped in the lithotomy position. Both a suprapubic tube and a urethral catheter are placed, and the scrotum is taped to the anterior abdominal wall. The bladder is filled with saline to mobilize the intraperitoneal contents away from the treatment zone.

Positioning of cryosurgery probes is performed with transrectal ultrasound guidance. A biplane 'side-fire' transducer is preferable, to allow more precise positioning of the probes (Figure 17.1). Using a perineal needle insertion guide, 18-gauge hollow-core needles are inserted into the prostate under real-time transrectal ultrasound guidance. Five or six needles are usually inserted: two anteromedially, two posterolaterally, and one or two posteriorly (Figure 17.2). Each needle is advanced to the planned location, usually near the base of the prostate. J-tipped guide wires are then advanced, followed by dilators and 12-F cannulas. The positioning of the needles and cannulas is confirmed sonographically.

Prior to initiating cryosurgery, the Foley catheter is replaced by a urethral warmer to guard against urethral damage. The cryotherapy probes are then 'stuck' into position by cooling to −50°C to −70°C (the so-called 'stick' temperature) to form

a small ice ball around the tip of the probe. When freezing, the anterior probes must be activated first. Once an ice ball has formed around a probe, tissue anterior to the ice ball is hidden by the acoustic shadow. The ice balls are monitored sonographically as they extend posteriorly and laterally (Figures 17.3 & 17.4). Once the anteriorly placed ice balls have reached the desired size, a thawing cycle is started for the anterior probes, and the posterior probes are activated. The posterior ice balls are monitored closely by sonography in order to avoid the complication of rectourethral fistula. In

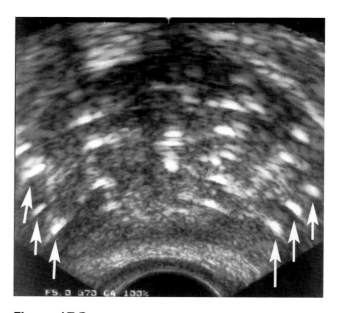

Figure 17.2

Transverse sonogram of the prostate with cryotherapy needles in position. Each needle appears as an echogenic focus (arrows). Courtesy of Dr. Jack Long.

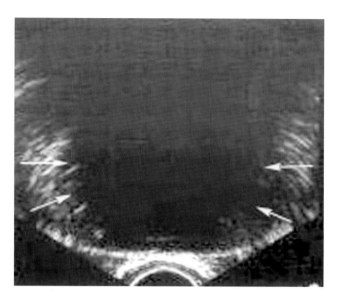

Figure 17.3
Transverse sonographic monitoring of the ice ball as it forms. The boundaries are indicated by arrows. Courtesy of Dr. Jack Long.

general, the average freezing time is approximately 10–15 minutes while the passive thaw time is approximately 40 minutes. Most centers utilize two freeze/thaw cycles. If the ice ball does not extend adequately to the apex of the prostate, cryoprobes may be pulled down toward the apex for an additional freezing cycle. If seminal vesicle involvement or extracapsular extension of the tumor is suspected, therapy

should be modified to ensure proper probe placement in these areas. Following therapy, patients may be discharged to home or admitted overnight with the suprapubic tube in place. Antibiotic coverage is continued for 2 weeks.

Indications and outcomes

Cryoablation of the prostate can be offered as an initial treatment option for clinically localized prostate cancer, or as a salvage therapy for standard treatment failure. Current uses for cryoablation of prostate cancer are shown in Table 17.4.

In 1993, Onik et al[1] described the percutaneous transperineal ultrasound-guided cryoablation technique and reported preliminary outcomes of cryoablation used in a primary setting to treat prostate cancer. In a group of 55 patients with 3-month follow-up, an overall rate of 17.4% of biopsy-proven residual disease was noted. In a more recent study with longer follow-up, Shinohara et al[2] reported rates of 48% and 60% for biochemical failure and biopsy failure respectively. A significant improvement in glandular ablation has been demonstrated using six to eight probes.[3] When used in a salvage setting, local recurrence rates of 14–23% have been reported, while biochemical failure rates range from 49% to 69%.[4–6]

Complications of prostate cryosurgery include urethrorectal fistula, sloughing urethral tissue, perineal ecchymosis, penile edema, and ileus. Other substantial complications include pelvic or rectal pain, incontinence, and impotence. The complications profile may be influenced by the use of ultrasound to guide the procedure, by operator expertise, and by the clinical setting – primary therapy vesus a salvage procedure. Historically, cryosurgery without ultrasound guidance was associated with higher rates of significant side-effects, mainly urethrocutaneous fistula formation[7,8] and a disease-specific death rate of up to 47% in a mean follow-up of 93.7 months.[9]

The use of ultrasound guidance and urethral warming devices has reduced morbidity. In a series of 63 patients who had cryosurgery as an initial treatment for their cancer,

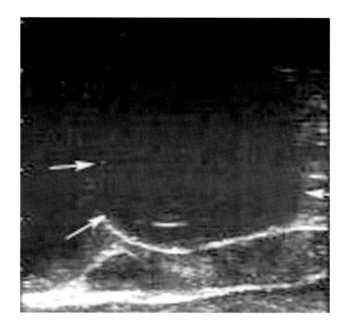

Figure 17.4
Sagittal sonographic monitoring of the ice ball as it forms. The boundaries are indicated by arrows. Courtesy of Dr. Jack Long.

Table 17.4   Current applications of cryosurgery for prostate cancer.
Initial therapy   • Clinically localized prostate cancer   **Salvage therapy**   • Local recurrence after radiation therapy   • Local recurrence after radical prostatectomy   • Local recurrence after previous cryosurgery   • Local progression after hormonal treatment

Cox and Crawford[10] reported the following complications rate: 3% urethrorectal fistula, 29% bladder outlet obstruction and 27% incontinence. When used in a salvage setting after radiation failure, significantly higher complication rates were noted. Rates of 11%, 67%, 95%, and 100% were reported for urethrorectal fistula, urinary obstructive symptoms, incontinence, and impotence, respectively.[2,4–6,11–14]

Conclusion

The early use of cryosurgery of the prostate without ultrasound guidance was fraught with complications. Although ultrasound-guided cryosurgical ablation of prostate cancer is associated with fewer complications, the complications rate is still considered unacceptably high by many urologic oncologists. In addition, treatment outcomes are inferior to those achieved using radical surgery or radiation, and data are lacking on long-term outcomes. Cryosurgery of the prostate is FDA-approved in the USA for both initial and salvage therapy of prostate cancer.

Many specialists in the field of prostate cancer consider cryosurgery of the prostate to be a promising technique. Centers of excellence have reported reasonable success while minimizing the side-effect profile. The use of multiple smaller probes placed in a fashion analogous to transperineal brachytherapy may allow more precise freezing of the gland with less morbidity.

Transurethral microwave thermotherapy (TUMT) for BPH

BPH is a common condition in older men. While many men are asymptomatic, others are affected by symptoms known as 'prostatism' or lower urinary tract symptoms (LUTS). Transurethral thermotherapy has gained in popularity as a minimally invasive therapy for symptomatic BPH.

Mechanisms of action

Microwaves comprise the 300–3000 MHz range of the electromagnetic spectrum.[15] As microwaves pass through biological tissue, energy is transformed into heat via electromagnetic oscillation of free charges (electrons and ions) and by polarization of small molecules (mainly water). The depth of penetration is influenced by wave frequency and tissue type. Microwave penetration is greater in low-water-content tissue

(fat) than in high-water-content tissue (muscle). Tissue penetration is inversely related to frequency. For prostate applications, the transurethral route is used to deliver the microwave energy through a flexible antenna. The goal of heating is to achieve temperatures that exceed the thermal threshold for cell death. For prostatic adenomatous tissue, this may be accomplished by heating at $45°C$ for 30 minutes. At all times, urethral temperature should not exceed $45°C$ (the thermal pain threshold of the urethra), otherwise the patient may experience severe pain and damage to the urethral mucosa. Accordingly, simultaneous urethral cooling is an essential part of this procedure. After treatment, pathological examination of the prostate typically demonstrates uniform hemorrhagic and coagulative necrosis with minimal inflammation.[16]

Technique

Patients referred for TUMT should have significant symptoms of bladder outlet obstruction (i.e. frequency, urgency, decreased stream, nocturia). Prior to TUMT, moderately severe symptoms of bladder outlet obstruction should be documented based on American Urologic Symptom (AUA) Score, decreased uroflowmetry, and the degree of post-void residual. Formal urodynamic studies are utilized when the diagnosis is unclear. Prospective TUMT candidates should be evaluated for clinically significant prostate cancer with a digital rectal examination and prostate-specific antigen (PSA) determination, followed by biopsy if indicated. Transrectal prostate imaging is mandatory. Patients with prostatic urethral lengths less than 20 mm and greater than 100 mm are not optimal candidates for TUMT. Cystourethroscopy is essential to evaluate for other pathology of the prostate and bladder and for the presence of median lobe hypertrophy. While median lobe hypertrophy has been a traditional contraindication to TUMT, catheter modifications such as the new Prostatron blue catheter place the energy source close to the bladder neck, permitting the treatment of patients with enlarged median lobes. Other contraindications include prior radiation therapy to the prostate or pelvis, active urinary tract infection, and urethral stricture disease.

Thermotherapy is usually performed in an outpatient setting without general anesthesia. Oral or parenteral sedation and analgesia with agents such as lorazepam, oxycodone, and/or toradol can be used, based on patient needs and physician preference. During the procedure, it is common for patients to experience mild perineal warmth, mild pain, and a sense of urinary urgency.

With the patient in a supine position, the urethra is anesthetized with lidocaine jelly and the bladder is emptied. The bladder is refilled with 50 ml of saline containing 10–20 ml of 1% lidocaine. A sterilized treatment catheter is then inserted and the balloon inflated with 20 ml of saline (Figure 17.5). The catheter is withdrawn until the balloon rests at the

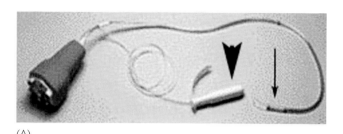

(A)

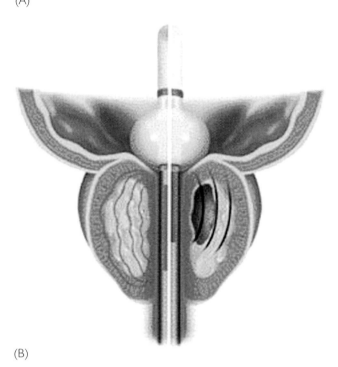

(B)

Figure 17.5

A. Transurethral microwave thermotherapy catheter. The arrowhead demonstrates the rectal probe that measures rectal temperature. The thin arrow demonstrates the urethral catheter with the treatment catheter. B. Schematic demonstrates the position of the microwave antenna relative to the prostate and bladder neck. Courtesy of Edap Technomed Inc; Norcross, GA.

bladder neck. The patient is turned on his side and a lubricated rectal temperature probe is inserted. It is essential to remind the patient that the rectal probe should not be forced from the rectum. The patient should inform the physician if the catheter becomes dislodged during the treatment. Using a transabdominal ultrasound probe, the integrity and position of the retention balloon are verified at the bladder neck (Figure 17.6).

Currently, several TUMT systems are available. We shall describe here the two most commonly used devices.

The Prostatron (Urologix Corp., Minneapolis, MN) uses a monopolar antenna and a urethral cooling device that circulates water at 20°C (Figure 17.7). The early Prostasoft 2.0 protocol was a low-energy protocol with a total treatment

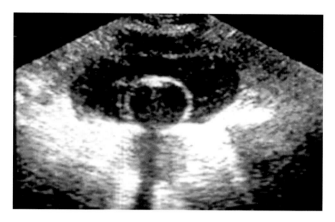

Figure 17.6

Ultrasound verification of the retention balloon at the bladder neck. Courtesy of Edap Technomed Inc; Norcross, GA.

time of 60 minutes. 'High-energy protocols', introduced with Prostasoft 2.5, utilize a stepwise increase in energy without interruptions, permitting prostate heating to 75°C over 60 minutes. According to the version of the software used (Prostasoft 2.0 or 2.5), the microwave power level is increased every 2 minutes to a maximum of 60 W or 70 W, and the rectal shut-off alarm is set at 42.5°C or 43.5°C, respectively. Prostasoft 3.5, the newest high-energy protocol, provides a maximum 80 W of power at the initiation of the treatment, and rapidly achieves intraprostatic temperatures of up to 75°C. The benefit of this protocol is a shorter 30-minute treatment time. However, there is a higher rate of urinary retention due to more intense prostatic edema. Patients treated with this rapid high-energy protocol may also require a higher level of sedation and analgesia.

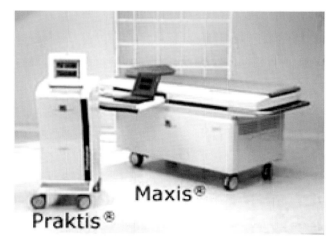

Figure 17.7

Transurethral microwave therapy systems. A portable system is demonstrated on the left side. A larger stationary unit is demonstrated on the right. Courtesy of Edap Technomed Inc; Norcross, GA.

The Targis system was introduced as a small, portable machine with treatment times ranging from 28.5 to 60 minutes, using power of up to 60 W. The Targis system uses a microwave frequency of 902–928 MHz. The treatment catheter is 21-F with either a 2.8 or 3.5 cm antenna. Catheter position is confirmed by transabdominal ultrasound. Next, the rectal thermosensing unit (RTU) is placed to monitor rectal wall temperature and provide an automatic shut-down if the rectal temperature reaches 42.5°C. The treatment antennae use a helical bipolar design that provides impedance matching with prostatic tissue, so that the thermal energy is delivered with minimal antenna heating. In addition, the shape allows preferential heating of the anterolateral prostate, resulting in fewer automatic shut-downs due to increased rectal temperatures. The computer-controlled treatment maintains a urethral temperature between 39°C and 41°C, with an automatic shut-off when the urethral temperature reaches 44.5°C. The Targis system employs prostate tissue temperatures of 60–80°C, while the urethral coolant circulates at 8°C, and produces a uniform area of coagulative necrosis of approximately 3.2 cm diameter.

After TUMT treatment, the urethral and rectal probes are removed. The patient may be discharged to home. Post-treatment edema of the prostate may result in urinary retention that can be treated with intermittent catheterization or an indwelling catheter. Urinary symptoms will usually worsen before they gradually improve.

Indications and outcomes

Although transurethral resection of the prostate (TURP) is the gold standard for management of BPH, medical therapy and minimally invasive modalities such as TUMT are more commonly used for initial treatment today. While considered by many to be a primary treatment option for symptomatic BPH, TUMT is usually offered to patients who have failed to improve on medical therapy. Controlled trials of low-energy TUMT (up to 50°C) have reported on its clinical efficacy.[17–19] Roehrborn et al[19] reported a decrease in the American Urological Association Symptom Index (AUA SI) from 23.6 to 12.7 points at 6 months in the active group (Urowave device), with significant improvements in peak flow rate, compared with a decrease in the AUA SI from 23.9 to 18.0 points in the sham-treated group ($p < 0.05$, between-group difference).[19] Blute et al[17] reported similar results, although others have reported conflicting results.[18] Although short-term outcomes of low-energy TUMT are favorable, the long-term efficacy is questionable. In one report, 31% of patients required invasive surgery and 23% required further medical therapy at 3 years' follow-up.[16]

Newer applications of high-energy TUMT (up to 75°C) have shown greater improvements in uroflow parameters than with low-energy TUMT. D'Ancona reported the results of a randomized trial comparing high-energy TUMT and TURP. At 1 year, the symptomatic improvement was 78% in the TURP group versus 68% in the TUMT group, with improvements in free flow rate of 100% and 69%, respectively. On the basis of their study findings, the authors concluded that high-energy TUMT is comparable to TURP. Investigations by de la Rosette et al[20] further substantiated the effectiveness of high-energy TUMT. However, the enhanced results of high-energy TUMT were achieved at the expense of higher morbidity rates, with significant urinary retention.[15] Pain, retrograde ejaculation, and irritative voiding symptoms were also reported to be higher with high-energy TUMT.[16]

Summary

TUMT is a safe and effective treatment for symptomatic BPH. Although high-energy TUMT may produce more pronounced improvement in uroflowmetry, it is associated with higher rates of adverse events. While the optimal TUMT treatment protocol and device are yet to be defined, the results with higher-energy therapies are very acceptable.

High-intensity focused ultrasound

The therapeutic application of high-energy ultrasound waves remains an investigational intervention for the treatment of prostate cancer in the USA.

Mechanisms of action

High-intensity focused ultrasound (HIFU) waves destroy tissue through mechanical, cavitational, and thermal effects, which are summarized in Table 17.5. Only a small, precisely defined volume of tissue is exposed to an extremely high temperature with HIFU (Figure 17.8). Other tissues lying in the path of the ultrasound waves are protected from high temperatures and cellular injury because of the rapid dissipation of the ultrasonic energy outside the focal zone. Modern piezoelectric ceramics allow for ultrasound transducers that contain high-power ablative elements as well as visualization elements (Figure 17.9). The frequency range for today's piezoelectric transducers varies from 0.5 to 10 MHz. Currently available HIFU devices include the Ablatherm (EDAP Technomed Inc., Norcross, GA) and the Sonablate system (Focus Surgery Inc., Indianapolis, IN) (Figure 17.10).

Table 17.5 Mechanisms of tissue destruction utilizing HIFU.

Mechanical effect
- Disruption of normal architecture between adjacent tissues due to radiation force.

Cavitational effect
- Cavitation bubbles form producing tremendous pressures (20–30 kbars) and extremely high temperatures (thousands degrees Celsius)

Thermal effect
- Coagulative necrosis is achieved when tissues are heated > 70°C

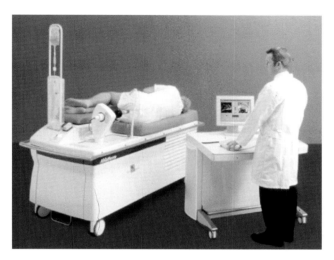

Figure 17.10
HIFU system. Courtesy of Dr. John Lynch.

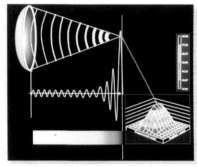

Focused transducer
Emitting ultrasound waves

Acoustical pressure

Tissue heating

Figure 17.8
Schematic presentation of high intensity focused ultrasound theory. The focused ultrasound yields high acoustical pressures that result in tissue heating. Courtesy of Dr. John Lynch.

Technique

In the USA, HIFU of the prostate is an investigational procedure performed on an outpatient basis. After administration of spinal anesthesia, a suprapubic catheter is placed. The patient is positioned in the right lateral decubitus position and the firing head is introduced manually into the rectum. The rectal balloon is filled with circulating cooled degassed coupling liquid. After placement of the firing head in the imaging position, the surgeon sets the target boundaries. Retraction of the biplane ultrasound probe and positioning of the HIFU transducer parallel to the posterior aspect of the rectum is software-controlled. To protect the rectum, the software detects the rectal wall and automatically allows a 3 mm margin ahead of the target zone. In addition, using a motion sensor, the computer will immediately interrupt treatment if patient movement is detected. Up to 1000 shots are administered to the prostate per session. Each shot lasts 4.5 seconds, with a 5-second delay between shots. In general, treatment sessions last from 2 to 4 hours. Once treatment has been competed, the balloon is deflated, the firing head is removed, and the rectal mucosa is inspected for any damage. Patients are discharged on antibiotics and oral pain medications with the suprapubic catheter in place. The catheter is usually removed on the seventh postoperative day.

Imaging Position

The targeted prostatic volume is localized with the bi-plan ultrasound imaging probe

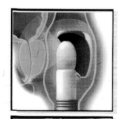

High-energy ultrasound waves are focused through the rectal wall to the targeted prostate area

Firing Position

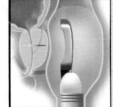

Figure 17.9
Piezoelectric ultrasound transducer with both ablative and visualization elements. Courtesy of Dr. John Lynch.

Indications and outcomes

HIFU was originally investigated as a treatment modality for BPH. Its more recent applications, however, have focused on prostate cancer. HIFU has been employed as an initial treatment for clinically localized prostate cancer as well as a salvage modality after external-beam radiation or early hormonal ablation.[21–23] Gelet et al[23] reported their initial experience using the Ablatherm device in a series of 82 patients with biopsy-proven localized (stage T1–T2) cancer who were not suitable for surgery. With a mean follow-up of 17.6 months (range 3–68 months), the authors noted an overall 62% progression-free rate 60 months after transrectal HIFU ablation. Of interest, for the low-risk group of 32 patients (PSA < 10 ng/ml and Gleason sum < 7), the disease-free survival rate was up to 83%. The authors concluded that transrectal HIFU prostate ablation is an effective therapeutic alternative for patients with localized prostatic adenocarcinoma. The use of HIFU in the salvage setting remains under investigations. In Europe, Thuroff and Chaussy[24] reported a negative biopsy rate of 78% using the Ablatherm device in a study of 28 patients with recurrent prostate cancer proven by biopsy and rising PSA levels.

In the USA, trials are being conducted with the Ablatherm and Sonablate devices in a salvage setting after failure of external-beam radiation therapy or radical prostatectomy. The preliminary results of the Ablatherm study indicated that at 12 months' follow-up, 5 of 8 (62%) patients had PSA levels below 1.0 ng/ml, and 7 of 8 (87.5%) had negative biopsies.[25] However, longer-term follow-up data are needed to define the role of HIFU as a salvage therapy. Potential complications of HIFU include urinary retention, incontinence, urinary infections, urethral stricture, rectal mucosa burns, and urethrorectal fistulas. Preliminary data from an ongoing study in the USA indicate complication rates of up to 50% for urinary infection, 45% for incontinence (stress/urge), and 9% for urethral stricture. In addition 14 of 22 patients (64%) experienced urinary retention, of whom 5 required transurethral resection of obstructive necrotic tissue. Thuroff and Chaussy[26] reported major adverse events of HIFU in 315 patients, including stress incontinence and rectourethral fistulas. The authors observed a drop in post-HIFU rectal mucosa burns from 15% in 1996 to 0% in 1999, as well as a drop in urinary tract infections (UTIs) rate from 58% to 8%.

Summary

The use of HIFU as a primary modality to treat low-risk patients with clinically localized prostate cancer has yielded encouraging outcomes with a relatively safe profile. Longer follow-up is mandatory to validate these preliminary results. As a salvage treatment modality, this technology is currently in its early investigational phase, with its ultimate role in treating recurrent prostate cancer yet to be defined.

Conclusion

In an era of sophisticated ultrasound technology, new treatment modalities for prostate diseases have evolved. The use of ultrasound technology to guide cryosurgical ablation of prostate cancer has resulted in reduced morbidity and an increased popularity of cryosurgery. TUMT is now a common procedure for treatment of BPH, although the optimal TUMT protocol has not yet been defined. The use of HIFU technology to treat prostate cancer is potentially promising, but long-term follow-up studies are needed to further define its ultimate role.

References

1. Onik GM et al. Transrectal ultrasound-guided percutaneous radical cryosurgical ablation of the prostate. Cancer 1993; 72: 1291–9.
2. Shinohara K et al. Cryosurgical ablation of prostate cancer: patterns of cancer recurrence. J Urol 1997; 158: 2206–9; discussion 2209–10.
3. Lee F et al. Cryosurgery for prostate cancer: improved glandular ablation by use of 6 to 8 cryoprobes. Urology 1999; 54: 135–40.
4. Pisters LL et al. The efficacy and complications of salvage cryotherapy of the prostate. J Urol 1997; 157: 921–5.
5. Miller RJ Jr et al. Percutaneous, transperineal cryosurgery of the prostate as salvage therapy for post radiation recurrence of adenocarcinoma. Cancer 1996; 77: 1510–14.
6. Bales GT et al. Short-term outcomes after cryosurgical ablation of the prostate in men with recurrent prostate carcinoma following radiation therapy. Urology 1995; 46: 676–80.
7. O'Brien JM, Carswell GF. A complication of cryoprostatectomy. Br J Urol 1972; 44: 713–15.
8. Ortved WE et al. Cryosurgical prostatectomy: a report of 100 cases. Br J Urol 1967; 39: 577–83.
9. Porter MP et al. Disease-free and overall survival after cryosurgical monotherapy for clinical stages B and C carcinoma of the prostate: a 20-year followup. J Urol 1997; 158: 1466–9.
10. Cox RL, Crawford ED. Complications of cryosurgical ablation of the prostate to treat localized adenocarcinoma of the prostate. Urology 1995; 45: 932–5.
11. Wieder J et al. Transrectal ultrasound-guided transperineal cryoablation in the treatment of prostate carcinoma: preliminary results. J Urol 1995; 154: 435–41.
12. Bahn DK et al. Prostate cancer: US-guided percutaneous cryoablation. Work in progress. Radiology 1995; 194: 551–6.
13. Lee F et al. Cryosurgery of prostate cancer. Use of adjuvant hormonal therapy and temperature monitoring – a one year follow-up. Anticancer Res 1997; 17: 1511–15.
14. Patel BG et al. Cryoablation for carcinoma of the prostate. J Surg Oncol 1996; 63: 256–64.
15. de la Rosette JJ et al. Current status of thermotherapy of the prostate. J Urol 1997; 157: 430–8.
16. Djavan B et al. Outcome analysis of minimally invasive treatments for benign prostatic hyperplasia. Tech Urol 1999; 5: 12–20.
17. Blute ML et al. Transurethral microwave thermotherapy v sham treatment: double-blind randomized study. J Endourol 1996; 10: 565–73.

18. Nawrocki JD et al. A randomized controlled trial of transurethral microwave thermotherapy. Br J Urol 1997; 79: 389–93.

19. Roehrborn CG et al. Microwave thermotherapy for benign prostatic hyperplasia with the Dornier Urowave: results of a randomized, double-blind, multicenter, sham-controlled trial. Urology 1998; 51: 19–28.

20. de la Rosette JJ et al. Pressure-flow study analyses in patients treated with high energy thermotherapy. J Urol 1996; 156: 1428–33.

21. Chaussy C, Thuroff S. High-intensity focused ultrasound in prostate cancer: results after 3 years. Mol Urol 2000; 4: 179–182.

22. Chaussy CG, Thuroff S. High-intensive focused ultrasound in localized prostate cancer. J Endourol 2000; 14: 293–9.

23. Gelet A et al. Transrectal high-intensity focused ultrasound: minimally invasive therapy of localized prostate cancer. J Endourol 2000; 14: 519–28.

24. Thuroff S, Chaussy C. Local recurrence of prostate cancer (rPCa) treated by high intensive local ultrasound(HIFU). Eur Urol 2000; 37 (2 Suppl): Abst 535.

25. Joel AB, Lynch J. HIFU: an emerging treatment for prostate cancer. Contemp Urol 2001; 13: 48–56

26. Thuroff S, Chaussy C. High-intensity focused ultrasound: complications and adverse events. Mol Urol 2000; 4: 183–87; discussion 189.

18

Imaging for prostate cancer radiation therapy

Richard K Valicenti

Although the optimal radiotherapeutic approach to treat clinically localized prostate cancer has yet to be established, planning and implementation of all modern radiation therapy to the prostate depends directly on ultrasound, computed tomography (CT), and magnetic resonance imaging (MRI). Current modern radiotherapeutic options involve either the primary use of external-beam radiation therapy or the delivery of interstitial brachytherapy. State-of-the-art techniques for external-beam therapy consist of three-dimensional conformal radiation therapy (3DCRT) or intensity-modulated radiation therapy (IMRT). The newest technique for delivery of interstitial brachytherapy is primarily image-guided transperineal brachytherapy (IGTPB).

Imaging in external-beam radiation therapy

For as long as megavoltage equipment has been used for the treatment of prostate cancer, imaging modalities have played a central role in the planning of treatment and in the identification of accurate treatment position for radiation therapy delivery. In the early days of external-beam radiation therapy, conventional kilovoltage X-rays and fluoroscopy constituted the simulation and treatment planning procedure, with megavoltage portal filming as a primary means of insuring precise and accurate treatment setup. Initially, these methods were suitable given that the techniques most commonly used consisted of parallel anteroposterior and lateral portals (box technique) or rotational fields. With these approaches, anatomical pelvic structures were not necessarily localized with other imaging modalities. Recently, 3DCRT and IMRT have become the state of the art. Consequently,

CT and MRI have become essential for accurate localization of the prostate and its relation to other anatomic structures in the pelvis. Compared with CT, MRI has superior soft tissue contrast and thus may allow improved definition of treatment volumes within the pelvis. Reports of the International Commission on Radiation Units (ICRU 50 and 62) provide guidelines for target-volume definitions from clinical evaluations involving radiographic imaging.[1,2]

Target definition

According to the ICRU 50 and 62 guidelines, the process of determining volumes for external-beam radiation therapy involves several distinct steps (Figure 18.1). The initial evaluation involves identification of the gross tumor volume (GTV)

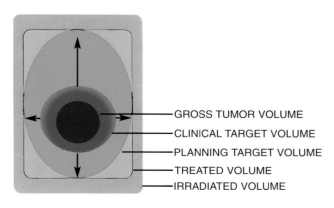

GROSS TUMOR VOLUME
CLINICAL TARGET VOLUME
PLANNING TARGET VOLUME
TREATED VOLUME
IRRADIATED VOLUME

Figure 18.1
The ICRU 50 graphical guidelines to three-dimensional conformal radiation-therapy treatment planning.

through acquisition of diagnostic information. Such information is obtained from various imaging modalities, typically CT scans and orthogonal X-ray films in the treatment position. A dedicated CT simulator is shown in Figure 18.2. The clinical target volume (CTV) is an anatomic–clinical concept that includes any observable tumor, including volumes with subclinical tumor extent. The planning target volume (PTV) is a geometrical concept that encompasses the CTV with additional margins accounting for internal organ motion and variations in patient–beam setup. The delineation of these structures as well as the bladder and rectum is illustrated in Figure 18.3. Sophisticated computer algorithms are used to create a three-dimensional reconstruction for dosimetric evaluation (Figure 18.4).

Accurate target-volume definition is a necessary condition for effective external-beam radiation therapy. It has been shown that the size of the radiation portal directly correlates with the probability of pelvic tumor control.[3] In conventional simulation, contrast medium is used to localize the prostate,

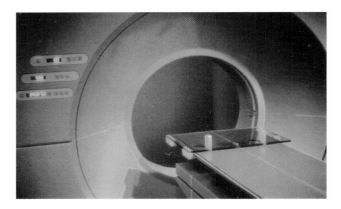

Figure 18.2
Dedicated CT simulator with registration device for patient repositioning.

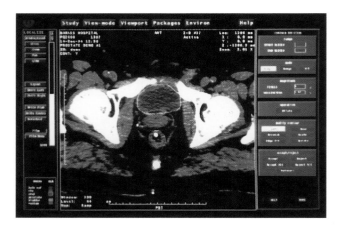

Figure 18.3
Computer workstation used for target-volume definition.

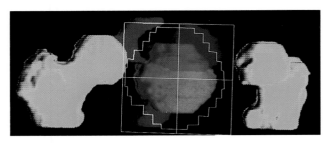

Figure 18.4
Computer reconstruction of pelvic anatomy for designing conformal portals.

rectum, and bladder. By carrying out a cystogram and retrograde urethrogram, it is possible to localize the prostate with a high degree of accuracy.[4] The urethrogram is effective in identifying the junction between the bulbous and prostatic urethra, which has been verified to lie within 1.5 cm of the prostatic apex.[5] Since urethrography appears more accurate than CT scanning in determining the inferior extent of the urogenital diaphragm, CT should not be used without contrast medium if patients are to receive minimal irradiation to the penile bulb.[6,7]

In a recent feasibility study, MRI appeared to provide improved definition of pelvic volumes for prostate radiation therapy compared with CT.[8] In this study, there was a trend for all transaxial MR sequences to provide better segmentation of the prostatic apex and rectum. Furthermore, MRI has additional advantages that allow for more accurate treatment planning and, when feasible, should be considered as a primary imaging modality for dose-escalated 3DCRT or IMRT. In a multi-observer study of prostate gland definition by CT and MRI, CT-derived prostate volumes were larger than MRI-derived volumes, especially toward the seminal vesicles and prostatic apex.[9] This has special implications for 3DCRT planning, since the volume of irradiated normal tissue receiving a given radiation dose may correlate with severe late rectal and urological toxicities.

Magnetic resonance spectroscopy (MRS) shows promise as a novel radiobiologic imaging modality.[10–12] This new technology has the potential advantage of identifying biologically active zones by identifying a higher cellular choline- and creatine-to-citrate ratios within tumor as compared with benign prostatic tissue. Future investigations will determine whether this information may benefit treatment planning algorithms for 3DCRT, IMRT, or IGTPB.

Treatment uncertainty

With modern radiation-therapy techniques, it is essential to encompass the entire prostate, with or without the seminal vesicles depending on risk of tumor involvement. Target localization is crucial for accurate prostate cancer treatment planning, and is a potential source of treatment uncertainty (systematic and random error in patient treatment setup, expressed as mean and standard deviation, respectively). These errors are important since they can lead to a 'marginal miss', which may decrease treatment efficacy or increase side-effects. In order to address these potential variations in patient setup, imaging modalities are routinely used and target localization accuracy is assessed throughout all phases of treatment planning and delivery. As described above, there is variation in CT and MRI imaging to radiographically localize the prostate and seminal vesicles accurately. Several authors have evaluated the precision of these two modalities by analyzing interobserver and intraobserver variations in prostate target-volume localization.[4,9,13,14] These authors have uniformly recognized that MRI and contrast materials improve upon target-volume definition, accuracy, and precision. In addition, by using MRI instead of CT, interobserver variation is less and thus localization more accurate. Perhaps, all patients undergoing 3DCRT, IMRT, or IGTPB for prostate cancer should undergo MRI for localization of the apex to assure accurate dose delivery.

Two other components of treatment uncertainty are organ motion and patient setup variation. Using CT images, megavoltage port films, or electronic portal imaging, several investigators have quantified this matter.[15–20] The frequency and range of motion of the prostate and seminal vesicles is important for accurate treatment delivery in prostate patients receiving 3DCRT or IMRT. Similar to target localization, patient setup variation has a component of systematic and random error. Generally, systematic error occurs from simulation to the first day of treatment, whereas random error is variation occurring daily without a specific cause. Precise information about these parameters provides direct guidelines for reliable estimations of the PTV.

In order to safely and effectively deliver dose-escalated 3DCRT or IMRT, it is important not only to understand the frequency and magnitude of the above variations but also to have an efficient means to make corrections. This should allow for a smaller PTV, since margins for organ motion can be reduced. To facilitate the tracking and changing of prostate position, portable ultrasound-based localization systems have been developed to stereotactically monitor prostate motion. In a pilot study, the prostate position in 35 consecutive men with prostate cancer was prospectively evaluated with daily CT and ultrasound.[21] The authors found a high correlation between the two modalities in all three dimensions. These data suggest that the application of ultrasound-directed stereotactic systems may allow for reduction in all treatment margins.

Imaging in transperineal brachytherapy

The use of transrectal ultrasound techniques and CT-based approaches with transperineal placement of seeds has greatly advanced the art of radioactive-source implantation over previously used retropubic methods. Technical limitations of the retropubic approach probably led to high local recurrence rates with this technique.[22] The use of current imaging modalities has played a central role in improving biochemical outcome for patients with favorable-risk prostate cancer.[23]

Several treatment-planning approaches are currently available for transperineal prostate implantation. Early in the evolution of permanent prostate implantation techniques, therapy relied on fluoroscopic visualization and CT images to guide an idealized seed distribution from a predetermined loading pattern.[24,25] The radioactive seeds are easily visualized on standard X-ray (Figure 18.5). However, this approach is seldom used today, and has been almost entirely replaced by techniques that rely primarily on ultrasonography. CT imaging is still used, but mainly for the estimation of pubic arch interference or for post-implant dosimetric evaluation (Figure 18.6).

The advantages of transrectal ultrasound include the ability to preplan implants based on the ultrasound images, and to verify the placement of both the needle and radioactive source with respect to the prostatic urethra (Figure 18.7). The planning process with transrectal ultrasound involves obtaining axial images of the prostate at 5 mm intervals. This information is critical, since it is used to determine treatment volume by summing the images and to carry out computerized isodose planning. The precise loading and source strength are determined on the basis of serial transaxial sonographic images. Sonography is also used to perform the needle and source placement with a needle-guidance template that is placed against the perineum. Radioactive sources are placed within the prostate under biplanar ultrasound guidance, with or without fluoroscopic guidance.

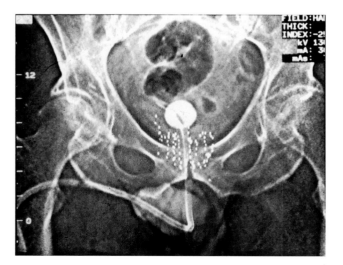

Figure 18.5
X-ray fluoroscopic view of radioactive seed placement.

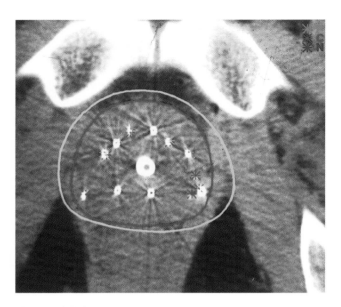

Figure 18.6

Axial image of prostate and radioactive seeds during post-implant dosimetric analysis.

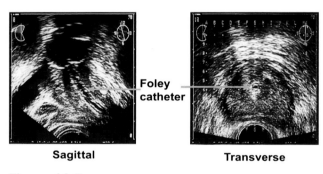

Sagittal   **Transverse**

Figure 18.7

Sagittal and axial views of the prostate during ultrasound-guided seed placement.

Recent advances in image-guided therapy

Recently, investigators have used an intraoperative computer-based optimization program to further optimize the target dose and minimize normal-tissue dose distribution.[26] These investigators have found that three-dimensional intraoperative computer-optimized IGTPB consistently provided superior target coverage, with significantly lower urethral doses as compared with preplanned CT-based or transrectal ultrasound approaches. In addition, intraoperative MRI systems are under evaluation to provide real-time guidance of needles and radioactive sources extrinsic to the patient. This treatment provides real-time dosimetry and assessment of the transperineal needle placement in the coronal as well as the sagittal and axial planes.[27]

References

1. International Commission on Radiation Units (ICRU). *Bulletin No. 50: Prescribing, Recording, and Reporting Photon Beam Therapy.* Washington, DC: International Commission on Radiation Units, 1993.

2. International Commission on Radiation Units (ICRU). *Bulletin No. 62: Prescribing, Recording, and Reporting Photon Beam Therapy (Supplement to ICRU Report 50).* Washington, DC: International Commission on Radiation Units, 1999.

3. Perez CA, Lee HK, Georgiou A et al. Technical and tumor-related factors affecting outcome of definitive irradiation for localized carcinoma of the prostate. Int J Radiat Oncol Biol Phys 1993; 26: 565–81.

4. Valicenti RK, Corn BW, Sweet JW et al. Variation of clinical target volume definition in 3 dimensional conformal radiation therapy for prostate cancer. Int J Radiat Oncol Biol Phys 1999; 44: 931–5.

5. Sandler HW, Bree RL, McLaughlin PW et al. Localization of the prostatic apex for radiation therapy using implant markers. Int J Radiat Oncol Biol Phys 1993; 27: 915–19.

6. Algan O, Hanks GE, Shaer AH. Localization of the prostatic apex for radiation treatment planning. Int J Radiat Oncol Biol Phys 1995; 33: 925–30.

7. Cox JA, Zagoria RJ, Raben M. Prostate cancer: comparison of retrograde urethrography and computed tomography in radiotherapy planning. Int J Radiat Oncol Biol Phys 1994; 29: 1119–23.

8. Khoo VS, Padhani AR, Tanner SF et al. Comparison of MRI with CT for the radiotherapy planning of prostate cancer: a feasibility study. Br J Radiol 1999; 72: 590–7.

9. Rasch C, Barillot I, Remiefer P et al. Definition of the prostate in CT and MRI: a multi-observer study. Int J Radiat Oncol Biol Phys 1999; 43: 57–66.

10. Yu KK, Scheidler J, Hricak H et al. Prostate cancer: prediction of extracapsular extension with endorectal MR imaging and three dimensional proton MR spectroscopic imaging. Radiology 1999; 213: 481–8.

11. Scheidler J, Hricak H, Vigneron DB et al. Prostate cancer: localization with three-dimensional proton MR spectroscopic imaging – clinicopathologic study. Radiology 1999; 213: 473–80.

12. Zelefsky M, Cohen G, Zakian KL et al. Intraoperative conformal optimization for transperineal prostate implantation using magnetic resonance spectroscopic imaging. Cancer J 2000; 6: 249–55.

13. Dubois DF, Prestidge BR, Hotchkiss LA et al. Intraobserver and interobserver variability of MR imaging- and CT-derived prostate volumes after transperineal interstitial permanent prostate brachytherapy. Radiology 1998; 207: 785–9.

14. Milosevic M, Voruganti S, Blend R et al. Magnetic resonance imaging (MRI) for localization of the prostatic apex: comparison to computed tomography (CT) and urethrography. Radiother Oncol 1998; 47: 277–84.

15. Beard CJ, Kijewski P, Bussierre M et al. Analysis of prostate and seminal vesicle motion: implications for treatment planning. Int J Radiat Oncol Biol Phys 1996; 34: 451–8.

16. Crook JM, Raymond Y, Salhani D et al. Prostate motion during standard radiotherapy as assessed by fiducial markers. Radiother Oncol 1995; 37: 35–42.

17. Valicenti RK, Waterman FM, Corn BW et al. A prospective, randomized study addressing the need for physical simulation following virtual simulation. Int J Radiat Oncol Biol Phys 1997; 39: 1131–5.

18. Michalski JM, Graham MV, Bosch WR et al. Prospective clinical evaluation of an electronic portal imaging device. Int J Radiat Oncol Biol Phys 1996; 34: 943–51.

19. Tinger A, Michalski JM, Bosch WR et al. An analysis of intratreatment and intertreatment variations in pelvic patient positioning using electronic portal imaging. Int J Radiat Oncol Biol Phys 1996; 34: 683–90.

20. Valicenti RK, Michalski JM, Bosch WR et al. Is weekly port filming adequate for verifying patient position in modern radiation therapy? Int J Radiat Oncol Biol Phys 1994; 30: 431–8.

21. Lattanzi J, McNeeley S, Hanlon A et al. Ultrasound-based stereotactic guidance of precision conformal external beam radiation therapy in clinically localized prostate cancer. Urology 2000; 55: 73–8.

22. Zelefsky MJ, Whitmore WF Jr. Long term results of retropubic permanent I-125 implantation of the prostate for clinically localized prostate cancer. J Urol 1997; 158: 23–30.

23. Ragde H, Elgama AA, Snow PB et al. Ten-year disease free survival after transperineal sonography-guided iodine-125 brachytherapy with or without 45 Gy external beam irradiation in the treatment of patients with clinically localized low to high Gleason grade prostate carcinoma. Cancer 1998; 83: 989–1001.

24. Wallner K, Roy J, Zelefsky MJ et al. Flouroscopic visualization of the prostatic urethra to guide transperineal prostate implantation. Int J Radiat Oncol Biol Phys 1994; 29: 863–8.

25. Wallner K, Roy J, Harrison L. Tumor control and morbidity following transperineal iodine 125 implantation for stage T1/T2 prostatic carcinoma. J Clin Oncol 1997; 14: 449–53.

26. Zelefsky MJ, Yamada Y, Cohen G et al. Postimplantation dosimetric analysis of permanent transperineal prostate implantation: improved dose distributions with an intraoperative computer-optimized conformal planning technique. Int J Radiat Oncol Biol Phys 2000; 48: 601–8.

27. D'Amico AV, Cormack RA, Tempany CM. MRI-guided diagnosis and treatment of prostate cancer. N Engl J Med 2001; 344: 776–7.

Index

abscess
    prostatic 151, 154–7
        CT imaging 79, 80
        Doppler ultrasound 44
        treatment 160
        tuberculous 159, 160
    seminal vesicle 179, 180
amyloidosis, seminal vesicle 177, 196
anesthesia, biopsy 53–4
antibiotic prophylaxis, transrectal biopsy 52, 53
arterial anatomy, prostate 39
atypical small acinal proliferation 24, 51
azoospermia 124, 192, 193

benign prostatic hypertrophy (hyperplasia) (BPH) 13, 129–47
    calcifications 136, 138, 140, 163, 165
    with cystic change 136, 138
        CT imaging 79, 80
    ejaculatory duct obstruction 184, 193
    imaging 130–1, 132–45
        bladder 132, 134
        computed tomography 79
        magnetic resonance 95–6
        prostate 135
        treatment studies 139, 141–4
        ultrasound 42–3, 130–1, 134–9, 141–5
        upper urinary tract 135
    lateral lobe hypertrophy 135, 136
    median lobe hypertrophy 11, 12, 130, 135, 136–8
    prevalence 129
    with renal failure 145
    symptoms 129–30
    treatment 139, 141
        transurethral microwave thermotherapy 204–6
        transurethral resection of prostate 143–4
        urethral stents 141–3
    urodynamic studies 131–2, 133
biopsy
    analgesia 53–4
    complications 52–3
    five-region approach 60, 61

follow-up 53
haematospermia 197
indications for 51–2
needle 59–60
preparation for 52
prostate cancer 21
    diagnosis 24–5
    Gleason scoring system 24
saturation 60
sextant 60
    modified approach 20–1, 60–1
targeted 61
transition zone 61
transperineal approach 54–8
    anaesthesia 53
transrectal approach 58–9
    anaesthesia 53–4
    strategies 60–1
ultrasound-guided 51–63
bladder
    after prostate biopsy 53
    cancer, haematospermia 197
    catheterization 145
    diverticula 134
    outlet obstruction
        benign prostatic hypertrophy 129–30
        CT imaging 79
    post-micturition volume 130–1
    trabeculated 134
bladder neck, post-prostatectomy ultrasound 35, 36
bladder wall thickening 134
bone marrow scintigraphy 108
bone metastases 102
    bone pain treatment 110
    bone scan index 107–8
    CT imaging 82, 83
    isotope bone scans 101–5, 106
        superscan 104, 107
    magnetic resonance imaging 104, 106
    single-photon emission computed tomography 107
bone pain, systemic treatment 110

bone scan index (BSI) 107–8
bone scan/scintigraphy 101
  flare phenomenon 105–6
  prostate cancer 101–7
    follow-up 107
    staging 101–2, 106–7
    superscan 104, 107
BPH *see* benign prostatic hypertrophy
brachytherapy 109
  CT evaluation for 84
  gray-scale ultrasound 35–6
  image-guided transperineal 213–14
BSI (bone scan index) 107–8

calculi/calcifications 14, 163–70
  benign prostatic hypertrophy 163
    CT imaging 79
    ultrasound imaging 136, 138, 140, 163, 165
  chronic prostatitis 149–50, 155, 157–8
    tuberculous 159, 160
  ejaculatory ducts 125, 183, 184, 185, 193, 196
  Müllerian duct cyst 122, 163
  parenchymal 166
  periurethral glands 163, 164
  post-radiotherapy 169
  prostate 167, 168, 169, 196
  prostate cancer 167, 168, 169
  prostatitis 163, 166–7, 169
    tuberculous 167, 168
  seminal vesicles 178–9, 180, 193, 196
  urethra 163, 165, 170
  vasa deferentia 178, 192
  verumontanum 164
cancer of prostate
  bone scans 101–7
    pre-treatment 107
  clinically significant, identification 65
  CT evaluation 80–4
    radiation therapy 84–5, 211–14
  detection/diagnosis 24–5, 65
    advanced sonographic techniques 65–75
    biopsy 51–63
    CT imaging 80–1
    Doppler ultrasound 39–50
    gray-scale sonography 27–34
    magnetic resonance imaging 89–91
  epidemiology 19
  follow-up, bone scans 107
  grading, Gleason scoring system 24
  haematospermia 196, 197
  histopathology 20–5
  magnetic resonance imaging 88–96
    radiation therapy 211–14
  magnetic resonance spectroscopy 91, 95, 96
  metastasis 22
    CT evaluation 81–2, 83
    nuclear evaluation and therapy 101–12
    to spine 47
    see also bone metastases

microvascular density in 24–5, 46
  contrast-enhanced sonography 67
  Doppler imaging and 47–8
radiation therapy, imaging for 35–6, 84–5, 211–15
recurrent
  CT evaluation 82, 84
  magnetic resonance imaging 97–8
  ultrasound imaging 34–5
screening 19, 20
seminal vesicle involvement 174–7
  magnetic resonance imaging 94–5, 96
sonography
  contrast-enhanced 67–73
  Doppler 39–50
  gray-scale 27–38
  post-prostatectomy 34–5, 36
  radiotherapy planning 35–6
  recurrent disease 34–5
  seminal vesicles 34
  signal-processing techniques 65–7
  transabdominal 27
  transperineal 27, 28
  transrectal 27–8
spread 20–1, 22
  CT evaluation 81–2, 83
  effect of zonal anatomy 13, 20
  magnetic resonance imaging 92–3
  perineural invasion 21
  seminal vesicles 34
staging 22–4
  bone scans 101–2, 106–7
  CT imaging 80–1
  immunoscintigraphy 108–9
  magnetic resonance imaging 91–5, 96, 97
  positron emission tomography 108
treatment
  cryosurgery 201–4
  high-intensity focused ultrasound 206–8
  MRI evaluation 97–8
  nuclear medicine 109–10
  radiation therapy 35–6, 84–5, 211–15
volume of tumor 21–2
capromab pendetide 108
catheterization
  benign prostatic hypertrophy 145
  high-intensity focused ultrasound 207
  prostatitis and 151, 154
  transurethral microwave thermotherapy 204–5, 206
color Doppler
  contrast-enhanced 67, 69–70, 72
  prostate 40, 44, 45–7, 48
    benign prostatic hypertrophy 43
    cancer detection 42, 48–9
computed tomography (CT)
  benign prostatic disorders 79–80, 81
  contrast-enhanced 78
  normal prostate 77–8
  prostate cancer 80–5
    radiation therapy 211–14

staging 81–4
prostate zones 14
seminal vesicles and vasa deferentia 172, 173
congenital anomalies
ejaculatory ducts 122–6
infertility and 193
prostate 8, 9–11, 116–22
seminal vesicles and vasa deferentia 184–7
infertility and 192–3
consent, informed, biopsy 52
contrast agents, microbubble, sonography 67–73
corpora amylacea 163
calcified 158, 163
cryosurgery
mechanisms of action 201–2
prostate cancer 201–4
complications 203–4
technique 202–3
CT *see* computed tomography
cystic fibrosis, vas deferens anomalies 192
cysts
ejaculatory duct 8, 10, 122–5, 183, 184
haematospermia 124, 196
epididymal 185, 192
Müllerian duct 10–11, 118–22
calculi 122, 163
complications 122
ejaculatory duct obstruction 182–3
haematospermia 196
infertility and 122, 193
parenchymal 126
periurethral 126
prostatic 31, 196
acquired 115–16
congenital 8, 9–11, 116–22, 126
CT imaging 79, 80
seminal vesicle 8, 9, 177–8, 193
utricular 10, 117
vasa deferentia 192

3DCTR (three-dimensional conformal radiation therapy) 211, 212, 213
Deconvilliers fascia 3
digital rectal examination 51
prostate cancer 20
prostatitis 151
DNA ploidy, prostate cancer 25
Doppler ultrasound
abscess 44
benign prostatic hypertrophy 42–3
contrast-enhanced 67–70, 72
prostate
focal zone settings 44, 46–7
frequency of insonation 43–4, 45
patient positioning 43, 44, 45
probe pressure in 44, 46
technical factors 43–7
prostate cancer 39–50
color vs power Doppler 48–9
microvascular considerations 47–8

prostatitis 43
see also color Doppler; power Doppler

ejaculatory ducts 182
anatomy 6, 7–8, 13
variations 8
anomalies, infertility and 193
calculi 163, 164, 166, 170, 183, 184, 185, 193
CT imaging 77, 78
congenital anomalies 125
cysts 8, 10, 122–5, 183, 184
haematospermia 124, 196
ductal ectasia 184
embryology 116
hypoplasia 183
obstruction 34, 125, 179–80, 182–4, 193
elastography, prostate cancer 66–7, 68
epididymal cysts 185, 192

Gleason scoring system, prostate cancer 24
gray-scale ultrasound
harmonic 70–1, 73
prostate, examination technique 27–9
prostate cancer 27–38
contrast-enhanced imaging 70–1, 73
examination technique 27–9
post-prostatectomy evaluation 34–5, 36
radiotherapy planning 35–6
recurrent 34–5
seminal vesicles 34
sonographic appearance 29–34, 36–7

haematospermia (haemospermia) 195–8
haematuria, post-ejaculatory 195, 197
high-intensity focused ultrasound (HIFU) 206–8
hyperaemia, prostatitis 151, 157, 158
hypoplasia, congenital, prostate 126–7
hypospadias, congenitally enlarged prostatic utricle 117

image-guided transperineal brachytherapy (IGTPB) 213–14
immunoscintigraphy 108–9
IMRT (intensity-modulated radiation therapy) 211, 212, 213
infertility, male 191–4
haematospermia and 197
seminal vesicle anomalies and 185, 192–3
seminal vesicle obstruction and 180
vas deferens abnormalities and 192
informed consent, biopsy 52
intensity-modulated radiation therapy (IMRT) 211, 212, 213
intravenous urography (IVU), benign prostatic hypertrophy 135, 136

lidocaine anesthesia, biopsy procedures 53–4

magnetic resonance imaging (MRI)
benign prostatic disease 95–7, 136, 140
cysts
ejaculatory duct 123
Müllerian duct 118–20
seminal vesicle 177, 178

magnetic resonance imaging (MRI) (*Continued*)
    ejaculatory ducts
        cysts 123
        obstruction 180
    post-therapy evaluation 97–8
    prostate cancer 89–91
        metastases 104, 106
        radiation therapy 211–14
        spread 21
        staging 91–5, 96, 97
    prostate volume measurement 139, 141
    prostate zones 14
    prostatitis
        acute 151, 153–5, 156
        granulomatous 159
    seminal vesicles 172, 173
        cysts 177, 178
        obstruction 180, 182, 184
        in prostate cancer 175–7
        tumors 188
    sequences and imaging planes 87
    T1–weighted 87–8
        benign disease 95, 96
        congenital anomalies 118–19
        prostate cancer 89–90, 91, 92
        prostatitis 151, 154, 156
        seminal vesicles 172
    T2–weighted 88–9
        benign disease 95, 96, 97
        congenital anomalies 118–20
        prostate cancer 90, 91, 92, 97
        prostatitis 151, 152–4, 156
        seminal vesicle/ejaculatory duct obstruction 180, 182
        seminal vesicles 172, 173, 176–7, 178, 188
    vasa deferentia 174
magnetic resonance spectroscopy (MRS) 89, 90
    prostate cancer 91, 95, 96
        radiation therapy 212
malakoplakia 159, 160
microvascular density, prostate cancer *see under* cancer of prostate
microwave thermotherapy 204–6
MRI *see* magnetic resonance imaging
MRS *see* magnetic resonance spectroscopy
Müllerian ducts
    cysts 10–11, 118–22
        calculi 122, 163
        complications 122
        ejaculatory duct obstruction 182–3
        haematospermia 196
        infertility and 122, 193
    embryology 116

neurovascular bundles 3, 5
nuclear medicine, prostate cancer
    bone metastases 101–7
    evaluation 101–9
    therapy 109–10

paramesonephric ducts *see* Müllerian ducts
pelvis, metastatic deposits 102

periurethral glands 12
    calculi 163, 164
PET (positron emission tomography) 108
PIN *see* prostatic intraepithelial neoplasia
planimetry, prostate volume measurement 29
positron emission tomography (PET) 108
power Doppler
    contrast-enhanced 67–9
    prostate 39, 40, 45, 48
        abscess 44, 45
        benign prostatic hypertrophy 42–3
        cancer detection 41–2, 48–9
prostadynia 151
prostate
    anatomy 3–15
        arterial 39
        historical perspective 11–12
        imaging 13–14
        venous 49
        zonal (McNeal's model) 12–13
    enlargement 3, 4, 6, 8, 13
        see also benign prostatic hypertrophy
    inner gland 14, 20
    outer gland 14, 20
    surgical capsule 14, 20
        calculi 165
    volume measurement 29, 131, 132, 136, 139, 141
prostate cancer *see* cancer of prostate
prostate-specific antigen (PSA) testing
    metastatic disease prediction 106–7
    prostate cancer screening 20, 51
    prostatitis 151
prostatectomy, gray-scale evaluation 34–5
    bladder neck 35, 36
prostatic capsule 13, 21
    tumor infiltration 20–1, 32, 33
prostatic intraepithelial neoplasia (PIN) 24
    biopsy 51
prostatism 129–30
prostatitis 149–62
    acute 149, 150
        imaging appearances 151–7
    calculi 163, 166–7, 169
    chronic 149–50
        imaging appearances 157–8
    diagnosis 151
    Doppler ultrasound 43
    granulomatous 150–1
        imaging appearances 159–60
        tuberculous 150, 159
    haematospermia 196
    iatrogenic 151
    imaging 79, 96–7, 151–60
    treatment, imaging in 160
    tuberculous 150, 159, 160
        calculi 167, 168
PSA *see* prostate-specific antigen

radiation therapy
    calcifications following 169

external-beam 110
    imaging in 211
    intensity-modulated 211, 212, 213
    role of imaging 35–6, 84, 211–15
        target definition 211–12
        treatment uncertainty 212–13
    three-dimensional conformal 211, 212, 213
radioimmunotherapy 110
radiopharmaceuticals, bone-seeking 110
renal anomalies, seminal vesicle anomalies and 192
renal failure, benign prostatic hypertrophy and 145
rete testis
    carcinoma 197
    ectasia 185, 192
ribs, metastatic deposits 102, 103, 105

schistosomiasis
    prostatic calcifications 167, 169
    seminal vesicles 179, 180
    vas deferentia/seminal vesicle calcifications 178
screening, prostate cancer 19, 20
seminal vesicles
    absence/hypoplasia 184–6
        infertility and 192
    amyloidosis 177, 196
    anatomy 6, 7, 13, 171
        variations 8
    calculi 178–9, 180, 193, 196
    cysts 8, 9, 177–8, 193
        infected 177, 178
    dilatation 186, 195
    ductal ectasia 8, 9, 34
        CT imaging 79, 81
    ectopia 186–7
    haematospermia and seminal vesicle pathology 195–6
    imaging 171–4
        computed tomography 77, 78
        ultrasound 34, 171–3, 177–80, 184–8
    infection (seminal vesiculitis) 179, 180, 196
    obstruction 179–81, 184
        infertility and 180, 193
    prostate cancer and 34, 174–7
        magnetic resonance imaging 94–5, 96
    reduplication 186
    tumors of 187–8
single-photon emission computed tomography (SPECT) 109
    bone metastases 107
sonography see ultrasound
SPECT see single-photon emission computed tomography
sphincter, preprostatic 12
spine, metastasis to 47, 102, 104
stents, urethral 141–3

testicular pathology, haematospermia and 197
therapy, image-guided 201–9
thermotherapy, transurethral microwave 204–6
three-dimensional conformal radiation therapy (3DCTR) 211, 212, 213
TNM staging system, prostate cancer 22–4
transurethral incision of prostate (TUIP) 143

transurethral microwave thermotherapy (TUMT) 204–6
    mechanisms of action 204
transurethral resection of prostate (TURP) 143–4
    defect following 8, 9
traumatic injury, haematospermia 197
tuberculosis
    prostatitis 150, 159, 160
        calcifications 167, 168
    seminal vesicles 179, 180
    vas deferentia/seminal vesicle calcifications 178
TUIP (transurethral incision of prostate) 143
TUMT (transurethral microwave thermotherapy) 204–6
TURP see transurethral resection of prostate

ultrasound 27–9, 70–1, 73
    benign prostatic hypertrophy
        bladder 130–1, 134
        prostate 135–9
        renal failure 145
        treatment studies 141–4
        upper urinary tract 135
        urine retention 145
    biopsy guidance 51–63
        transperineal approach 53, 54–8
        transrectal approach 53–4, 58–9, 60–1
    brachytherapy delivery 213–14
    calculi 164–70, 178–9
    contrast-enhanced
        harmonic imaging and 70, 71, 72–3
        intermittent (transient response) imaging 70, 71, 72–3
        prostate cancer 67–73
    cysts
        acquired prostatic 115–16
        ejaculatory duct 123–5
        Müllerian duct 118–22
        urethral 126
    Doppler see Doppler ultrasound
    ejaculatory ducts 182
        obstruction 182–4
    gray-scale 27–9, 70–1, 73
        prostate cancer 27–38, 70–1, 73
        for detailed entry see gray-scale ultrasound
    high-intensity focused 206–8
    image-processing techniques and 65
    prostate
        harmonic imaging 29, 70–1, 73
        three-dimensional imaging 29, 36
        transabdominal approach 27
        transperineal approach 27, 28
        transrectal approach 27–8
        zones 14
    prostate cancer
        advanced techniques 65–75
        Doppler imaging 39–50
        gray-scale evaluation 27–38
        recurrent 34–5
        screening 20
        spread 21
    in prostate disease therapy 201–9
    prostate volume measurement 139, 141

ultrasound (*Continued*)
  prostatitis
    acute 151, 152, 155, 157
    chronic 157–8
    granulomatous 159–60
    treatment 160
  seminal vesicles 34, 171–3
    abscess 179, 180
    calculi 178–9
    congenital anomalies 184–6
    cysts 177
    obstruction 180, 181, 184
    in prostate cancer 175, 176
    tumors 187–8
  signal-processing techniques, prostate cancer 65–7
  spectral analysis 66
  three-dimensional
    prostate 29, 36
    prostate cancer 29
    prostate volume measurement 141
ureter, ectopic 125
  entering vas deferens 187
urethra
  anatomy 5–6
  calculi 163, 165, 170
  catheterization, prostatitis and 151, 154
  cysts 126
  diverticuli 126
  haematospermia and urethral pathology 197
  polyps 197
  preprostatic 12
  stents 141–3

urethrography
  calculi 170
  prostate localization, radiation therapy 212
  urethral cysts/anomalies 126, 127
urinary tract, upper, benign prostatic hypertrophy 135
urine flow rate 131, 132
urine retention
  acute, imaging in 145
  following biopsy 53
urodynamic studies, benign prostatic hypertrophy 131–2, 133
urography, intravenous, benign prostatic hypertrophy 135, 136
utricle, prostatic 5–6
  congenital enlargement 117–18
  cysts 10, 117
  embryology 116

vasa deferentia
  absence/hypoplasia 184–6
    infertility and 192
  anatomy 6, 7
  calcifications 178, 192
  CT imaging, normal anatomy 77, 78
  cysts 192
  ectopia 186–7
  magnetic resonance imaging 174
  obstruction 192
vasography, seminal vesicles 172, 174
venous anatomy, prostate 47
venous plexus of Santorini 3, 5
verumontanum 5, 12
  calculi 164
vesiculography, seminal 174, 175